Techniques in Bedside Hemodynamic Monitoring

Techniques in Bedside Hemodynamic Monitoring

ELAINE KIESS DAILY RN, BS
Clinical Cardiovascular Research Nurse
University of California–San Diego Medical Center
San Diego, California

JOHN SPEER SCHROEDER MD
Professor of Medicine (Cardiology)
Cardiology Division, Department of Medicine
Stanford University School of Medicine
Stanford, California

FOURTH EDITION

*with **212** illustrations*

THE C. V. MOSBY COMPANY

ST. LOUIS • BALTIMORE • PHILADELPHIA • TORONTO   1989

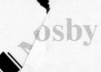

osby

or: **Don Ladig**
velopmental Editor: **Sally Adkisson**
Manager: **Suzanne Seeley**
tion Editor: **Jolynn Gower**
ner: **Liz Fett**

FOURTH EDITION

The C.V. Mosby Company
11830 Westline Industrial Drive, St. Louis, Missouri 63146

Library of Congress Cataloging-in-Publication Data

Daily, Elaine Kiess.
   Techniques in bedside hemodynamic monitoring.

   Includes bibliographies and index.
   1. Hemodynamic monitoring.   I.   Schroeder, John
Speer, 1937-   . II.   Title. [DNLM: 1. Hemodynamics.
2. Monitoring, Physiologic. WG 106 D133t]
RC670.5.H45D35 1989   616.1'075   89-3063
ISBN 0-8016-5758-X

C/VH/VH   9   8   7   6   5   4   3   2   1

CONTRIBUTOR

MARY FRAN HAZINSKI RN, MSN
Pediatric Critical Care Clinical Specialist
Vanderbilt University Medical Center
Nashville, Tennessee

TO AUBURN

Preface

Revising and updating a book for its fourth edition is quite revealing when viewed in terms of historical changes and progress. The advances made in the last two decades of hemodynamic monitoring relate not only to the myriad technologic changes but, more dramatically, to the more aggressive medical management of the critically ill patient. Invasive hemodynamic monitoring has become more standardized and widely used as medical and pharmacologic interventions have expanded. Monitoring hemodynamic parameters has become essential for the immediate assessment of the effectiveness and appropriateness of selected therapeutic interventions.

Technologic advances in hemodynamic monitoring have provided the clinician with expanded ability to rapidly determine and monitor numerous cardiopulmonary parameters at the bedside. The critical care nurse plays a pivotal role in determining whether these expanded data are helpful or harmful to the care and outcome of critically ill patients. A clear understanding of the physiologic and technologic principles of hemodynamic monitoring forms the cornerstone of safe, appropriate, and helpful hemodynamic monitoring, while standardized techniques promote accuracy as well as efficiency.

We have updated and expanded the technical aspects of this book by including the principles and methods of continuous monitoring of oxygenation through the use of the fiberoptic pulmonary artery catheter to monitor Svo_2 and the pulse oximeter to monitor Sao_2.

In recognition of the increased practice and unique demands of monitoring infants and children, who are not just small adults, Mary Fran Hazinski has expertly revised and expanded the chapter on hemodynamic monitoring of children.

A chapter on clinical management based on hemodynamic parameters has been added to provide a necessary understanding of the ways in which those determinants of cardiac output are pharmacologically or mechanically manipulated in critically ill patients. Frequently, it is the critical care nurse at the bedside who must make these minute-to-minute decisions about which infusions to increase, decrease, discontinue, or add to optimize cardiac output and oxygen delivery.

The cardiac output chapter has been expanded to include more troubleshooting steps and information to help the clinician obtain the most accurate data possible. The remaining chapters have been updated and revised to reflect the current practices of bedside monitoring.

Our goal in this revised edition continues to be to present the principles and techniques of hemodynamic monitoring in a simple, practical way that will ensure its utility to all health care personnel involved in hemodynamic monitoring. Any book that remains on a shelf, unused or unread, is just so much ink on paper. This book, we hope, is one that will be used, and used again, to help both the novice and the experienced nurse overcome some of the obstacles that frequently accompany hemodynamic monitoring.

ELAINE KIESS DAILY
JOHN SPEER SCHROEDER

Contents

Chapter 1

The Heart as a Pump

The function of the heart is to pump blood returning from other parts of the body to the lungs and into the aorta. This process serves to deliver oxygenated blood and nutrients to peripheral tissues via the vascular system and to remove metabolic waste products. Bedside hemodynamic monitoring permits minute-to-minute surveillance of the cardiovascular system and provides the physiologic data to guide therapy. This chapter reviews basic principles of cardiac physiology and anatomy as they pertain to hemodynamic monitoring.

FUNCTIONAL ULTRASTRUCTURE OF THE MYOCARDIAL CELL

The myocardial cell, or myocardial fiber, is the basic unit of the ventricular myocardium (Fig. 1-1). Composed of multiple linearly arranged myocardial fibrils and a cell nucleus, it is separated from other myocardial fibers by intercalated disks. These intercalated disks are true cell boundaries but have very low electrial impedance, so that electrical impulses can travel rapidly throughout the myocardium. The myocardial fibril, or myofibril, is composed of *sarcomeres,* the basic functional unit of the myocardium. These sarcomeres are composed of contractile proteins called *myofilaments,* specifically *myosin filaments* and *actin filaments.* Mitochondria are distributed in the myocardial cell between myofibrils and, by the process of oxidative phosphorylation, are the major source of energy for cell function. The last major component of the myocardial cell is the *sarcoplasmic reticulum,* which surrounds the cell. The sarcoplasmic reticulum is a complex network that interconnects between myofibrils, so that it is adjacent to the surfaces of individual sarcomeres. Not only is it in direct relationship to the sarcomere, but it is also in continuity with the extracellular space and serves as the transport mechanism for ionic movement and ionic control of contraction. Individual myocardial fibers are also surrounded by cell surface membranes, the *sarcolemma.*

The sarcomere is the contractile unit of the heart and is similar to the contractile unit of skeletal muscle. The thicker myofilaments of the sarcomere are the myosin filaments and are limited to the A band of the sarcomere. The thinner actin filaments begin at the Z band and interdigitate with the myosin filaments (see Fig. 1-1, *C*). The relationship between the actin and myosin filaments depends on the sarcomere length, which is determined by the amount of stretch of the myocardial fibers. There is maximal contact between the actin and myosin filaments when the sarcomere is 2.2 μ in length. If the sarcomere is shorter or longer than 2.2 μ, force

1

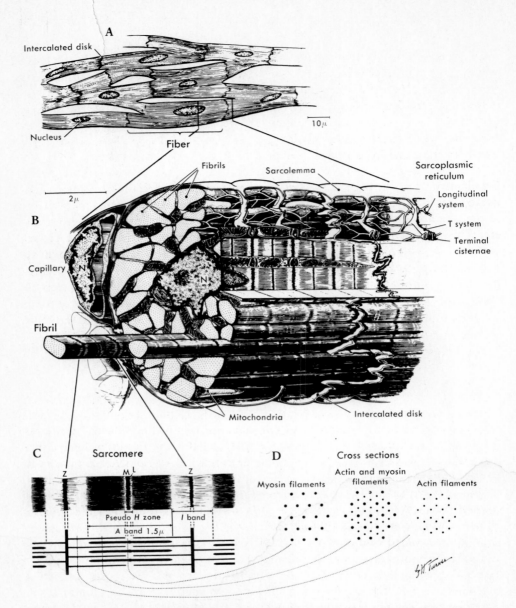

A

Intercalated disk

Nucleus

Fiber

10 μ

B

Fibrils

Sarcolemma

Sarcoplasmic reticulum

Longitudinal system

T system

Terminal cisternae

2 μ

Capillary

N

Fibril

Mitochondria

Intercalated disk

C   Sarcomere

Z   M L   Z

Pseudo *H* zone   *I* band

A band 1.5 μ

D   Cross sections

Actin and myosin filaments

Myosin filaments   Actin filaments

Fig. 1-1. Microscopic structure of heart muscle. **A,** Myocardium as seen under the light microscope. Branching of fibers is evident; each fiber contains a centrally located nucleus. **B,** Myocardial cell or fiber reconstructed from electron micrographs; the arrangements of the multiple parallel fibrils composing the cell and of the serially connected sarcomeres composing the fibrils are apparent (*N*, nucleus). **C,** Arrangement of myofilaments making up an individual sarcomere from a myofibril with nucleus). **C,** Arrangement of myofilaments making up an individual sarcomere from a myofibril with thick (myosin) filaments 1.5 μ in length, forming the A band, and thin (actin) filaments 1.0 μ in length, extending from the Z band through the I band into the A band, ending at the edges of the H zone. (An H zone exists in the central area of the A band, where thin filaments are absent; overlapping of thick and thin filaments is seen only in the A band.) **D,** Cross sections of the sarcomere indicating the specific lattice arrangements of the myofilaments. In the center of the sarcomere *(left)* only thick filaments arranged in a hexagon are seen; in the distal portions of the A band *(center)* both thick and thin filaments are found (each thick filament is surrounded by six thin filaments); in the I band *(right)* only thin filaments are present. (From Braunwald E, et al: N Engl J Med 277[15]:794-800, 1967. Reprinted, by permission from the New England Journal of Medicine.)

development decreases (Fig. 1-2). When the sarcomere is stretched to approximately 3.6 μ, tension development no longer exists, because there is no contact between the actin and myosin filaments. In contrast, when the sarcomere is shorter than 2 μ before contraction, tension development is less, since the filaments bypass one another and overlap. As the volume and radius of the ventricle increase in response to either increased diastolic filling pressure or volume, the myocardial fibers lengthen, reflecting an increase in sarcomere length.

Huxley and others have explained the shortening of the sarcomere by the sliding filament or ratcheting mechanism. It is believed that, when the sarcomere is activated electrically, interaction between the actin and myosin filaments takes place, so that the filaments actually slide or ratchet by each other, shortening the sarcomere. This contractile process requires adenosine triphosphate (ATP) and proper concentrations of calcium, magnesium, and other ions. The sarcoplasmic reticulum plays a critical role in initiation, control, and reversal of reactions between the actin and myosin filaments. This basic function of the sarcomere serves as the basis for length-tension curves and for the Frank-Starling law. Studies by Braunwald, Ross, and Sonnenblick on the relationship of the sarcomere to cardiac performance have been reviewed.

To explain relaxation of the sarcomere, Hill proposed a model involving a series elastic element that is stretched during contraction and results in return of the original sarcomere length during relaxation (Fig. 1-3). This model also considers viscous elements to explain changes in the sarcomere's rapidity of relaxation when it returns to its original length. More recently, Sonnenblick and associates have proposed other models to explain certain characteristics of the isolated heart muscle. The elastic element is probably not a separate anatomic entity in the sarcomere; rather, it serves primarily as a model to explain characteristics of relaxation and resting tension.

In summary, the basic functional unit of contraction is the sarcomere, which is composed of myofilaments, contractile proteins that interdigitate and slide by one another during contraction, shortening the sarcomere. Physiologic and pharmacologic agents used to change contraction operate to affect this interaction.

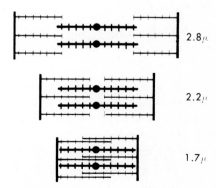

Fig. 1-2. As the sarcomere is shortened or lengthened from 2.2 μ, actin-myosin interactions are fewer and less contractile force is generated.

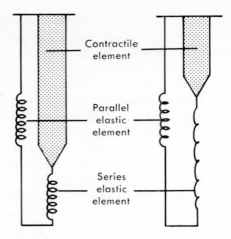

Fig. 1-3. Hill model for muscle contraction-relaxation. As the contractile element contracts, the series elastic element is stretched. When the contractile element relaxes, the series elastic element returns the contractile element to its resting length. The parallel elastic element is primarily responsible for resting tension and viscosity (resistance to sudden stretch).

FUNCTIONAL GROSS ANATOMY OF THE CARDIOVASCULAR SYSTEM

It is beyond the purpose of this book to describe the basic anatomy of the heart and vascular system. The following is a review of several aspects of the functional anatomy of the cardiovascular system that are pertinent to the understanding of hemodynamic changes in the critically ill patient.

Cardiac Innervation

Autonomic innervation to the heart is extensive. Sympathetic nerve fibers are found throughout the atria and the ventricles, including the sinoatrial (SA) and atrioventricular (AV) nodes. Parasympathetic fibers are found primarily in the atria and SA and AV nodes but extend into the ventricles as well. The autonomic nervous system has a significant influence on regulation of impulse formation and on conduction of the excitation impulse. It also influences contractility of both the atria and the ventricles.

Sympathetic innervation arises in the upper thoracic spinal cord and reaches the heart via cervical ganglia, giving rise to the cardiac nerves. These nerves form the cardiac plexus, which surrounds the root of the aorta and has fibers extending to the SA and AV nodes and to the right and left coronary arteries.

Parasympathetic innervation orginates in the medulla oblongata and goes to the heart via the vagus nerve, joining sympathetic fibers in the cardiac plexus. Stimulation of the vagus nerve produces cardiac slowing and inhibits AV conduction. Since there are few parasympathetic nerve fibers in the ventricular myocardium, the vagus nerve has little effect on contractility except by its indirect effect on heart rate.

Sensory pain fibers are present in the pericardium, connective tissue adventitia, and myocardium and pass via sympathetic plexuses through thoracic dorsal ganglia. The impulses then ascend via the ventral spinal thalamic tract, terminating in the posteroventral nucleus of the thalamus. These fibers may be important for reflex responses of the heart to ischemia and injury.

Regulation of the Peripheral Vascular System

Peripheral blood flow is controlled by local autoregulation and the nervous system. The exact function of autoregulation is poorly understood but may depend on several mechanisms:

1. Local metabolic tissue demands. Blood flow is regulated to meet the oxygen requirements of the tissues. With decreased flow, metabolic byproducts increase, causing vasodilation and increased blood flow.
2. Intraluminal stretch and pressure. Autonomic constriction of smooth muscle of the vessel wall occurs in response to increased intraluminal stretch and pressure. With decreased stretch and pressure, the vessel relaxes and dilates.
3. Turgor. Increased luminal pressure causes increased fluid in surrounding local tissue (turgor), which compresses small, thin-walled vessels and reduces blood flow.

Nervous system control is accomplished primarily by sympathetic effects on peripheral vessels from a vasomotor center in the medulla oblongata. This sympathetic activity mainly affects the arterioles, capillaries, and venules. The vasomotor center operates in conjunction with a vagal parasympathetic center, which affects cardiac performance and some capacitance vessels. The vasomotor center is influenced by many autonomic, reflex, and supratentorial factors, including baroreceptors, chemoreceptors, the hypothalamus, and the cerebral cortex.

Baroreceptors are pressure and stretch receptors that are located in the carotid sinus and aortic arch. As arterial blood pressure rises, these receptors sense the pressure rise and respond with an increased rate of firing signals, which inhibit the vasomotor center, with a resultant fall in vessel tone and pressure. Reflex vagal-induced bradycardia contributes to this response. In arterial hypotension the reverse effect occurs, and increased vasoconstriction causes the blood pressure to rise.

Chemoreceptors in the carotid sinus and elsewhere regulate respiration by responding to changes in Pa_{CO_2} and Pa_{O_2}. These changes also influence the vasomotor center.

The *hypothalamus* affects the vasomotor center principally in response to temperature-regulating mechanisms, resulting in changes in peripheral circulation.

The *cerebral cortex* influence on the vasomotor center can be noted during excitement (blushing may occur) or emotionally induced syncope.

In summary, circulatory homeostasis is maintained by complex interactions of autoregulation and neural influences. Built into this system are highly protective mechanisms to provide sufficient cerebral and coronary blood flow to maintain life.

Pulmonary Circulation

The pulmonary arterial vessels differ markedly from the systemic vessels; they have thinner walls, less medial muscle, and a resistance to flow that is approximately six times less than that of the systemic vessels. For example, in patients with left-to-right shunts there can be a threefold to fourfold increase in flow before there is any significant rise in pressure or resistance. The pressure in the systemic capillaries is 25 to 35 mm Hg: the pressure in the pulmonary capillaries is 7 to 10 mm Hg. Thus there is relatively little interstitial fluid in the lung at these pressures, and pulmonary edema does not occur until a pulmonary capillary pressure of 25 to 30 mm Hg is reached.

Coronary Circulation

The right and left coronary arteries are epicardial arteries with perforating branches that enter the myocardium and septum, terminating on the endocardial surface. Approximately 75% of coronary blood flow occurs during diastole, when the heart is in a relaxation phase. Control of coronary flow is inadequately understood, but autoregulation is a primary factor of this control when the diastolic pressure is greater than 80 mm Hg. From 80 to 40 mm Hg there is a more direct relationship between coronary blood flow and perfusion pressure at the coronary ostia. At approximtely 40 mm Hg the coronary arteries actually collapse, and there is essentially no flow. Therefore it is essential to maintain a mean arterial diastolic pressure of 60 to 80 mm Hg in the patient with cardiovascular disease.

When occlusive disease is present, there may be multiple pressure gradients across areas of stenosis because of atheromatous plaques. Experiments in animals have demonstrated that the coronary artery must be 75% occluded before there is any significant decrease in coronary flow. This finding is also seen at the time that patients who have severe three-vessel coronary artery disease first develop symptoms.

CARDIAC CYCLE

The sequence of events occurring during the cardiac cycle are best divided into systole and diastole, as described by Wigger's classic diagram (Fig. 1-4). *Isovolumic contraction* is the first phase of systole and results in mitral and tricuspid valve closure, which produces the first heart sound. With a continuing rise in ventricular pressure the aortic and pulmonic valves open, and blood is ejected from the ventricles. As the volume of ejecting blood falls, the pressure decreases until the aortic and pulmonic valves close, producing the second sound. *Isovolumic relaxaton* then follows as the pressure continues to fall in the ventricles until it is lower than the pressure in the atria; at this time there is *rapid ventricular filling,* which is initiated by the opening of the mitral and tricuspid valves. If the mitral valve is stenotic, there may be an opening snap at this point. As blood rushes into the ventricles, the ventricular walls suddenly expand; if there is decreased compliance because of disease or hypertrophy, an S_3 sound, or gallop, may occur. As diastolic filling continues, ventricular diastolic pressure rises until atrial systole occurs, which causes further ejection of blood from the atria into the ventricles. This rapid filling can produce an S_4 sound if there is resistance to filling or if atrial systole is vigorous.

Abnormalities in impulse conduction patterns may result in one ventricle contracting and relaxing before the other, causing abnormalities in the relationship between the first and second sound. Abnormalities in flow across valves, either during diastole or systole, result in murmurs caused by turbulence of blood flow. These murmurs and sounds are described more completely in Chapter 2.

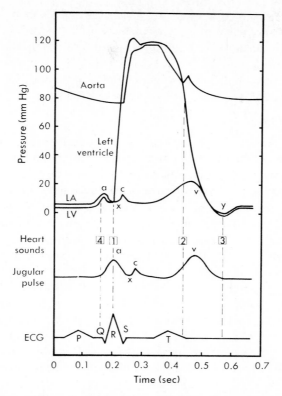

Fig. 1-4. Modification of Wigger's classic diagram dividing the cardiac cycle into systole and diastole. Simultaneous ECG, jugular pulse, heart sounds, and left-sided pressure events are diagramed. RA and RV pressure tracings are omitted for the sake of simplicity. The *a* wave of the LA pressure follows electrical atrial systole (the P wave) and may produce an S_4 heart sound. As ventricular systole occurs, the mitral valve closes, causing part of the first heart sound and producing a *c* wave in the atrial pressure tracing. As isovolumic contraction continues, pressure rises in the left ventricle until it exceeds the aortic pressure and opens the aortic valve. In late systole a *v* wave in the left atrium and jugular venous tracing reflects bulging of the AV valve into the atrium. As the LV pressure falls, the aortic pressure exceeds it, closing the aortic valve and producing part of the second heart sound. The LV pressure continues to fall until the LA pressure exceeds it, opening the mitral valve. As blood rushes into the left ventricle from the left atrium, an S_3 sound may occur. Note the delay in transmission of pressure waves to the jugular pulse in comparison with LA or ECG timing. (Modified from Hurst JW, and Logue RB, editors: The heart, New York, 1974, McGraw-Hill Book Co.)

CONTROL OF CARDIAC PERFORMANCE

Homeostatic mechanisms regulating cardiac output involve not only factors controlling performance of the pump but also factors affecting the peripheral vascular system and resistance. Normally, the heart can vary its cardiac output up to five or six times the resting level, depending on the age and physical condition of the person. Some aspects of the regulatory mechanism vary continuously; for example, sinus arrhythmia during the respiratory cycle is a result of continuous change in the balance between parasympathetic and sympathetic tone on the sinus node. Other regulatory mechanisms vary little until challenged by disease or a demand for increased cardiac output. This section briefly describes regulatory mechanisms affecting the hemodynamic performance of the heart as they relate to cardiovascular monitoring.

There are two basic methods by which the heart regulates cardiac output in response to stress or disease. Since cardiac output equals heart rate times stroke volume, the heart may respond by altering either of these factors to maintain or increase the output.

Changes in Heart Rate

Because of the rapidity of its response, a change in heart rate is the most effective method of changing cardiac output. An increase in heart rate can double or triple the cardiac output, particularly in a healthy person, who could develop a heart rate of 170 or 180. In the patient with cardiac disease, however, a heart rate over 120 may have deleterious effects because of the resultant increased myocardial oxygen demand and the decreased time for diastolic coronary blood flow. Rapid or instantaneous changes in heart rate are effected by the autonomic nervous system via its influence on the SA pacemaker. In addition, the heart rate can increase in response to circulating catecholamines, as can be seen in the denervated heart during exercise. When the heart rate increases, there is a slight increase in ventricular contractility (Bowditch's law).

Decreases in heart rate to approximately 50 beats/min may not decrease cardiac output, because there is increased diastolic filling time, which increases stroke volume. However, below this rate cardiac performance may be affected, particularly in the diseased heart.

Changes in Stroke Volume

The stroke volume of an intact ventricle is influenced by three factors: (1) ventricular end-diastolic volume (preload), (2) ventricular afterload, and (3) contractility. Although these three factors operate simultaneously to determine the stroke volume, they are discussed separately as they relate to the hemodynamic performance of the heart.

Ventricular end-diastolic volume (preload). Since the end-diastolic volume profoundly influences the myocardial fiber length and ultimately the sarcomere length (as discussed earlier), it also has a great influence on myocardial performance. The Frank-Starling law describes the principle for this factor and was based on work by Wiggers and Straub, who concluded that the mechanical energies set free when the sarcomere moves from a relaxed to a constricted state depend on the area of chemically interactive surfaces between the actin and myosin filaments; therefore, these energies depend on the length of the muscle fibers. Since a change in myocardial fiber length affects sarcomere shortening and stroke volume, the Frank-Starling law accounts for minute-to-minute changes in stroke volume of both the right and the left ventricles. In response to disease, rises in end-diastolic pressure and volume will also aid in a compensatory increase in stroke volume because of the increase in the myocardial fiber length of the remaining functioning myocardial cells. However, the diseased and markedly dilated heart can actually have a decreased stroke volume because of areas of fibrosis and slippage of myocardial fibers past one another.

Fig. 1-5 shows the relationship between left ventricular (LV) end-diastolic fiber length and stroke work or volume. As fiber length increases, stroke work will increase until the sarcomere is stretched past the optimal length of 2.2 μ, at which point there is maximal contact between actin and myosin filaments. A change in the relationship between end-diastolic fiber length and stroke volume therefore reflects a change in contractility.

In the normally functioning heart the end-diastolic volume is determined by four major factors: (1) diastolic filling pressure, (2) total blood volume, (3) distribution of blood volume, and (4) atrial systole. The major determinants of *diastolic filling pressure* are central venous return, blood volume, and pressure generated in the atria. In general, an increase in diastolic filling pressure results in increased myocardial stretch and, by the Frank-Starling law, increased shortening. If the *total blood volume* is depleted, as during hemorrhage, diastolic-filling pressures may fall and affect stroke volume. The *distribution of blood volume* is of critical importance, because it affects central venous return to the right side of the heart. Such factors as body position, intrathoracic pressure, intrapericardial pressure (as in cardiac tamponade), and venous tone will affect blood return from the body to the right side of the heart and will thus affect stroke volume. *Atrial systole* results in an increase in atrial pressure and increased diastolic filling of the left ventricle at the end of diastole just before ventricular systole. This mechanism is particularly important for increasing end-diastolic volume in the patient with decreased ventricular compliance, such as that seen with LV hypertrophy. These patients may have a disastrous fall in stroke volume and cardiac output when atrial fibrillation occurs because of the loss of atrial systole.

Ventricular afterload. The ventricular stroke volume is critically determined by the extent of myocardial fiber shortening during systole. The primary factor that will determine the extent of shortening, in addition to the fiber's initial length, is the *afterload* or resistance to flow from the ventricle. Thus, as the LV outflow pressure increases because of hypertension or other factors (such as aortic stenosis), there may be a gradual decrease in stroke volume because of increased resistance to

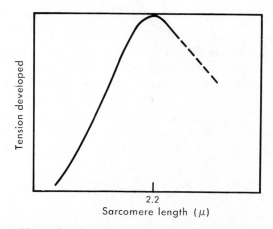

Fig. 1-5. Ultrastructural basis for the Frank-Starling curve showing that peak tension development occurs at a sarcomere length of 2.2 μ; whether a downslope of the curve after peak tension exists is questionable.

systolic ejection of blood from the ventricle. Conversely, as resistance falls (during exercise, sepsis, or therapeutically induced afterload reduction), there is increased stroke volume at the same level of myocardial contractility. The concept of decreasing afterload or resistance to flow during systole is important and can be applied pharmacologically or mechanically to treat the failing ventricle.

Contractility. The level or degree of ventricular performance at any given end-diastolic volume and afterload depends on the contractile state of the ventricle. There are multiple influences that will modify the simple relationship between ventricular end-diastolic volume and performance (Fig. 1-6). Each of these influences may shift the ventricular performance to a different curve or change the relationship between end-distolic volume and performance or stroke volume.

Sympathetic influence is one of the most important regulatory factors for myocardial contractility. Rapid changes may be initiated via the sympathetic nervous system or more slowly via catecholamines circulating from the adrenal medulla and other sympathetic ganglia outside the heart. The heart rate has a slight effect on contractility (Bowditch's law), as previously discussed, but changes in rhythm can have a marked effect on the relationship between end-diastolic volume and performance.

Metabolic abnormalities, such as hypoxemia, hypercapnia, or metabolic acidosis, decrease myocardial contractility regardless of the cause. Loss of myocardial viability can decrease performance of the remaining normal myocardium because of changes in ventricular diameter and wall stress.

Finally, pharmacologic agents that can alter the contractile state of the ventricle can be administered. Positive inotropic agents include epinephrine, digitalis, isoproterenol, dopamine, and dobutamine. There are also multiple agents that can decrease the contractile state of the ventricle. These agents include antiarrhythmic agents, such as procainamide, and drugs that cause beta-receptor blockade, such as propranolol.

Other factors, such as the ionic state and abnormalities in metabolism, may influence the intrinsic contractile state of the ventricle, but these factors are poorly understood at this time.

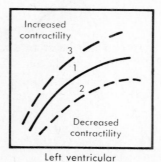

Left ventricular
end-diastolic fiber length

Fig. 1-6. Relationship between LV end-diastolic fiber length (sarcomere length) and LV work. Curve 1 represents normal function; curve 2 shows depressed function (negative inotropy or contractility); and curve 3 shows increased function (positive inotropy or contractility) at the same fiber length.

DETERMINANTS OF MYOCARDIAL OXYGEN CONSUMPTION

As an aerobically pumping organ, the heart requires a continuous supply of oxygen to develop sufficient energy to maintain its pumping function. The primary determinants of the amount of oxygen needed or consumed by the myocardium ($M\dot{V}O_2$) are wall tension, contractility and heart rate.

Factors that cannot be influenced as much by pharmacologic or mechanical means are (1) the basal resting metabolism of the myocardium, (2) the external work performed by the heart, and (3) the energy required for activation-relaxation of the ventricle. This section concerns only those factors that can be easily altered during hemodynamic monitoring.

Myocardial Tension

It is now recognized that wall tension is a major factor in determining myocardial oxygen demands. The myocardial tension of the ventricle is a direct function of the intraventricular pressure (systolic pressure) and the ventricle's radius and is inversely related to wall thickness. This is expressed by the LaPlace Law:

$$T = \frac{Pr}{2h}$$

where: T = Wall tension
P = Intraventricular pressure
r = Radius of the ventricle
h = Thickness of the ventricle

From this formula, it is clear that wall tension and therefore myocardial oxygen consumption ($M\dot{V}O_2$) increases with increases in heart size and intraventricular pressure, but decreases with hypertrophy.

Monitoring of systolic arterial blood pressure and heart rate (Rate Pressure Product) provides a global reflection of myocardial oxygen demands.

Contractile State

There is a direct relationship between an increase in the contractile state and myocardial oxygen demands. Changes in the contractile state must be differentiated from other effects of changes in the heart rate and preload or afterload.

Heart Rate

There is a direct relationship between heart rate and myocardial oxygen demands, primarily because of the increase in the number of times tension is being exerted per minute. This relationship is a major factor in determining oxygen consumption and is important in the treatment of the patient with myocardial ischemia, particularly since the increased heart rate also decreases the diastolic period and therefore myocardial oxygen delivery.

Summary

In summary, stroke volume may be affected by factors influencing total blood volume and central venous return, resistance to forward systolic ejection of the blood in the ventricle, and the contractile state of the myocardium, which responds to multiple factors, including autonomic tone, disease, and drug intervention. The relationships between these factors during myocardial insult, such as infarction, are discussed in subsequent chapters. Their physiologic relationships must be kept in mind during hemodynamic monitoring of the critically ill patient with cardiovascular disease.

REFERENCES

Benzig G III et al: Evaluation of left ventricular performance: circumferential fiber shortening and tension, Circ 49:925-932, 1974.

Braunwald E: Regulation of the circulation, N Engl J Med 290:1124-1129, 1974.

Braunwald E, Ross J, Jr, and Sonnenblick EH: Mechanisms of contraction of the normal and failing heart, N Engl J Med 277:795-800, 1967.

Guyton AC: Regulation of cardiac output, N Engl J Med 277:805-812, 1967.

Hill AV: Heat of shortening and dynamic constants of muscle, Proc R Soc Lond Biol 126:136-195, 1938.

Huxley HE: Structural arrangements and contraction mechanism in striated muscle, Proc R Soc Lond Biol 160:442, 1964.

Huxley HE: The mechanism of muscular contraction, Sci Am 213:18-27, 1965.

Ricci DR, Orlick AE, and Alderman EL: Influence of heart rate on left ventricular ejection fraction in human beings, Am J Cardiol 44:447-451, 1979.

Sarnoff S: Myocardial contractility as described by ventricular function curves: observations on Starling's law of the heart, Physiol Rev 35:107, 1955.

Sarnoff S et al: Homeometric autoregulation in the heart, Cir Res 8:1077-1091, 1960.

Schlart RC: Normal anatomy and function of the cardiovascular system. In Hurst JW, and Logue RB, editors: The heart, New York, 1974, McGraw-Hill Book Co.

Sonnenblick EH: Myocardial ultrastructure in the normal and failing heart, Hosp Pract 5:35-43, April 1970.

Sonnenblick EH, and Shelton CL: Myocardial energetics: basic principles and clinical implications, N Engl J Med 285:668-675, 1971.

Starling EH: The Linacre lecture on the law of the heart, given at Cambridge, 1915, London, 1918, Longman Group, Ltd.

Straub H: Dynamik des Saugetierherzens. I. Duetsche Arch Klin Med 115:531, 1914. II. 116:409, 1914.

Strobeck JE, Krueger J, and Sonnenblick EH: Load and time considerations in the force-length relation of cardiac muscle, Fed Proc 39:175-182, 1980.

Strobeck JE, and Sonnenblick EH: Myocardial and ventricular function, Cardiovasc Rev Rep 4:568-581, 1983.

Wiggers CJ: Some factors controlling the shape of the pressure curve in the right ventricle, Am J Physiol 33:382, 1914.

Chapter 2

Monitoring Signs and Symptoms

The patient's history and physical examination are critical components in monitoring minute-to-minute and day-to-day cardiovascular status. The use of invasive and noninvasive monitoring procedures augments and complements rather than replaces these basic techniques. This chapter reviews the techniques of history-taking and physical examination that are applicable to cardiovascular monitoring.

HISTORY AND ANALYSIS OF SYMPTOMS

The patient's complaint, whether it is the severe chest pain of an acute myocardial infarction or transient dizziness during an episode of ventricular tachycardia, is frequently the precipitating factor in initiating medical care. Symptoms can reflect spontaneous changes in cardiovascular status or response to therapy. For example, a patient may complain of progressive dyspnea before any x-ray or auscultatory findings of pulmonary edema are actually detected. Another patient may develop uneasiness or a sense of doom before a major catastrophic event. However, because symptoms may be common to many problems or diseases, a careful analysis of each symptom is necessary to relate its importance to the current illness.

Depending on both the severity of the illness and the patient's individual personality, an open-ended question may provide helpful information. More frequently, however, the person caring for the patient will need to direct the patient's answers through skilled questioning based on the questioner's knowledge of the problem and disease process, triggering responses about certain aspects of the illness. The following is a procedure for clarifying the characteristics of symptoms:

Location: Define the location and origin of the pain, discomfort, or unusual sensation. Radiation to other areas is particularly important.

Severity: Attempt to quantitate the extent and severity of the symptoms in relation to the patient's attitudes and pain or complaint threshold.

Character: Determine the descriptive quality of the symptoms. Is the pain sharp, dull, or burning?

Associated symptoms: Determine whether there are other sensations that accompany the primary symptom. For example, aching in the left arm associated with transient epigastric pressure is much more suggestive of angina than of gastroitestinal problems.

Timing: Determine the duration of the symptoms in comparison with previous episodes. Does the pain last for a longer or shorter time?

Factors altering the symptoms: Determine what factors affect the symptoms. What initiated the symptoms? Do they occur during activity, rest, or sleep? What relieves or partially relieves them? What aggravates them?

These descriptions of a patient's symptoms may allow one to assess progression of disease or development of a new problem or provide a guide for requesting further diagnostic information.

PHYSICAL EXAMINATION
General Inspection

General inspection of the patient may sometimes be overlooked during intensive invasive hemodynamic monitoring. Its importance cannot be overemphasized, because the inspection may provide important information concerning the cardiovascular status of the patient.

Does the patient appear to be the stated age? Physical appearance may be a better indication of the physiologic status of the patient than is the chronologic age.

Does the patient appear to be in distress? The patient complaining of dyspnea while lying comfortably in bed may have a low complaint threshold. On the other hand, the denying patient may have obvious tachypnea and respiratory distress yet not complain about it.

Does the patient respond appropriately to your questioning and care? Lack of cooperation may reflect a changing mental status caused by either physiologic or psychologic factors.

Is the patient cyanotic or pale? Careful, continued observation for cyanosis may provide the first clue to a diagnosis of decreased peripheral perfusion or pulmonary embolus.

The restless, anxious patient who cannot get comfortable or who is constantly tossing and turning may reflect a deteriorating cardiovascular status. Not only is the distress disconcerting, but the resulting anxiety and movements may demand increased cardiac output and cause further deterioration of the patient's cardiovascular condition.

Mental Status

A changing mental status in the critically ill patient with cardiovascular disease may indicate the development of a postoperative psychosis or a decrease in cardiac output. Depending on the patient's status, the examination might include evaluation of the following mental abilities:

1. Appropriateness of responses
2. Orientation to time, place, and person
3. Memory for recent and past events

4. Retentive ability, such as the ability to repeat five random numbers from memory

5. Ability to do calculations, such as serially subtracting 7 from 100

6. Understanding of the meaning of proverbs

Venous Pulses

Examination of the neck veins is one of the easiest components of the cardiovascular examination and may yield important information regarding a patient's cardiovascular status. Fig. 2-1 shows the distended external jugular vein, which is easiest to examine because it is superficial to the sternocleidomastoid muscles. When distended, it accurately reflects the venous pressure of the right atrium, although apparent lack of distention may be caused by obesity or fibrosis of the vein. At times the external jugular vein can be so distended that it does not pulsate and is actually not noticed until the patient assumes a semiupright or upright position. The anterior jugular vein is of a smaller caliber but can usually be seen when distended. The internal jugular vein is more difficult to examine because of its position below the sternocleidomastoid muscles and next to the carotid artery.

If the venous pressure is normal or near normal, the patient's head and trunk can be elevated just slightly above the horizontal. The patient's head should be rotated away from the examiner's side of the bed and examined for distention of the external jugular vein. A bedside lamp arranged to shine tangentially across the area being inspected may help to detect a slightly distended vein. If there is no distention, the examiner's finger should be placed horizontally across the base of the sus-

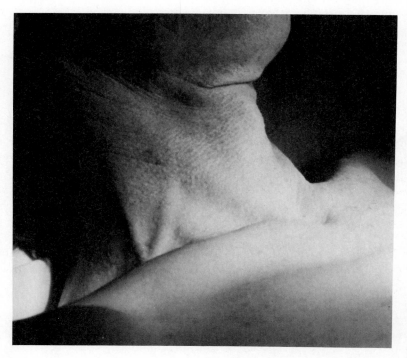

Fig. 2-1. Distended external jugular neck vein of a patient with right-sided heart failure.

pected location of the external jugular vein (Fig. 2-2). If the external jugular vein fills during pressure application and collapses when pressure is released, the examiner can be sure that the venous pressure is low. The patient's head can then be lowered further to determine the actual venous pressure. Conversely, if the venous pressure is very high, the external jugular veins may be markedly distended without visible pulsation when the patient is in a flat or only slightly upright position. The patient's head should be raised until visible pulsations can be seen in the external jugular vein. A patient with cardiac tamponade, constrictive pericarditis, or severe right heart failure may have a venous pressure higher than 30 cm H_2O, resulting in distended neck veins above the level of the upper neck when the patient is in an upright or standing position. In these patients the veins may be distended even in the temporal area or the forehead.

Venous Pressure

The right-sided venous pressure reflects the right atrial (RA) pressure and right ventricular (RV) end-diastolic pressure. This venous pressure can be measured directly by a central venous catheter or estimated by examination of the neck veins. Although the central venous pressure (CVP) has been shown to have a poor correlation with the more accurate pulmonary arterial wedge (PAW) or left atrial (LA) pressure (which reflects LV diastolic filling pressure), the trend of changes in the

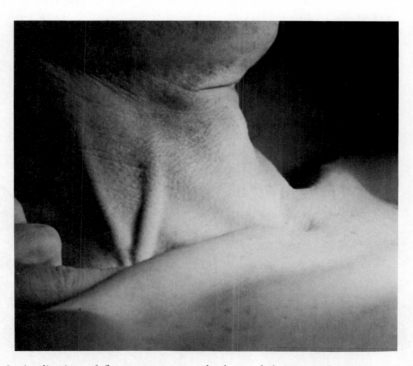

Fig. 2-2. Application of finger pressure at the base of the external jugular vein causing venous distention. When the finger pressure is released, the venous pressure will fall and can be estimated.

CVP during monitoring of the seriously ill patient can provide important information concerning the patient's hemodynamic status.

Noninvasive assessment of the venous pressure is particularly important when there are contraindications to invasive measurement or when there is difficulty using or inserting the central venous catheter. In these situations estimation of the pressure from examination of the neck veins may be invaluable in deciding whether pressure measurements are correct or whether the central venous catheter requires replacement.

Method of measurement. An accurate noninvasive measurement of the CVP (RA pressure) is contingent on the following criteria: (1) that there is no obstruction to venous flow from the neck veins to the right atrium and (2) that one can approximate the location of the right atrium in the chest. If these criteria are met, CVP can be accurately estimated by the following procedure (Fig. 2-3):

1. Raise the patient's head to a semiupright position. If the patient is in severe RV failure, raise the patient's head to an upright position.
2. Examine the neck for pulsating and distended internal or external jugular veins. If the patient is able to cooperate, have the patient breathe in; look for a fall in the amount of venous distention.
   a. If the neck vein is completely distended, increase the elevation of the patient's head or have the patient stand beside the bed.
   b. If there is no venous distention, lower the patient's head until you can see filling of the vein.
3. Estimate the level at the top of the fluid column within the vein.
4. Estimate the location of the middle of the right atrium.
5. Using a centimeter rule, measure the *vertical* distance between the two.

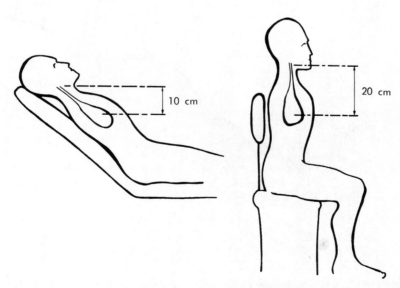

Fig. 2-3. Estimate of venous pressure by measuring the *vertical* height between the level of the right side of the heart and the meniscus of the distended neck veins.

Sources of error. The following are sources of error in the noninvasive measurements of CVP:

1. Inability to visualize the vein in a short, fact neck or in one without a visible external jugular vein
2. Inability to see the neck veins because of marked distention when the patient is in a supine or semiupright position (This error is a common one in patients who have constrictive pericarditis or cardiac tamponade and extremely high venous pressures.)
3. Inability to estimate the top of the fluid column because the patient's head cannot be raised
4. Confusion in identification of venous versus arterial pulsations (Venous pulsations are easily obliterated by pressure on the neck at the level of the clavicle.)
5. Hypovolemia causing poor distention of neck veins in a supine position
6. Neck surgery or previous procedures on the neck veins causing local venous distention, which does not reflect true central venous pressure

Clinical application

Case 1

A 49-year-old man was admitted to the coronary care unit with an extensive anterior myocardial infarction. Except for frequent premature ventricular contractions that were suppressed by lidocaine hydrochloride, he appeared to be doing well on hospital day 1. Routine CVP ranged from 2 to 6 cm H_2O. On hospital day 3 his CVP steadily rose to as high as 17 cm H_2O. This rise in CVP was accompanied by a slight rise in heart rate, but there was no change in respiratory rate or blood pressure. Blood had been difficult to withdraw from the inserted catheter, although the IV infused fairly well.

Examination of his neck veins revealed no venous distention, and it was suspected that the readings were inaccurate. A new catheter was inserted by Seldinger's technique, and a CVP of 3 cm H_2O was confirmed. This simple examination of the neck veins prevented inappropriate treatment based on artifactual, high venous pressures.

Case 2

A 35-year-old woman with severe RV and LV failure caused by an idiopathic cardiomyopathy was admitted to the hospital because of increasing dyspnea. Examination revealed severe dyspnea and marked venous distention. With bed rest, oxygen therapy, and repeated IV injections of furosemide, she had an excellent diuresis and showed marked improvement. On hospital day 5 she complained of fatigue and had a resting heart rate of 100 beats/minute. Despite continued treatment, she became worse and developed a narrowed pulse pressure and hypotension. The use of IV diuretics effected no improvement. It was then noted that her neck veins were barely distended, even in a supine position. A diagnosis of iatrogenic hypovolemia resulting from excessive diuresis was made. Diuretics and salt restriction were stopped, and 500 ml of 0.2% NaCl with 5% dextrose in water were administered, resulting in striking improvement.

Venous waves. Venous neck pulsations of the patient with normal sinus rhythm reflect the same waves seen in RA pressure tracings (Fig. 2-4). The *a* wave is produced by atrial contraction and in timing just precedes the arterial pulsation that can be timed by simultaneous palpation of the other side of the neck. The *a* wave precedes the first heart sound if the heart is simultaneously auscultated. When atrial fibrillation is present, atrial contraction does not occur, and no *a* wave will be visible.

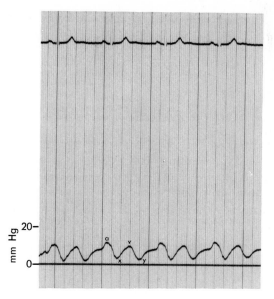

Fig. 2-4. Central venous or RA pressure tracing showing *a* and *v* waves with *x* and *y* descents. No *c* wave is seen in this pressure tracing.

The second wave seen in the neck is the *c* wave, which is small in amplitude and frequently not seen. This wave reflects the closing of the tricuspid valve at the beginning of ventricular systole.

The third wave is the *v* wave, which reflects changes of pressure in the right atrium as the AV valve bulges into the right atrium during ventricular systole. The descent of the *a* wave is termed the *x* descent, and the descent of the *v* wave is termed the *y* descent.

VENOUS WAVE ABNORMALITIES. Elevations of right-sided pressures, for any reason, will result in increased RA and venous pressure; likewise, abnormalities of the tricuspid valve (either stenosis or insufficiency) will result in abnormalities in venous pulsation.

Rhythm disturbances may also result in abnormalities of venous waves. For example, AV dissociation results in a lack of synchronization between atrial and ventricular systole, and atrial contraction may take place at a time when ventricular systole is occurring. This atrial contraction against a closed tricuspid valve results in giant *a* waves (called cannon waves) in the right atrium and neck veins. Similar abnormalities can be seen in complete heart block and ventricular pacing.

Patients with mitral stenosis and pulmonary hypertension, pulmonic valvular stenosis, and tricuspid stenosis have abnormally high *a* waves.

An exaggerated *v* wave is seen from tricuspid insufficiency, whether it results from RV hypertension and dilatation of the annulus or is caused by valvular disease.

Severe constrictive pericarditis, or cardiac tamponade, can cause a marked elevation of the necks veins that may be overlooked during superficial examination. This distention of the neck veins is one of the most valuable diagnostic clues to this life-threatening problem. In constrictive pericarditis and tamponade, both the *a* and v waves are prominent and have rapid x and y descents (Fig. 2-5). In chronic constrictive pericarditis, Kussmaul's sign occurs with a rise, instead of a fall, in the venous pressure during inspiration.

Arterial Pulses

Examination of arterial pulsations provides monitoring of the patient's heart rate and information regarding the stroke volume. During the initial examination, it is important to palpate all major pulses, that is, the carotid, radial, brachial, femoral, popliteal, dorsalis pedis, and posterior tibial pulses. Although not all of these pulses need to be monitored continuously, regular observation of their presence or absence and their character is helpful for making an accurate assessment of changes in the critically ill patient.

Simultaneous assessment of both the brachial and radial pulses is an efficient and useful method of assessing both pulsations. In younger patients, or patients with well developed biceps, the brachial artery may be hidden beneath the belly of the biceps muscle, requiring heavier pressure or some manipulation of the arm for accurate assessment. Elderly patients with arterial tortuosity may have lateral displacement of the artery. Various amounts of elbow flexion are necessary to properly palpate the brachial arterial pulses in these patients.

During the initial examination or periodic reevaluation, taking the patient's hand can be extremely valuable, not only for palpation of the radial pulse but also for an overall assessment of the patient's mental and physical status. The patient's response to this action may provide clues about his mental status. A desperate grasp of the examiner's hand may indicate anxiety or fear that the patient may not be able to express verbally. A sweaty, moist hand may indicate anxiety or a diffuse,

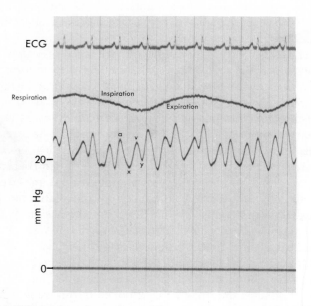

Fig. 2-5. Elevated CVP tracing of a patient with constrictive pericarditis showing prominent a and v waves.

hypersympathetic state. A cool, limp hand may indicate a low cardiac output in a patient with cardiovascular disease. Examination of the nail beds for color and arterial pulsation can provide information about the arterial system. Finally, palpation of the radial pulse not only measures the heart rate but also determines the character of the pulse, which may indicate a changing stroke volume. In addition to providing information, taking the patient's hand provides a physical contact that gives the patient important psychologic support.

This section deals with the common cardiovascular abnormalities that affect arterial pulsations.

Absent or weak pulsations.. Determining the presence or absence of arterial pulses during the initial examination and thereafter is vital in monitoring the critically ill patient with cardiac disease. Diffuse atherosclerosis may result in absence of the dorsalis pedis or posterior tibial pulse before the patient is admitted to the hospital. It is helpful to document this absence to differentiate it from a new catastrophic event, such as an arterial embolus. After a cardiac procedure involving catheterization of femoral or brachial arteries, monitoring of distal pulses is critical for the early detection of local thrombosis or distal embolization, either of which might require urgent thrombectomy or Fogarty catheterization. Finally, the sudden disappearance of a pulse may be indicative of a systemic embolus. The source of this embolus may be a thrombus in the left ventricle from an artificial valve, from the left atrium (particularly in atrial fibrillation or mitral valvular disease), or more rarely from a myxomatous tumor in the left atrium. Arterial embolization is usually accompanied by pain and frequently by pallor of the extremity distal to the embolus. There may be a difference in temperature between the two extremities. Arterial pulsations may be weak because of low stroke volume or abnormalities of the arterial vessel. Patients who have had previous coronary arteriography by the Sones technique may have a diminished or absent brachial artery pulse. Information concerning a previous arteriogram can be obtained through the history; an arteriotomy scar may also be present in the antecubital area. Some disease states, such as dissecting aortic aneurysms, may result in cessation of arterial pulsation and should be considered an emergency. Patients with diffuse atherosclerosis may have diminished or absent femoral pulses and absent distal pulses in the legs. Whereas this disease process is bilateral, one pulse may well be stronger than the other. Similar abnormalities may occur in the carotid vessels in elderly patients. In these situations palpation of the carotid arteries should be performed carefully to prevent complete occlusion of flow for any period of time.

Auscultation of the artery. Bruits may be heard over arteries (particularly the femoral and carotid arteries) with diminished pulsation caused by occlusive atherosclerotic disease. Auscultation of the carotid arteries is performed while the patient is suspending respiration, so that bruits can be differentiated from inspiratory or expiratory noises. Abdominal bruits may also be heard but do not hold the same significance, since approximately 25% of young normal people have a systolic bruit during auscultation of the abdomen.

Rapid upstroke of the arterial pulse. The upstroke of the arterial pulse normally becomes more rapid, the more peripherally it is palpated. A quick uptake of the arterial pulse can be ascertained by the experienced examiner. This quick upstroke may indicate nothing more than an anxious patient, but it may also reflect cardiac disease. A rapid upstroke of the pulse accompanied by a rapid fall (that is, a spiking arterial pulse) may reflect mitral insufficiency with a rapid initial ejection from the ventricle followed by regurgitation into the left atrium and early closure of the aortic valve. Aortic insufficiency, when not accompanied by significant stenosis, will also be reflected by a rapid upstroke of the arterial pulse and a widened pulse pressure of as much as 100 mm Hg. One can clinically see this markedly widened pulse pressure by placing a light under the patient's finger pad and observing the pulsating nail beds while applying slight pressure to the nail. Other diseases that may result in a rapid upstroke of the pulse are systemic diseases, such as thyrotoxicosis and anemia, and arteriovenous shunts with high cardiac output and rapid distal runoff. The pulse of an elderly patient may have a seemingly rapid upstroke because of generalized arteriosclerosis and rigidity of the arterial system. Another disease resulting in a prominent early pulse is hypertrophic obstructive cardiomyopathy or hypertrophic subaortic stenosis; in this case the arterial pulse has a rapid, early peak, and there is either a bifid pulse (double-peaked) or absence of the second half of the systolic pulse because of LV outflow obstruction during late systole.

Slow upstroke of the arterial pulse. A slow upstroke of the arterial pulse is associated with aortic stenosis, in which a prolonged ejection time and late appearance of the peak systolic pressure occur. Although the character of the pulse may allow differentiation between mild and severe aortic stenosis, changes in compliance of the arterial system (particularly in the elderly patient) may make this estimation difficult. A slow upstroke of the pulse may also be the result of severe congestive heart failure and a small stroke volume.

Pulsus paradoxus. During inspiration, the systolic arterial pressure may fall as much as 10 mm Hg. This normal decline is caused by decreased LV stroke volume and transmission of the negative intrathoracic pressure to the great vessels during systole. A decrease in systolic pressure greater than 10 mm Hg during inspiration is called pulsus paradoxus (Fig. 2-6) and reflects either severe cardiac decompensation or, classically, cardiac tamponade. Pulsus paradoxus also occurs in about 50% of patients with constrictive pericarditis as well as in patients with obstructive airway disease. Kussmaul first described this condition as paradoxical as the disappearance of the peripheral pulse occurred in the face of obvious apical pulsations.

The character and variations of the pulse during inspiration should be noted during palpation of the pulse. In the patient with a critically severe cardiac tamponade, the pulse may nearly disappear during inspiration and reappear during expiration. This condition is an exaggerated pulsus paradoxus that can be more easily demonstrated with a stethoscope and blood pressure cuff.

Pulsus alternans. Pulsus alternans is an alternation of peak systolic pressure and usually reflects severe LV failure. If the finding is exaggerated, the examiner may even detect the variation during palpation of the pulse. These alternating stronger and weaker pulsations of the distal pulse can be confirmed by a blood pressure cuff or intra-arterial monitoring.

Arrhythmias. Abnormalities in cardiac rhythm result in abnormalities of pulsation. For example atrial fibrillation may result in shorter R-R intervals that prevent adequate time for diastolic filling of the ventricle. When this situation occurs, even though mechanical systole occurs, there is insufficient volume or pressure gener-

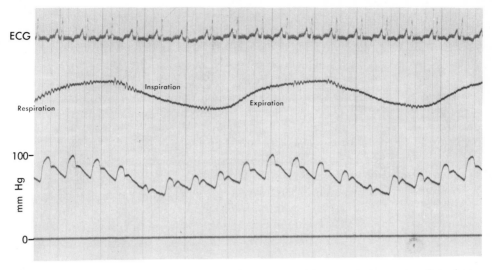

ECG

Inspiration

Respiration   Expiration

100—

mm Hg

0—

Fig. 2-6. Brachial artery pressure tracing of a patient with constrictive pericarditis during normal respiration. Systolic pressure falls from 100 mm Hg during expiration to 70 mm Hg during inspiration. This exaggerated fall in pressure is termed pulsus paradoxus.

ated by the ventricle to open the aortic valve and produce a pulse. For this reason the peripheral pulse may be an inaccurate determinant of the true ventricular rate in atrial fibrillation. The occurrence of premature ventricular contractions (PVCs) or ventricular bigeminy may result in palpation of only the normal sinus beats. In these instances correlation of the peripheral pulse with the ECG monitor will prevent a misdiagnosis or an inaccurate measurement of the cardiac rate.

The Lungs

Examination of the lungs and respiratory status provides information regarding pulmonary problems that may be aggravating or causing serious cardiovascular difficulties. A daily chest x-ray examination cannot substitute for frequent evaluation of the respiratory rate and character, the character of breath sounds during auscultation, and the presence or absence of rales. This section briefly discusses the techniques of percussion and auscultation of the chest as they relate to monitoring the critically ill patient with cardiovascular disease.

Percussion. Percussion of the anterior chest consists of defining areas of cardiac dullness and areas of dullness from the liver and possibly the spleen. Percussion of the posterior chest is performed with the patient in a sitting position, which is not always feasible in the critically ill patient. When it is possible, the patient should be relaxed and leaning forward slightly. It is best to begin percussion at the top of the chest and proceed downward, comparing the sounds produced on each side of the chest and from top to bottom. Examination is hampered by obesity, wasting of the upper chest, asthma, distention of the bowel or stomach by gas, and incorrect positioning of the patient. Examination by percussion requires practice and skill. Since the amount of resonance obtained at any point depends on the strength of the stroke delivered, minor variations in technique can cause considerable differences in the percussion note produced.

Percussion sounds are divided into normal vesicular resonance, hyperresonance, dull or flat sounds, and tympanic resonance. Normal vesicular resonance is a low-pitched, vibrant sound that occurs over healthy, air-containing lungs. Overinflation of the lungs results in a louder and more vibrant note referred to as hyperresonance. Areas not containing air produce a dull or flat sound that is short, higher pitched, and without a vibrant quality. Tympanic sounds occur over hollow organs distended with air. These sounds are high pitched and similar to the sound produced by the kettledrum. Percussion to define areas of fluid in the lung is performed with the patient in an upright position. Fluid-filled areas are characterized by a dull sound occurring abnormally high above the usual diaphragmatic area or unequally from one side of the chest to the other.

Auscultation. Auscultation of the lungs is easily performed and should be a component of each cardiovascular examination. Before auscultation is begun, the patient should be observed carefully to characterize the respirations. Are they labored or quiet? Are they regular or irregular? Does the patient make audible noise during respiration that will be heard during auscultation? Characterizing these features of the patient's respiration will prevent initial confusion during examination.

Examination of the lungs is traditionally performed with the diaphragm component of the binaural stethoscope, because if detects higher-pitched sounds. The earpieces should be applied properly to exclude extraneous room noise, and the diaphragm of the stethoscope should be placed firmly on the patient's chest. Skillful use of the stethoscope requires knowledge of what to listen for and what to ignore and the ability to concentrate on various components of the respiratory cycle while listening for particular sounds. A quiet room is preferred but is usually not possible when the critically ill patient is being examined. A great deal of information can be obtained in a less than perfect environment. Care must be taken to disregard noise from movement of the diaphragm on the skin. This noise can be avoided by maintaining firm, light pressure of the diaphragm against the skin. In very thin patients the bell component of the stethoscope may be needed for listening between the ribs.

Normal breath sounds. The three types of sounds heard during examination of the normal lungs are vesicular, tracheal, and bronchovesicular. Experience gained from the examination of many normal people is needed so that minor deviations from normal can be detected and applied to the care of the critically ill patient Vesicular breath sounds are heard best during inspiration and have a breathy quality. Tracheal breath sounds occur more frequently during expiration and have tubular, harsher quality. Bronchovesicular breath sounds are a mixture of trache and vesicular elements and are heard best over the central areas of the chest ov lying the large bronchi.

Abnormal breath sounds. Diminished vesicular breath sounds relate either t change in the flow of air to the alveoli or to abnormalities of the pleural ca such as the presence of fluid, air, or scar tissue. Restriction of air movement, e because of chest wall disease or bronchial disease such as asthma, can mar decrease vesicular breath sounds. Tubular or bronchial breath sounds are he diseases where there is excessive transmission of sound from the bronchi chest, as in consolidation caused by pneumonia. Asthmatic breath sounds are acterized by a markedly prolonged expiratory phase with wheezing or gr sounds and a short inspiratory phase with minimal vesicular breath sounds

Rales are the sounds produced when air passes through bronchi that contain fluid of any kind. Rales vary greatly from patient to patient, depending on the cause and extent of the underlying cardiac or pulmonary disease. It is best to have the patient cough before auscultation, so that the lungs are cleared of any minimal hypostatic fluids. Moist rales can be coarse and gurgling (rhonchi) and occur when there is excessive secretion in the trachea and large bronchi that the patient is unable to cough up. Rhonchi usually occur in patients with decreased mental status or a critical illness. Medium crepitant rales are small and bubbling and occur over areas of pneumonia or pulmonary congestion. Fine rales are sometimes described as crackling and occur in conditions where pulmonary venous congestion is present. Dry rales are caused by a small amount of thickened exudate in the bronchioles and are occasionally heard in patients with chronic bronchial disease. These rales are almost always associated with bronchial breath sounds or asthmatic sounds.

Pleural friction rubs. Sound of a friction rub may be heard during the respiratory cycle, particularly during inspiration. The rubbing sound seems very superficial, as though it were right under the diaphragm of the stethoscope. Pleural rubs are variously described as grating, rubbing, or creaking and may even have a leathery characteristic. They frequently alter with a change in the patient's position or state of inspiration. A friction rub may be important to identify because it can be caused by an underlying pulmonary infection or infarcted area.

The Heart

Inspection and palpation of the anterior chest. Diagnostic information can be obtained from brief but careful inspection and palpation of the anterior chest during monitoring of the critically ill patient with cardiac disease. This section describes briefly the technique and some of the more common abnormalities found in specific areas of the precordium. Abnormalities detected during inspection or palpation must be correlated with the cardiac cycle and auscultation. This examination is carried out in the aortic area, the pulmonic area, the lower left sternal border, and the apical area.

AORTIC AREA. Although abnormal pulsations in the aortic area may be produced by marked dilatation of the ascending aorta, its position near the sternum usually prevents any visible pulsation. During palpation, a vibratory thrill may be felt in the patient with aortic stenosis and is associated with a loud systolic murmur. The aortic valve closure can occasionally be palpated in the patient with severe hypertension.

PULMONIC AREA. Abnormalities of pulsation in the pulmonic area are rare except in the patient with marked dilatation of the pulmonary artery because of either pulmonary hypertension or pulmonary ectasia. During palpation, a thrill may be felt in the patient with pulmonic stenosis. A loud pulmonic second sound may be palpated in severe pulmonary hypertension, and a pulmonic systolic tap may be palpated in patients with a dilated pulmonary artery.

LOWER LEFT STERNAL BORDER. Palpation in the lower left sternal border area may reveal a palpable thrill in patients with a ventricular septal defect. Abnormalities of pulsation in this area are most commonly found in conditions associated with RV hypertrophy, such as pulmonary hypertension (with or without severe mitral stenosis). When RV hypertrophy is present, the sternum can be felt to move anteriorly during systole; this movement is referred to as a *substernal heave.*

APICAL AREA. The LV apical impulse can be identified and actually pinpointed within a 1 cm area. It is normally located in the fifth intercostal space in the midclavicular line. Displacement of the point of maximal impulse (PMI) lateral to the midclavicular line is indicative of cardiac enlargement. Not only is the location of the PMI important, but its character may reflect LV contractility. A poorly palpable apical impulse may indicate poor LV contraction and stroke volume if the apex is near the chest wall. However, a very muscular chest or emphysema will obscure this finding. A systolic thrill may be palpated in this area because of mitral insufficiency from any cause. Occasionally, a very loud, rumbling diastolic murmur can be palpated. A forceful or sustained apical impulse generally reflects LV hypertrophy associated with aortic stenosis or arterial hypertension. In patients with mitral insufficiency or rapid peripheral runoff (as in AV fistula), a rapid damping of the apical impulse during systole may be palpated.

Events occurring in the left ventricle during diastolic filling can also be appreciated. Palpation of an early diastolic gallop, associated with outward movement of the left ventricle during early filling, usually reflects LV failure. An early diastolic gallop may also be palpated in patients with a hyperadrenergic state and large cardiac outputs. Rarely, during late diastole, a systolic gallop or "atrial kick" may be palpated. In patients with mitral valvular disease, palpation of an opening snap in early diastole can occasionally be appreciated, but this snap is much easier to hear than to palpate.

EPIGASTRIC AREA. Visible or palpable pulsations of the aorta in the epigastric area are normal findings. Many people are also slightly tender in this area. For these reasons palpation in the epigastric area generally does not yield further information about cardiac events, although aneurysmal dilatation of the abdominal aorta may be detected.

Auscultation. Although cardiac auscultation is traditionally thought of as a diagnostic tool, components of this part of the cardiac examination may be used to assess the current cardiovascular status of the heart and to monitor hemodynamic changes. Ideally, auscultation of the heart should be carried out in a quiet room with a cooperative patient. The stethoscope should be equipped with both a diaphragm and a bell. In general, the diaphragm is used for high-frequency sounds, such as aortic or mitral insufficiency murmurs, and the bell for low-frequency sounds, particularly diastolic gallops and the rumbling murmur of mitral stenosis. It is important to place the bell on the skin with just enough pressure to seal out extraneous noise. With further pressure on the bell the skin itself becomes a diaphragm and accentuates any high-frequency sounds.

Auscultation of the heart involves selectively listening for each component of the cardiac cycle separately, that is, the first sound, the second sound, the period of systole, and the period of diastole. This listening should be done systematically in at least four cardiac areas: the aortic area, the pulmonic area, the lower left sternal border, and the apical regions of the precordium (Fig. 2-7). These areas do not correspond exactly to their anatomic location but to the area in which the particular valve sounds are best heard. Although each examiner develops a personal system, optimal auscultation is usually begun at the aortic area to determine cardiac cycle time and to identify the first and second heart sounds. Once these sounds are firmly

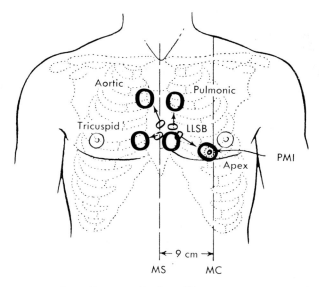

Fig. 2-7. Primary areas of cardiac auscultation. These areas correspond to the locations where sounds and murmurs are best heard rather than to an anatomic valve location. *MS,* Midsternum; *MC,*midclavicle; *PMI,* point of maximal impulse; *LLSB,* lower left sternal border.

identified, the listener may then move to other areas of the precordium, mentally noting murmurs and changes in heart sounds.

The character of heart sounds should be noted carefully, and specific attention should be directed to differences in intensity and constancy. Each heart sound is identified and characterized separately. The presence of extra heart sounds should then be identified, particularly in midsystole and in early and late diastole. Once they are noted, more exact timing can be ascertained in relation to the first and second heart sounds. Whenever difficulty develops in the timing of the sounds, the examiner may wish to return to the aortic area to confirm the first and second sounds, since these sounds indicate systole and diastole and can be used as a timing reference. When possible, the patient should assume other positions, including sitting upright or even standing, so that changes in heart sounds and murmurs that otherwise might not be heard may be detected.

Heart sounds. The *first heart sound* (S$_1$) is produced by closure of the mitral and tricuspid valves (Fig. 2-8). These AV valves open at the initiation of diastole and allow filling of the ventricles. The valves float partially closed during ventricular filling, then reopen during atrial systole. At the onset of ventricular systole, the pressures in the two ventricles quickly exceed the pressures in the atria and result in forceful closure of both valves. This closure results in vibrations that are transmitted through tissues of the body and are heard through a stethoscope as the first heart sound. Changes in conduction time and blood volume can cause alterations in the timing of valve closure, resulting in a separate sound for closure of each valve. This process is termed *splitting of the first sound.*

Conditions that accentuate the first heart sound are hyperthyroidism, anemia, tachycardia, and mitral stenosis.

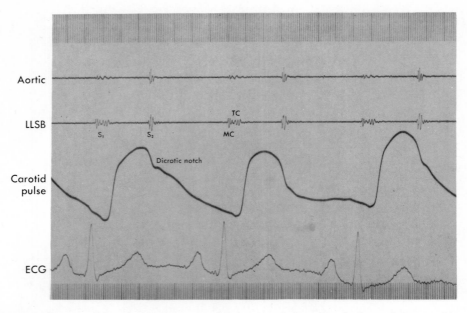

Fig. 2-8. Phonocardiogram showing normal heart sounds heard at the lower left sternal border *(LLSB)* and aortic area. Split first sound (S_1) is composed of mitral valve closure *(MC)* and tricuspid valve closure *(TC)*. Dicrotic notch in the carotid artery tracing indicates aortic valve closure.

The *second heart sound* (S_2) is associated with closure of the aortic and pulmonic valves and represents the onset of ventricular diastole (Fig. 2-9). Closure of the aortic valve usually precedes closure of the pulmonic valve. The aortic component of the second heart sound may be accentuated in systemic hypertension and diminished or absent in aortic stenosis, where there is restricted movement of the valve. The pulmonic component will be accentuated in pulmonary hypertension from any cause.

Splitting of the second sound normally occurs during inspiration as increased blood flow to the right side of the heart prolongs RV systole and delays pulmonic valve closure. An atrial septal defect results in wide splitting of the second sound, which varies little with respiration because of the balancing of the central venous return between the right and left atria through the atrial septal defect.

Paradoxical splitting of the second sound (pulmonic valve closure preceding aortic valve closure) occurs with (1) left bundle branch block caused by delay of LV systole and (2) severe aortic stenosis caused by prolonged LV ejection time and restricted movement of the aortic valve.

The *third heart sound* (S_3) occurs at the end of rapid diastolic ventricular filling and probably results from vibrations of the ventricular wall and by tensing of the papillary muscles. It may originate in either the right or the left ventricle and is heard best at the apex with the bell of the stethoscope. The presence of a third heart sound may be normal in adolescents, in patients with ventricular dilatation from any cause, and in patients with decreased ventricular compliance (Fig. 2-10).

The *fourth heart sound* (S_4) occurs during atrial systole and is produced by the forceful movement of blood from the left atrium into the ventricle near the end of

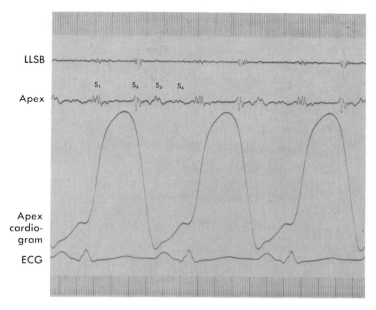

Fig. 2-9. Phonocardiogram of a patient with severe congestive heart failure showing an S_3 and S_4 gallop. Apex cardiogram records systolic outward bulging of the ventricle during systole.

diastole. Usually it is not heard in normal patients, although it may be recorded by a phonocardiograph. This sound is also heard at the apex in patients with decreased LV compliance, which may occur with coronary artery disease, LV hypertrophy, and cardiac failure.

Systolic sounds. Ejection clicks may occur when a partially stenotic aortic or pulmonic valve opens at the initiation of ventricular systole. Ejection clicks may result from sudden expansion of the pulmonary or aortic wall at the initiation of systole and are heard frequently in midsystole and late systole. The best-known syndrome is the midsystolic click that initiates a late systolic murmur of mitral insufficiency caused by prolapse of the mitral valve.

Diastolic sounds. Opening snaps can be heard when a stenotic mitral or tricuspid valve is forced open at the start of diastole. The sound has a snapping quality and is heard best at the left sternal border, where it may be confused with the widely split second sound. Early diastolic sounds without an opening snap may occur in pericardial disease because of sudden distention of the thickened pericardium during diastole.

Gallop rhythms. Gallop rhythms (Fig. 2-10) occur when the third or fourth heart sounds become pathologically accentuated. The summation of the third and fourth sounds during tachycardia is called a *summation gallop* and usually represents severe cardiac decompensation.

Heart murmurs. Heart murmurs are produced by turbulent blood flow through stenotic or abnormal valves or vessels, resulting in audible vibrations that can be heard with a stethoscope. Blood flow is laminar, and valve movement normally occurs in such a way as to provide unimpeded flow. When stenosis or insufficiency of a valve occurs, blood flow becomes turbulent, producing audible vibrations.

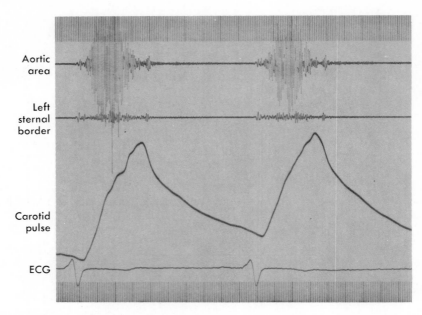

Fig. 2-10. Phonocardiogram of a patient with aortic stenosis showing a crescendo-decrescendo systolic murmur. Slow-rising carotid pulse also suggests aortic stenosis.

When all cardiac sounds have been identified and their timing ascertained, the presence of murmurs or other heart sounds can be identified. When a murmur is heard, it should be characterized in relation to the cardiac cycle and changes in intensity (holosystolic or crescendo-decrescendo murmurs).

Systolic murmurs. Systolic murmurs can generally be categorized as either ejection or regurgitant murmurs. Ejection murmurs result from aortic or pulmonic stenosis or increased flow through a normal valve and have a crescendo-decrescendo character (Fig. 2-10). The systolic ejection murmur of aortic stenosis is heard best at the aortic area and radiates to the suprasternal notch and carotid artery and to the apex. Regurgitant systolic murmurs begin immediately after the first sound and extend through the entire systolic period. They are termed *holosystolic,* which means they last through all of systole. Holosystolic murmurs occur with mitral insufficiency, tricuspid insufficiency, ventricular septal defects, or other AV communications.

At times it may be difficult to differentiate between ejection and regurgitant systolic murmurs. A number of maneuvers can be performed to cause alterations in the character and intensity of the murmur, and these alterations may help the examiner to identify the correct valve and the cause of the murmur. Table 2-1 outlines some commonly used methods to characterize systolic murmurs.

The occurrence of a new systolic murmur can be an extremely important development during monitoring of the critically ill patient. It may indicate papillary muscle dysfunction resulting in mitral insufficiency, or it may indicate the development of a ventricular septal defect caused by perforation of an infarcted ventricular septum.

Table 2-1. Effect of maneuvers on systolic murmurs

Maneuver	Ejection murmur	Mitral regurgitation	Tricuspid regurgitation	Ventricular septal defect	Hypertropic sub-aortic stenosis
Inspiration	—*	—	↑	—	—
Straining	↓	↓	↓	—	↑
Valsalva's release	↑	↑	↑	—	↓
Postextrasystolic beat	↑	↓ or —	—	—	↑
Amyl nitrite	↑	↓	↑ or ↓		↑

*—, No change; ↓, murmur decreases; ↑, murmur increases.

Diastolic murmurs. As the pressure in the relaxing ventricles falls to a level below the pressure in the atria, the AV valves open and diastolic filling is initiated. If either the mitral or tricuspid valve is stenotic, low-pitched, rumbling murmurs occur as the result of the turbulence of the blood flow through these valves. In typical mitral stenosis the diastolic murmur is initiated by the opening snap of the stenotic valve. Placing the patient in the left lateral position brings the apex of the heart nearer to the chest wall and optimizes detection of a mitral diastolic rumble.

The other major diastolic murmurs occur in relation to insufficient aortic or pulmonic valves that produce a soft, high-frequency murmur. Diastolic murmurs may be initially listened for at the base of the heart or in the aortic and pulmonic areas. These murmurs are soft and of very high frequency when they are caused by aortic insufficiency or pulmonic insufficiency. Rather than being caused by organic valvular disease, pulmonic insufficiency usually is caused by severe pulmonary hypertension and results from dilatation of the pulmonary artery and valve ring. Aortic insufficiency may be caused by aortic valvular disease or dilatation of the ascending aorta and valvular ring from systemic hypertension. The appearance of a new murmur of aortic insufficiency in a patient with a suspected aneurysm or dissection of the descending aorta is an important physical sign of further proximal dissection that may be life threatening.

Continuous murmurs and sounds. Continuous murmurs are unusual but may be encountered with patent ductus arteriosus; these murmurs have a systolic and diastolic accentuation. Occasionally, a continuous murmur can be heard over an arteriovenous fistula anywhere in the body.

Venous hums. Venous hums are benign murmurs that may be heard in the neck and confused with organic murmurs. Differentiation is made by the application of slight pressure to the neck to stop the venous flow, resulting in complete disappearance of the hum.

Extracardiac sounds

Pericardial rubs. Pericardial disease (particularly pericarditis) may result in both systolic and diastolic sounds. These sounds are scratching and high pitched and vary considerably during the respiratory cycle. The development of a pericardial rub is an important sign to monitor, because it may reveal the cause of chest pain in the patient with diffuse ST elevation on an ECG. Its presence may also be a contraindication for anticoagulation therapy.

Mediastinal crunches. Mediastinal crunches occur when there is air in the mediastinum and are produced by movements of the heart in the mediastinum against these small air pockets. The sounds are random or occur during ventricular systole. They may be associated with crepitation in the neck caused by subcutaneous air collection. These sounds may be heard after cardiac surgery; however, they can also be an ominous sign in an accident victim, since they can be caused by rupture of the trachea or tracheobronchial tree.

The Abdomen

Examination of the abdomen during continuous monitoring provides some information about the cardiovascular status of the critically ill patient. An enlarged, tender liver in the right upper quadrant of the abdomen may signify elevated right-sided pressures and, if pulsatile, indicates serious tricuspid insufficiency. As this situation is usually a long-standing one, it does not reflect a changing cardiovascular status.

Recurring abdominal pain may be caused by ischemia of the bowel as a result of a low cardic output. This diagnosis is extremely difficult to ascertain; however, when excruciating abdominal pain accompanied by a rigid abdomen occurs in the patient with a low cardiac output, ischemia of the bowel must be considered. Differential diagnosis includes a peripheral embolus to one of the mesenteric arteries or to the kidneys.

Extremities

Examination of the hand and wrist is discussed in the section on arterial pulses. Pedal edema in the ambulatory patient with cardiac disease usually reflects right heart failure with retention of salt and water. However, in the bedridden patient, this fluid moves to the most dependent part of the body and should be looked for in the sacral and gluteal areas.

Peripheral cyanosis is evident when the arterial oxygen saturation falls below 75% as a result of an increase (>5 g) in the amount of unsaturated hemoglobin. Whereas its presence indicates severe hypoxia, its absence does not indicate the converse. The cause of this hypoxia may be pulmonary or cardiac:

Pulmonary	Cardiac
Emphysema	Congenital heart disease with
Atelectasis	right-to-left shunt
Pulmonary edema	Low cardiac output
Pulmonary shunts	
Pulmonary emboli	

The occurrence of cyanosis in the patient with cardiac disease is usually an ominous sign and requires prompt treatment. Recognition of this sign may be impaired by poor room lighting, anemia, or the patient's skin pigmentation. An arterial blood gas analysis is needed for a differential diagnosis.

REFERENCES

American Heart Association: Examination of the heart: a series of booklets. Part I: Data collection: the clinical history; part II: Inspection and palpation of venous and arterial pulses; part III: Inspection and palpation of the anterior chest; part IV: Auscultation, New York, 1972, The Association.

Constant J: Diagnostic information from palpation of arterial pulses, Med Times 116:87-98, 1988.

Fowler NO: Examination of the heart. Part II: Inspection and palpation of venous and arterial pulses, New York, 1972, American Heart Association.

Hardman V, and Butterworth J: Auscultation of the heart. Parts I and II, Mod Concepts Cardiovasc Dis 30:645-649, 651-656, 1961.

Luisada AA, MacCanon DM, Kumar S, and Feigen LP: Changing views on the mechanism of the first and second heart sounds, Am Heart J 88:503-514, 1974.

Rivin, AU: Abdominal vascular sounds, JAMA 221:688-690, 1972.

Romhilt DW, and Fowler NO: Physical signs in acute myocardial infarction, Heart Lung 2:74-80, 1973.

Silverman ME, and Hurst JW: The hand and the heart, Am J Cardiol 22:718-728, 1968.

Tilkian AG, and Conover MB: Understanding heart sounds and murmurs, Philadelphia, 1979, WB Saunders Co.

Chapter 3

Principles and Hazards of Monitoring Equipment

I n 1903 William Einthoven introduced the string galvanometer, which served as the basis for the ECG. Since then, electronic instrumentation has become an integral part of medicine. Biomedical instrumentation provides the tools for physiologic measurements in both the research laboratory and the clinical setting. Although some forms of biomedical instruments are unique to the medical field, most are applications of widely used methods for physical measurements, and an understanding of the basic principles of physiologic measurements is needed for cardiovascular monitoring with biomedical equipment to be both safe and effective.

Before discussing the components of hemodynamic monitoring equipment, let us look briefly at the characteristics of hemodynamic pressures. These consist of the following (Fig. 3-1):
1. The *residual, or static, pressure* inside the fluid-filled vessel
2. The *dynamic pressure,* which is caused by the imparted kinetic energy of the moving fluid (This component is encountered in arterial pressures when the catheter tip directly faces the flow of fluid.)
3. The *hydrostatic pressure head,* which results from the difference in height between the ends of the fluid-filled tube (that is, the catheter tip and the air-reference port of the transducer)

In hemodynamic monitoring the most commonly obtained measurement is the residual, or static, pressure within the vessel. To do this, both the dynamic and hydrostatic pressure components must be eliminated. As mentioned, dynamic pressures are only encountered in high flow rates when the catheter tip points into the flow. This additional component is difficult to eliminate completely but can be reduced by changing the direction of the catheter tip or by applying a damping device.

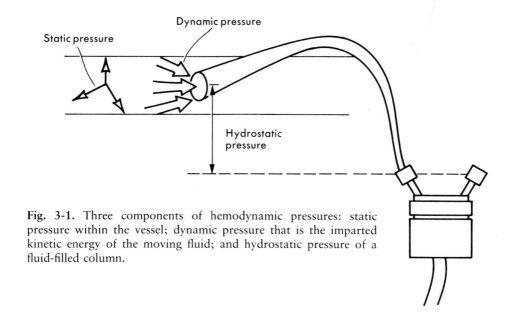

Fig. 3-1. Three components of hemodynamic pressures: static pressure within the vessel; dynamic pressure that is the imparted kinetic energy of the moving fluid; and hydrostatic pressure of a fluid-filled column.

The hydrostatic pressure component is eliminated by leveling the air-reference port of the transducer with the estimated level of the patient's right atrium. See p. 37 for further discussion of this procedure.

PRESSURE-RECORDING DEVICES
Principle

All biomedical recording instruments have three basic components: (1) a transducer or device to detect the physiologic event; (2) an amplifier to increase the magnitude of the signal from the transducer; and (3) a recorder, meter, or oscilloscope to display the resultant signal (Fig. 3-2).

Pressure measurement requires the transformation of a biophysical event into an electric signal that can be displayed, recorded on paper or magnetic tape, and quantified. This transformation is done with a transducer, which converts one type of energy or signal into another. Physiologic events are able to be transduced, but appropriate transducer selection is needed for results to be successful (Table 3-1).

Transducers

Transduction involves the sensing of a particular biophysical event and its conversion to a usable electric signal. Transducers can sense changes in flow, color,

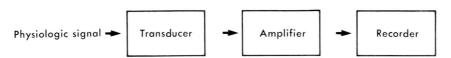

Fig. 3-2. Three basic components of a biomedical recording instrument.

Table 3-1. Characteristics of cardiovascular parameters

Parameter	Range/unit	Frequency response (cps or Hz)	Type of transducer
ECG	10 μV to 5 mV	0.05 to 85	Skin electrodes
Blood pressure	0 to 300 mm Hg	0 to 60	Strain gauge
			Pressure gauge
Cardiac output	2 to 15 L/min	0 to 60	Oximeter (dye) or thermistor
Temperature	25° to 40° C	Variable	Thermistor
Heart rate	45 to 180 beats/min	0.75 to 3	From ECG or pulse
Phonocardiogram	—	2 to 2000	Microphone
Echocardiogram	—	20,000	Piezoelectric

temperature, concentration, pressure, displacement, light intensity, frequency, and sound, and other physiologic changes. Transducers are classified according to the type of energy to which they are sensitive and the method of energy coupling used. The pressure transducer most commonly used in biomedical instrumentation is a mechanical, or displacement, transducer, so called because it consists of a mechanical element that is displaced as a result of changes in pressure. Although there are many types of transducers employing different physical principles to measure displacement, the strain gauge transducer is the most widely used.

The principle of operation of the strain gauge transducer involves the measurement of pressure on wires that function as a Wheatstone bridge. These wires are mounted beneath the diaphragm material in the dome of the transducer (Fig. 3-3). The amplifier provides the energizing current to the Wheatstone bridge. As pressure is applied to the strain gauge, the wires increase in length and decrease in diameter, changing the resistance to the flow of current through the wires of the Wheatstone bridge. This change in the wires' electrical resistance causes a voltage change that can be quantitated to reflect the amount of pressure that changed the wires' length and diameter. The electrical signal can then be amplified and measured; when calibrated, it is proportional to the pressure change.

One of the most recent advances in transducers is the development of the disposable pressure transducer, consisting of a silicon pressure-sensor chip. The ⅛-inch square chip has a thin, etched diaphragm with a single, transverse voltage, strain gauge, piezoresistive element. Temperature compensation is done directly on the chip. The chip is mounted on an electrically isolated carrier and backplate assembly with a bonded flow-through dome (Fig. 3-4). Some disposable transducers can be directly attached to an amplifier via a reusable electrical cable, whereas others require an electronic interface unit for attachment. Connector compatibility among different brands of monitors should be a consideration if a variety of equipment is to be used. Disposable transduces provide accuracy and sensitivity comparable to reusable transducers and eliminate the need for sterilization between patients.

External pressure transducers are most commonly used in the clinical setting to measure blood pressure through a fluid column (fluid-filled catheter). However, they can also be used internally, with the transducer placed at the tip of a catheter.

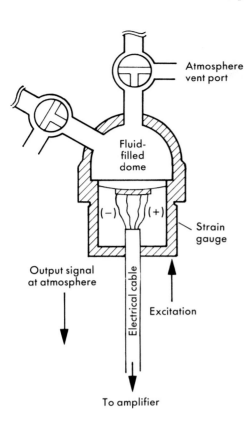

Fig. 3-3. Strain gauge pressure transducer showing interaction of pressure applied to the dome and the effect on the four resistance wires forming the Wheatstone bridge. Changes in pressure cause increases or decreases in the length of the wires; these changes unbalance the Wheatstone bridge, causing a voltage change.

Fig. 3-5 illustrates several pressure transducers used in measuring hemodynamic pressures. The Wheatstone bridge is in the base between the diaphragm of the transducer and the cable connection to the amplifier. The transducer has two openings, each with Luer-Lok fittings. One opening connects the catheter to the transducer; the other opening may be used for zero-pressure reference to atmospheric pressure and for flushing of the transducer or to connect to the second port of the catheter. A clear plastic dome over the transducer allows detection of air bubbles or blood in the fluid, either of which distorts the pressure measurements.

Pressure transducers are usually mounted on an IV pole near the patient's bed or secured directly to the patient (Fig. 3-6). Since the pressure is being measured through a fluid-filled column, any difference between the level of the cardiac chamber where the catheter tip is positioned and the air reference port of the transducer will result in an incorrect pressure. The pressure exerted by the weight of the fluid within the catheter and connecting tubing is termed hydrostatic pressure and is proportional to the height of the fluid column. If the tip of the catheter within the heart is higher than the level of the reference port, the pressure reading will be erroneously high because of the contribution of hydrostatic pressure. Conversely, if the reference port is placed higher than the catheter tip, the pressure reading will be erroneously low. To negate the effects of the hydrostatic pressure of the fluid, it is essential that both "ends" of the system be at the same level (Fig. 3-7). In this instance, the two "ends" are (1) the tip of the catheter and (2) the air-fluid junction

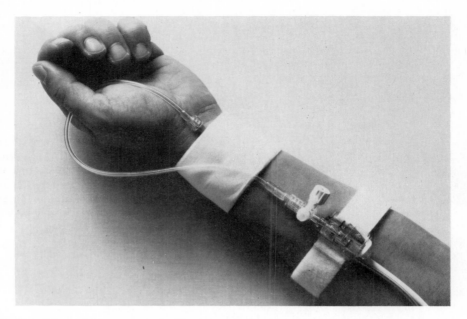

Fig. 3-4. Disposable pressure transducer attached to the patient's arm with a Velcro strap. (Courtesy Gould, Inc, Oxnard, Calif.)

of the transducer (the air-reference stopcock). Although the exact anatomic location of the catheter tip is not known, it is generally considered to be in the midchest position. To obtain the patient's midchest position, measure the distance from the posterior chest to the anterior chest and place a midway mark on the patient's lateral chest wall. Another method is to measure 10 cm up from the top of the mattress and mark the patient's lateral chest wall at this point. Yet another method uses the phlebostatic axis at the junction of the fourth intercostal space and an imagined midaxillary line. (Since no exact anatomic site can identify the actual position of the catheter tip, any of the methods can be used to approximate its position.) The transducer reference level should then be set to correspond to the estimated midchest level. This reference point must be used consistently to obtain accurate pressure measurements. If the patient moves or is elevated, the reference port of the transducer must also be moved to the same midchest level and the system re-zeroed.

Although the above directions are applicable to catheters located centrally, at the level of the heart, confusion often exists regarding appropriate "leveling" with peripheral arterial catheters. Placement of the air-reference port of the transducer at the level of the tip of the arterial catheter eliminates the effect of hydrostatic pressure within the fluid-filled column, therefore providing an accurate measurement of the static pressure within the peripheral artery itself. However, many clinicians, interested in a closer approximation of the aortic root pressure (as a reflection of coronary perfusion pressure), place both the catheter tip (that is, the patient's arm) *and* the transducer port at the right atrium level, thereby eliminating the effects of hydrostatic pressure between the transducer and the catheter tip and between the catheter tip and the aorta. This method, however, does not eliminate the normal amplification of arterial pressure that occurs distally from the aorta.

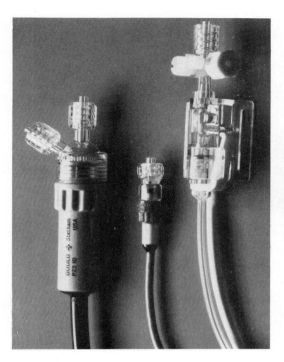

Fig. 3-5. Three types of pressure transducers: external nondisposable strain gauge pressure transducer *(left)*; miniaturized external pressure transducer *(center)*; and disposable pressure transducer *(right)*. (Courtesy Gould, Inc, Oxnard, Calif.)

The electrical signal from the transducer is transmitted by the cable to an amplifier. The amplifier modifies this electrical signal by increasing voltage and filtering it for display on an oscilloscope or suitable recording device.

Strain gauge transducers are sensitive to temperature changes (typically 0.1 mm Hg/1° C) and require frequent checking of the zero-pressure baseline for drift. The room in which they are used should be kept at a fairly constant temperature. Solutions flushed through the transducers will also cause a temperature change and baseline drift.

Transducers placed at the tip of a catheter and introduced directly into the vascular system usually operate on the same principle as external displacement strain gauge transducers. These transducer-tipped catheters have the advantage of not being dependent on a fluid-filled column for transmitting the pressure events at the catheter tip to the transducer. This feature eliminates problems with delay of pressure change transmittance and, more importantly, errors in the pressure tracing caused by inherent characteristics of the diameter and compliance of the catheter. It also avoids artifacts in the pressure tracing caused by movements of the catheter as well as those errors involved in estimating correct placement of the external transducer.

Amplifiers

Biomedical parameters are difficult to measure because of the relatively low energy levels generated within the body and the similarity of signals from organ to organ (for example, heart and skeletal muscle); this similarity makes discrimination of a particular signal difficult. Not only does the transducer have a certain frequency response and sensitivity to detect a particular signal accurately, but the sig-

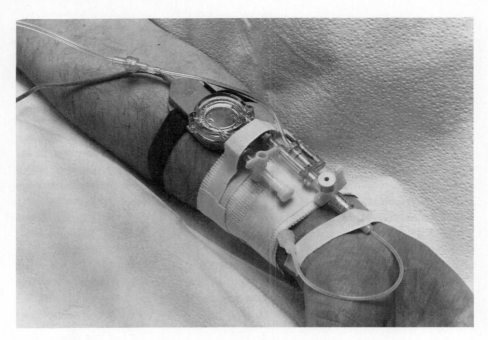

Fig. 3-6. Quartz pressure transducer attached directly to the patient's arm. (Courtesy Hewlett-Packard Co, Santa Clara, Calif.)

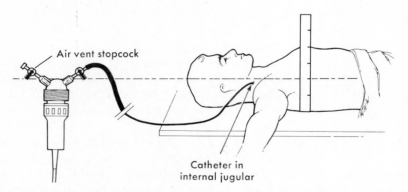

Fig. 3-7. Illustration showing measurement of the patient's chest to determine the midchest position and placement of the transducer reference port at this level. In this way the two open "ends" (the air vent stopcock and the catheter tip) are at the same level and negate the effects of hydrostatic pressure.

nal generated by the transducer usually requires processing (for example, impedance matching or filtering of noise) and amplification.

Most modern transducers produce only about 6 mV above their "zero level" output when reproducing the systolic arterial pressure, whereas most monitor displays require several *volts* of signal to operate. Consequently, an amplifier is necessary to boost the size of the signal by approximately a factor of 1000 before display.

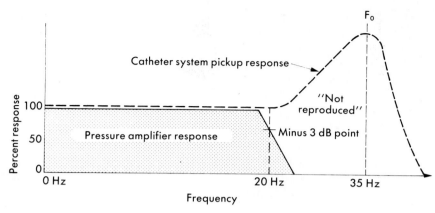

Fig. 3-8. Pressure amplifier response curve and catheter (plumbing) system response curve. Note the accuracy of amplifier response (100%) up to an upper limit cutoff frequency of approximately 20 Hz. Although the plumbing system can add distortion to the signal, if its characteristic resonant frequency is above the upper limit cutoff frequency (20 Hz), it will not be processed by the amplifier.

Amplifiers can be straightforward electronic devices that simply energize the Wheatstone bridge in the transducer and amplify the signal from the transducer, or they can be highly complex devices that process, filter, and amplify the signal for display on an oscilloscope recorder. The signal can also be fed into a computer for further digital processing and analysis.

Amplifiers for cardiovascular measurements are designed to meet specific requirements. They must be easy to use with clearly labeled controls, and they should filter out other physiologic signals and undesired environmental noise detected by the transducer (Fig. 3-8). The amplifier's ability to increase signal level and faithfulness in reproduction of signals from input to output should not add significant distortion (termed linear response). Calibration, stability, and temperature drift should minimally affect the signal. Good electronic design can accommodate all of these requirements and result in an extremely sensitive and precise diagnostic instrument.

Display devices. Physiologic pressures can be displayed on oscilloscopes and digital readout devices or on permanent recording devices using graphic recordings. The modified electrical output from the amplifier can be meaningful only when it is converted into readable form in a display or recording device. Since a display device has an upper and lower frequency limit, it is essential for faithful reproduction that the frequency response range match that of the input signal.

The *oscilloscope* is a display device that provides a visual image of voltage changes as a function of time. The basic component of an oscilloscope is a cathode-ray vacuum tube that produces an electron beam focused on a screen. The electron beam is visible because the interior of the screen is painted with phosphorescent chemicals that transiently emit visible light when excited by the electron beam. The brightness and persistence of the light depend on the type of phosphorescent chemical used. The horizontal sweep of the beam indicates the amount of time required for the signal to go from left to right and can be adjusted on most oscilloscopes. The vertical deflection of the beam reflects voltage changes from the amplifier and transducer. Plotting can be adjusted for optimal display of the voltage change, termed *sensitivity,* which is determined by *calibration,* the insertion of a signal of known quantity and the adjustment of the amplifier and readout device to reproduce this known change accurately. Oscilloscopes can display one or more signals simultaneously, depending on the purpose of the unit. Some oscilloscopes allow the signal to remain on the scope until it is erased by a new sweep of signals. This nonfade display allows more time for study of the waveform during monitoring of patients.

Digital readout devices provide numeric values of pressure changes during specific times of the cardiac cycle. Selection of systolic, diastolic, or mean pressure values is available on most digital display devices.

To obtain a permanent record of a physiologic signal and to accurately measure pressures at end-expiration, a paper-recording device with a galvanometer is often used. The galvanometer's motion is proportional to the amount of current flowing through a wire. This flow of current generates a magnetic field, causing movement of the suspended mirror on optical recorders or movement of a writing pen on direct-writing recorders. The *direct-writing recorder* uses a stylus to record the pressure tracing on moving paper. The stylus is driven by an attached galvanometer coil. These direct-writing recorders are termed *strip chart recorders* and are used for the measurement of low-frequency parameters. Recording of high-frequency events requires an *optical recorder,* which uses a suspended mirror on the galvanometer coil to direct a light beam across moving photographic or light-sensitive paper. Ultraviolet, light-sensitive recording paper allows immediate development for review of recordings. Some recording systems use a pressurized system that squirts ink through a nozzle located in the center of the galvanometer coil and onto recording paper. This system has a very high frequency response and provides an immediate permanent recording of events.

Zero reference. The weight of air or atmospheric pressure exerts a certain force dependent on altitude and environmental factors (usually about 760 mm Hg at standard temperature and pressure at sea level). Physiologic measurements are made relative to atmospheric pressure by opening the transducer to air and adjusting the display system to read zero. In this way all pressure contributions from the atmosphere are negated, and only pressure values that exist within the heart chamber or vessel will be measured.

Calibration. Accurate quantitation of recorded pressure measurements requires precise calibration of both the transducer and its associated amplifying electrical components. Most monitor systems have a built-in electrical calibration that yields a known pressure value. This calibration should be checked before hemodynamic monitoring is initiated. To avoid electronic drift, the instruments should be allowed to warm up for approximately 15 minutes. The steps for checking the electrical calibration of the monitoring system are as follows:

1. Depress the "cal" button on the monitor system.
2. After the readout stabilizes, adjust the control knob to obtain the appropriate readout value (for example, 200 mm Hg).
3. Release the "cal" button and make sure the reading returns to zero.

Although this procedure checks the electrical calibration of the system, it does not check the actual calibration of the transducer. Since transducers are sensitive instruments and can easily be damaged, the calibration of each nondisposable transducer should be checked before pressure monitoring is initiated. The following steps should be taken to calibrate each transducer (Fig. 3-9):

1. Attach a dome to the transducer head (there should be no fluid in the system). Do not use the dome that is or will be attached to the patient.
2. Zero and calibrate following the three steps for electrical calibration.
3. Attach a mercury manometer to one of the Luer-Lok fittings of the transducer dome using a short plastic tubing.
4. Attach a hand bulb to the remaining Luer-Lok fitting of the transducer dome using another short piece of plastic tubing.
5. Squeeze the hand bulb to elevate the mercury column to 200 mm Hg. The digital readout on the manometer should be 200. Deviations of ±2 mm Hg are acceptable at this pressure range.
6. Release the hand bulb and check for a return of the digital readout to zero.
7. To check the transducer at lower pressure levels, elevate the mercury column to only 10 mm Hg. At this level the digital readout should be within 1 mm Hg of 10 mm Hg.

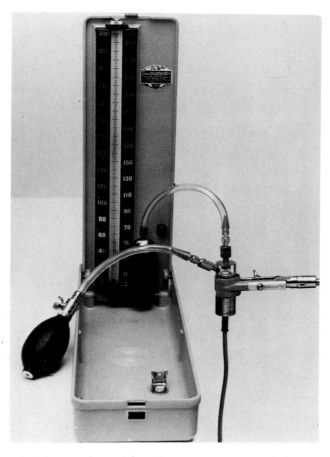

Fig. 3-9. Connections between a mercury sphygmomanometer and the pressure transducer for calibration of the transducer.

If the digital readouts correspond to the applied mercury pressure, the monitor and transducer are functioning correctly and may be reliably used for hemodynamic monitoring. If discrepancies occur greater than those within the specifications listed, the nondisposable transducer is out of calibration and should be repaired and recalibrated. Disposable transducers are precalibrated and coded by the manufacturer and are less likely to be out of calibration. However, if there is any question concerning the integrity or reliability of the transducer during the monitoring period, calibration checks can be performed.

An alternative method of calibration uses fluid-filled tubing extended vertically above the transducer to produce a water manometer (Fig. 3-10). Use of a 3-foot length of tubing filled with fluid exerts a pressure equivalent to 67 mm Hg, whereas a 4-foot length of fluid-filled tubing exerts 90 mm Hg. This method has the advantage of allowing rapid calibration checks without disman-

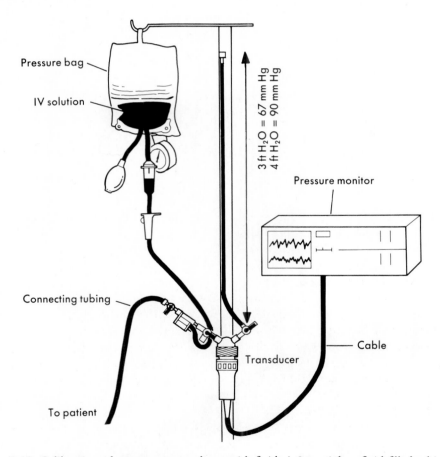

Fig. 3-10. Calibration of a pressure transducer with fluid. A 3- or 4-foot fluid-filled tubing is extended vertically above the transducer. Pressure monitoring of the patient is temporarily discontinued by turning the transducer stopcock off to the patient. The air-reference stopcock is then turned open to the vertical column of fluid. The appropriate values should be observed on the monitor. This tubing can remain attached to the IV pole for additional calibration checks if necessary. As with all tubing, it should be changed every 24 to 48 hours.

tling the system and eliminates the possibility of introducing air into the system. The primary disadvantage is the inability to calibrate with high pressures because of the awkwardness of vertically mounting longer tubing lengths. For this reason, verification of higher pressures may require a mercury manometer.

Plumbing System

Transmission of a pressure signal from the patient to a transducer occurs through fluid-filled tubing. However, there are inherent properties of the fluid-filled system which can distort the true pressure signal. The characteristics of a fluid-filled system that affect pressure wave accuracy during transmission are the resonant (or natural) frequency and the damping coefficient. Because of the inertia of the fluid in the system, the pressure changes of the fluid column may differ in amplitude and time from the action within the vessel. Because of this, pressure waves can be distorted before reaching the transducer. (This principle applies more to arterial pressures, which vary continuously, than to venous pressures, which are more static.) Since the transducer will faithfully reproduce the pressure it senses (no matter what the degree of distortion), inaccurate pressure readings can be obtained. Several factors can create pressure distortion in the plumbing system. These include the following:
1. Catheter and tubing length
2. Catheter and tubing stiffness
3. Catheter and tubing diameter
4. Air bubbles or blood clots

Resonant frequency

The responsiveness of a plumbing system (including catheter, tubing, and stopcocks) depends on the *resonant frequency* of the system (see Fig. 3-8). This refers to the frequency at which the oscillations have their maximum amplitude. This resonance is quite separate from the frequency of the pressure waveform itself and is determined by the size, shape, and material of the plumbing system. If the pressure waveform being transmitted contains a frequency component that is the same as or near the system's resonant frequency, the system will tend to vibrate or resonate (analogous to a bell after being struck). This results in an overshoot of the systolic pressures (accentuation), lowered diastolic pressures (attenuation), and the appearance of numerous small oscillations in the waveform (Fig. 3-11). This can be avoided by constructing a plumbing system whose natural, or resonant, frequency is as far away from the frequency of the signals as possible (see Fig. 3-8). This contruction includes the following:
1. **Keeping catheter and tubing length to a minimum (no longer than 3 to 4 feet).** Increased length of tubing reduces the resonant frequency of the system to a point at or near the frequency components of the pressure signal. As mentioned, this can result in accentuation and resonating of the signal.
2. **Using stiff, noncompliant tubing.** Soft, compliant catheters and tubing are compressible by the transmitted pressure wave. This compression absorbs some of the pressure's energy and results in distortion and reduced amplitude of the pressure waveform (attenuation).

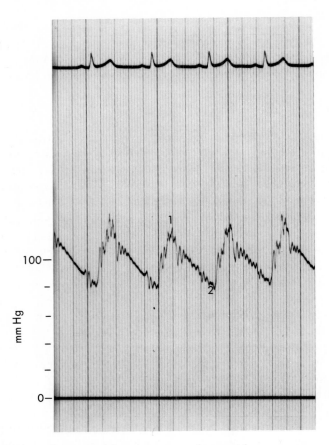

Fig. 3-11. Distortion of an arterial pressure waveform with numerous small oscillations caused by decreased resonant frequency of the plumbing system. (From Daily EK, and Schroeder JS: Hemodynamic waveforms: exercises in identification and analysis, St Louis, 1983, The CV Mosby Co.)

3. **Using large diameter catheters (7 Fr or larger in adults; as large as possible in infants and children).** Small catheters increase the frictional resistance to movement. To overcome this, energy from the pressure wave is lost. This generally results in reduced amplitude of the frequency components of the pressure signal. It must be mentioned that in the clinical setting it is necessary to strike a balance between using the smallest size catheter possible to minimize the risks of thrombosis and using the largest size catheter possible for faithful transmission of the physiologic signal.

4. **Eliminating all air bubbles from the system and preventing blood clot formation.** Air bubbles and blood clots are compressible. As with soft tubing, this compression of the bubble(s) by the transmitted pressure wave causes loss of the pressure wave's energy. The more energy that is lost or absorbed, the greater the amplitude reduction and distortion of the waveform. The extent of wave distortion is directly proportional to the size of the air bubble. This distortion can also occur with the formation of even small clots in the catheter tip or the

stopcocks. Elimination of unnecessary stopcocks reduces the number of possible places for air bubbles or blood clots to lodge. Basically, the system should be kept as simple and streamlined as possible. The judicious use of anticoagulants and a continuous low-volume infusion can reduce the likelihood of clot formation.

Damping coefficient

In addition to having low natural or resonant frequencies, most catheter, tubing, and plumbing systems are *underdamped*, possessing high damping coefficients. The damping coefficient describes how quickly an oscillating system comes to rest.

Visual inspection of the displayed waveform sometimes reveals the dynamic qualities of the monitoring system. Underdamping is often associated with amplified pressure changes ("ringing" or "fling"), or a narrow, high, very peaked systolic pressure followed by a second, less peaked, systolic curve. An overdamped system often produces a waveform possessing a low upstroke and a very rounded appearance of the curve. Frequently, however, alterations in the pressure signal, as a result of a low resonant frequency of the plumbing system, or incorrect damping (either over or under), are less obvious, and incorrect pressures may be used as a basis for inappropriate therapeutic interventions.

Both the natural frequency and damping coefficient can be measured quite easily at the bedside with the use of the in-line fast flush device. Activation of the fast flush produces a square wave followed by one or two oscillations that then revert to the pressure wave. Actual measurement of components of the oscillations following the square wave are used to determine both the natural frequency and the damping coefficient of the system.

The resonant or natural frequency is determined by measuring the distance between consecutive peaks of two oscillations following the square wave. This measurement is then divided into the speed of the paper recording (e.g., 25 mm/sec) to estimate the natural frequency of the system (Fig. 3-12).

The damping coefficient can be obtained by measuring the amplitude, or height of two consecutive oscillations following the square wave. The smaller number is then divided by the larger (Fig. 3-12). This ratio can then be converted to the estimated damping coefficient by a complex formula, or, more easily, with use of a graphic solution as shown in Fig. 3-13.

Fig. 3-14 plots the relationships between the natural frequency and the damping coefficient as well as the ranges that are necessary to prevent distortion of the pressure waveform. The best dynamic responses are obtained with a high natural frequency (20 Hz or higher) and optimum damping (with a damping coefficient between 0.5 and 0.75). As depicted in Fig. 3-14, the lower the natural frequency (particularly at or below 25 Hz), the higher the required damping coefficient (up to an approximated damping coefficient of 1.0).

Because optimum damping is difficult to achieve, all efforts should be made to increase the system's natural frequency. However, if the natural frequency of the plumbing system cannot be increased by minimizing the length of the tubing between the patient and the transducer, as well as meticulous removal of any air bubbles, attempts should be made to increase the damping coefficient. (Even very tiny air bubbles can significantly lower the natural frequency to 10 Hz or less, resulting

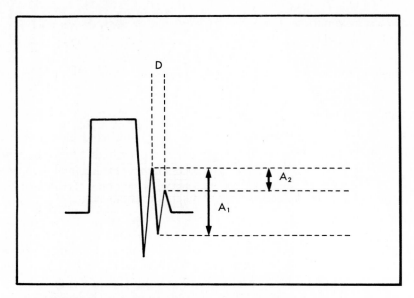

Fig. 3-12. Schematic illustration of a square wave (fast-flush) response to demonstrate measurement of the *natural frequency* (fn) and *damping coefficient* (ζ). The natural frequency is estimated by dividing the measured distance (d) between two consecutive peaks following the square wave into the speed at which the paper was run (usually 25 or 50 mm/sec). The damping coefficient can be estimated by calculating the ratio between the amplitude of two consecutive peaks (*A2/A1*) and then plotting that ratio on the graphical equation in Fig. 3-13, or on the scale in Fig. 3-14 to determine the corresponding damping coefficient.

in gross over-estimation of the actual pressure.) The damping coefficient can be mechanically altered with the addition of damping devices such as Corrector or Accudynamic. These damping devices are attached to the plumbing system and permit adjustment of resistance to increase the damping coefficient without changing the natural frequency.

If the systolic and diastolic pressures are considered important parameters to measure, the resonant frequency and damping coefficient of the system should be measured to ensure their accuracy. (The MAP is less likely to be affected by amplitude distortion.) The dynamic response of the monitoring system should be checked on a regular basis (at least once a shift) and any time the system has been opened to permit introduction of air or blood accumulation at some point in the system. The best way to avoid overshoot, peaking, or ringing in a recording system is to be sure that the natural frequency is far out into the high frequency range— far beyond those of any frequency of interest.

Figs. 3-15 to 3-17 illustrate several examples of dynamic response tests performed in several monitoring situations.

ELECTRICAL HAZARDS

The proliferation of electrically powered equipment for monitoring the critically ill patient increases the possibility of electrical shock. Death of patients by electrocution probably occurs more frequently than is actually reported, because

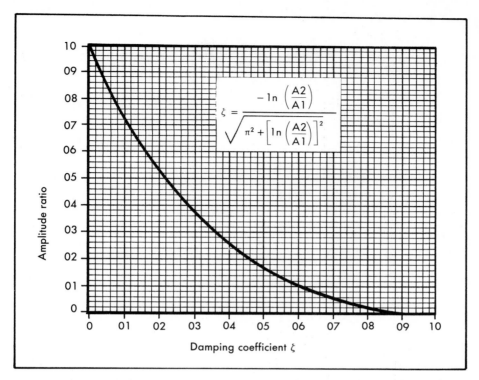

Fig. 3-13. Graphic solution for the damping coefficient according to the equation:

$$\text{Damping coefficient} = \frac{-\ln\left(\frac{A2}{A1}\right)}{\sqrt{\pi^2 + \left[\ln\left(\frac{A2}{A1}\right)\right]^2}}$$

where: A1 = Amplitude of 1st peak
       A2 = Amplitude of 2nd peak
       ln = Natural logarithm

Optimal damping occurs with a damping coefficient of approximately 0.7 to 1.0. (From Gardner RM: Direct blood pressure measurement—dynamic response requirements, Anesthesiology 54:227-236, 1981.)

this cause of sudden lethal arrhythmias is not easily traced to faulty electrical equipment. Penetration of the skin by needle electrodes, catheters, and wires may provide a low-resistance pathway to the heart through which current leaking from an electrical device or bed may flow. The resulting hazard to the patient may cause muscle stimulation, cardiac arrhythmias, or ventricular fibrillation.

Principle

Electrical current flows through a pathway when the circuit is completed or closed and when a difference in electrical potential exists between the two points. This current may be direct (DC), which is continuous, or alternating (AC). Most electrical devices in the clinical setting use alternating current. The amount of cur-

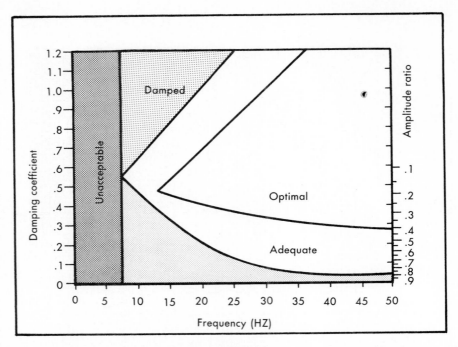

Fig. 3-14. Natural frequency plotted against the damping coefficient, illustrating the five areas into which catheter-tubing-transducer systems fall. Systems in the optimal area will reproduce even the most demanding (fast heart rate and rapid systolic upstroke) arterial or pulmonary artery waveforms without distortion. Systems in the adequate area will reproduce most typical patient waveforms with little or no distortion. All other areas will cause serious and clinically important waveform distortion. Note the scale on the right can be used to estimate the damping coefficient from the amplitutde ratio determined during fast flushing. (From Gardner RM, and Hollingsworth KW: Optimizing the electrocardiogram and pressure monitoring, Crit Care Med 14:651-658, 1986.)

rent flowing between two points of different electrical potential varies inversely with the resistance encountered by that flow. If the resistance is low, the current flow is large, and vice versa. Dry skin provides a high-resistance barrier to externally applied current. Skin that is wet (because of sweat, saline, or electrode gel) can reduce this resistance by a factor of 1000.

The basic characteristics of electricity in a circuit are described by Ohm's law:

$$V = I \times R$$

where V = Voltage, the unit of potential difference in an electrical field
      I = Current, the number of electrical charges moving from one place to another per unit time, measured in amperes
      R = Resistance, the opposition to the conduction of electric current, a function of the length, cross-sectional area, and nature of the conductive material, measured in ohms

Fig. 3-18 is a schematic drawing of current (amperes) flowing through a wire offering resistance (ohms) to flow. Ohm's law can be applied to determine the amount of voltage drop across the resistor.

Electric power is the amount of work per unit time and is measured in watts:

$$P = V \times I$$

where P = Power (watts)
   V = Voltage
   I = Current (amperes)

One can understand the relationships between volts, amperes, and watts by applying Ohm's law to an ordinary 100 W light bulb. The power source is a 120 V outlet, and the amount of work performed by this bulb cannot be more than 100 W.

$$P = V \times I \text{ or } I = \frac{P}{V} = \frac{100}{120} = 0.83A$$

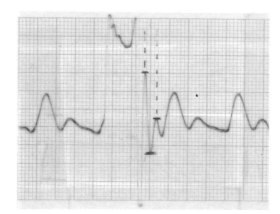

Fig. 3-15. An arterial pressure waveform with a superimposed square wave from activation of the fast flush device. With the paper run at 25 mm/sec, and the distance (d) between two consecutive peaks of 2.5 mm, the calculated fn is 10 Hz (25 ÷ 2.5). The amplitude of A_1 is 22 mm and A_2 is 9 mm, yielding an amplitude ratio of 0.4. When this is plotted according to the graphic solution in Fig. 3-13, the damping coefficient is determined to be 0.28. This represents an underdamped waveform, and efforts should be made to increase the natural frequency of the system.

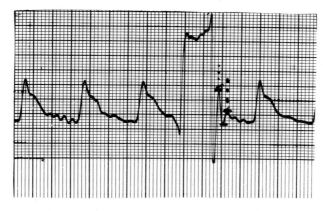

Fig. 3-16. Underdamped arterial waveform confirmed by the fast-flush mechanism with a calculated fn of 10 Hz and a damping coefficient of 0.31.

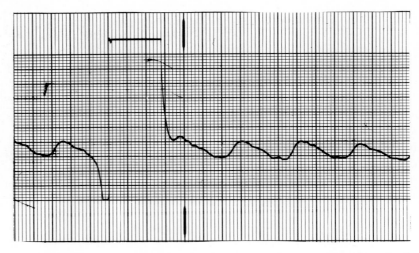

Fig. 3-17. Excessively damped arterial waveform by appearance confirmed by the fast-flush test, which has no downward spike and slowly returns to the waveform signal.

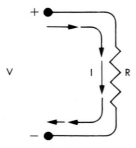

Fig. 3-18. Amount of electrical current (I) flowing from positive (+) to negative (−) is determined by the resistance (R) to flow. Large amounts of current can flow when resistance is low; small amounts flow when resistance is high.

As shown in Table 3-2, these 830 mA are much greater than the current required to cause ventricular fibrillation when the current is applied to the skin.

Wires or catheters placed in the heart via veins or arteries provide a direct, very low-resistance pathway through which the passage of a minute amount of current may be lethal. Because of its high resistance and greater dispersion, the skin can tolerate greater amounts of current than can the myocardial muscle. Table 3-2 illustrates the response to various levels of current applied to the skin. Current as low as 100 mA when applied to the skin can cause ventricular fibrillation. However, this same result can occur with current as low as 0.1 mA (100 μA) when applied directly to the heart through a catheter or wire.

Safety Precautions

Nearly all electrical equipment has some leakage of current from the circuitry to the frame (chassis). For safety, maximal leakage of current should be 0.01 mA (100 μA) for exposed metal surfaces and 0.001 mA (10 μA) for patient connec-

Table 3-2. Response to current applied to the skin

Current (mA)	Response
1	Tingling sensation
10 to 20	Muscular contraction
50	Pain
100 to 300	Ventricular fibrillation

tions. Proper grounding of electrical equipment protects the patient from this current leakage by allowing the current to flow from the chassis to the ground wire. Grounding is based on the principle that electrical charges lose their energy in earth, which has an infinite capacity to receive these charges. For grounding, a three-pronged electrical outlet and plug are required; one prong leads to the ground (Fig. 3-19). This three-pronged safety feature also eliminates the possibility of causing a reversal of power flow, which could be lethal, by reversing the hot and neutral wires of an electrical plug when inserting it into a power outlet.

A major problem in monitoring the patient with cardiac disease concerns the patient's frequent connection to multiple electrical devices. To provide safety through proper grounding, *each* device should be attached to a *common* ground wire, which will drain all current leakage to a single ground point. A single ground reference eliminates current flow caused by slight variances in ground potential. This type of wiring is termed "equipotential grounding." A panel of outlets near the patient work area, connected to a common ground, should be the only outlets used for patient monitoring. Connection to remote or separated outlets is to be avoided, since current flow from one electrical device to another with a slightly different potential or ground can pass through the patient. Looping or kinking of electrical cables is also to be avoided to prevent resistive and capacitance leakage. Grounding by attaching a wire from a piece of equipment to a water pipe is not safe for patient care.

Caution is essential in the use of electrical devices. The three-pronged plug, as well as the ground connection, should be routinely checked. Whereas this is usually the responsibility of the hospital engineering department, the person using the equipment must be alert in detecting and reporting any defects. A common occurrence is the presence of 60-cycle interference on a standard ECG tracing (Fig. 3-20). The presence of this interference usually represents inadequate grounding and should be reported to the electrical safety engineer. When electrical interference such as minor tactile sensations, is detected, the defect must be corrected before the device is used further.

Direct grounding of the patient can impose an electrical shock hazard by placing the patient in a low-resistance pathway through which accumulating current leakage from electrical equipment may drain. If a patient is grounded, precautions should be taken to prevent the patient from touching any metal object, switch, or device that might expose the patient to electrical current. A staff member may also place the patient in this hazardous situation by simultaneously touching a poorly grounded device and the patient. Isolation transformers or optically coupled isolation amplifiers attached to electrical monitoring devices limit the flow of current and are preferable to directly grounding the patient.

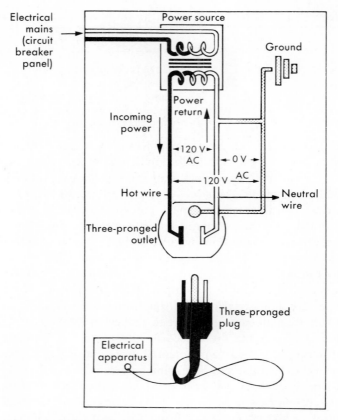

Fig. 3-19. Three-pronged plug and outlet; electrical potential between hot wire to neutral wire and ground wire is the same.

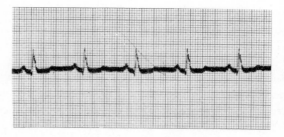

Fig. 3-20. ECG tracing showing 60-cycle interference, possibly indicating inadequate grounding and electrical hazard.

Sources of Error

Improper use of equipment and defective equipment are the greatest sources of electrical hazards. Use of corroded electrodes, inappropriate application of electrodes, and failure to use a properly grounded, three-pronged plug are only some of the common errors. Fig. 3-21 illustrates on example of a potential electrical hazard.

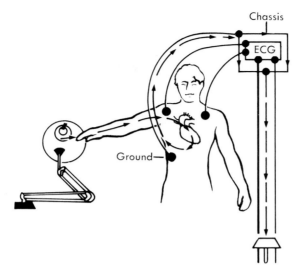

Fig. 3-21. Electrical hazard presented by a patient touching an ungrounded bedside lamp. Leaking current flows from the lamp, through the body, and out the ground lead to the ECG chassis, which is grounded with the three-pronged plug. If the lamp had the same ground, there would be no current differential and no current flow through the patient.

REFERENCES

Abrams JH, Olson ML, Marino JA and Cerra FB: Use of a needle valve resistor to improve invasive blood pressure monitoring, Crit Care Med 12:978-982, 1984.

American Association of Medical Instrumentation: ANSI standard: safe current limits for electromedical apparatus, 1982, AAMI.

Boutros A, and Albert S: Effect of the dynamic response of transducer tubing system on accuracy of direct pressure measurement in patients, Crit Care Med 11:124-127, 1983.

Chandraratna, PAN: Determination of zero-reference level for left atrial pressure by echocardiography, Am Heart J 89:159-162, 1975.

Cromwell L, Weibell FJ, Pfeiffer EA, and Usselman LB: Biomedical instrumentation and measurements, Englewood Cliffs, NJ, 1973, Prentice-Hall, Inc.

Falsetti HL et al: Analysis and correction of pressure wave distortion in fluid-filled catheter systems, Circ XLIX:165-173, 1974.

Donovan KD: Invasive monitoring and support of the circulation, Clinics in Anesthesiology 3:909-953, 1985.

Gardner R: Direct blood pressure measurement-dynamic response requirements, Anesthesiology 54:227-236, 1981.

Gardner RM, and Hollingsworth KW: Optimizing the electrocardiogram and pressure monitoring, Crit Care Med 14:651-658, 1986.

Geddes LA: The direct and indirect measurement of blood pressure, Chicago, 1970, Year Book Medical Publishers, Inc.

Geddes LA, and Baker, LE: Principles of applied biomedical instrumentation, New York, 1968, John Wiley & Sons, Inc.

Gibbs NC, and Gardner RM: Dynamics of invasive pressure monitoring systems: clinical and laboratory evaluation, Heart & Lung 17:43-51, 1988.

Goldman MJ: Principles of clinical electrocardiography, Los Altos, Calif, 1979, Lange Medical Publications.

The heart and electrical hazards. In Directions in cardiovascular medicine, Somerville, NJ, 1973, Hoechst Pharmaceuticals, Inc.

Hewlett-Packard Co.: Guide to physiological pressure monitoring, Waltham, Mass, 1977, Hewlett-Packard Co.

Hunziker P: Accuracy and dynamic response of disposable pressure transducer-tubing systems, Can J Anaesth 34:400-414, 1987.

Kantrowitz P: Blood pressure measurement: state of the art, Med Electronics Data, pp. 59-65, Jan.-Feb. 1974.

Landin Z, Trautman, E, and Teplick R: Contribution of measurement system artifacts to systolic spikes, Med Instr 17:110-112, 1983.

Luskin RL et al: Extended use of disposable pressure transducers, JAMA 255:916-920, 1986.

Manktelow RT, and Baird RJ: A practical approach to accurate pressure measurements, J Thorac Cardiovasc Surg 58:122-127, 1969.

Morton BC: Basic equipment requirements for hemodynamic monitoring, Can Med Assoc J 121:879-892, 1979.

Morton BC: Basic requirements for hemodynamic monitoring, CMA Journal 121:879-885, 1979.

Shapiro GG, and Krovetz LJ: Damped and undamped frequency responses of underdamped catheter manometer systems, Am Heart J 80:226-236, 1970.

Shinozaki T, Deane RS, and Mazuzan JE: The dynamic responses of liquid-filled catheter systems for direct measurements of blood pressure, Anesthesiology 53:498-504, 1980.

Tojik RAN: Measurement of intracardiac pressure, Herz 11:283-290, 1986.

Yanof HM: Biomedical electronics, Philadelphia, 1972, FA Davis Co.

Chapter 4

Vascular Access

A ccess into either the venous or arterial system can be done via the percutaneous or surgical cutdown approach. Both techniques should be performed under aseptic conditions (exception emergency situations), with adequate administration of local anesthesia. The procedure should be explained to the patient (and family, if appropriate) and informed consent obtained.

VENOUS ACCESS
Access Sites

Access to the venous system for insertion of a CVP or PA catheter can be obtained via peripheral arm veins (basilic, cephalic, median, cubital, or axillary), peripheral leg veins (femoral, saphenous), the peripheral neck vein (external jugular), the central neck vein (internal jugular), and the central chest vein (subclavian). Selection of a particular site depends on the patient's needs, individual anatomical considerations, and the operator's experience. Most clinicians have experience with cannulation of the arm veins; however, this site is less suitable for pacing or long-term monitoring purposes. Nonetheless, in an emergency situation the first choice is any site that is available for rapid cannulation with the least amount of harm. Successful cannulation has been shown to closely correlate with the amount of operator experience. Table 4-1 lists some of the advantages and disadvantages for each venous insertion site.

Skin Preparation

Infection may be prevented by proper preparation of the skin surface before catheter insertion via percutaneous or venous cutdown routes. The site should be shaved, and an iodine preparation such as povidone-iodine complex (Betadine) should be applied for 1 minute and allowed to dry. A solution of 70% alcohol should then be applied and allowed to dry, and sterile drapes with a small opening placed around the area. Sterile gloves should be worn and sterile technique should be maintained throughout the procedure.

Catheter Preparation

For insertion of a CVP, the length of catheter insertion required for proper positioning of the tip in the SVC, just above the RA junction, should be estimated. This can be done by holding the packaged or protected catheter over the patient

Table 4-1. Advantages and disadvantages of venous insertion sites

Site	Advantages	Disadvantages
Internal jugular vein	Less risk of pleural puncture and pneumothorax Easier insertion with constant landmarks If hematoma occurs, it is visible and can usually be compressed Malposition of central venous catheter is rare with direct path to right side of the heart from right internal jugular vein Best approach for emergency transvenous pacing during chest and abdominal surgery (most accessible direct route to right side of the heart)	Difficult to cannulate in hypovolemic patients "Blind" puncture Restriction of patient's neck mobility Increased risk of catheter movement or kinking with head movements Trendelenburg position for catheter insertion may not be possible for some patients Risk of carotid artery puncture
Subclavian vein	Remains open even in profound circulatory collapse Catheter fixation more secure Less restricting for patient Direct route to right side of the heart	Pleural space easily entered "Blind" puncture Risk of subclavian artery puncture Difficult to apply compression if the subclavian artery is inadvertently punctured Higher incidence of catheter malposition
Femoral vein	Easy to cannulate Fewer major complications Accessible during CPR, but may not be best route	Increased risk of infection Increased risk of thrombosis and pulmonary embolism "Blind" puncture Less mobility for the patient Risk of femoral artery puncture Malposition of the central venous catheter unless fluoroscopy is used
External jugular vein	Fewer major complications "Nonblind" puncture Accessible during operation	Increased difficulty negotiating catheter for central venous placement Increased risk of central venous catheter malposition Vein not always visible
Basilic and median cubital veins	Easy to cannulate when visible or palpable Safe Preferred route during CPR	Vein not always visible or palpable Difficult to cannulate in hypovolemic patients High rate of malposition if fluoroscopy is not used for central catheter placement Not optimal for rapid fluid infusion or emergency transvenous pacing
Cephalic vein	Same as for basilic and median cubital veins	Same as for basilic and median cubital veins Sharp angle at shoulder may preclude entry into central vein without use of a guidewire

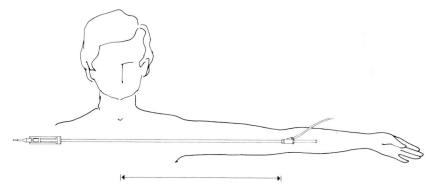

Fig. 4-1. CVP catheter is measured from the proposed insertion site to the sternal notch. This measurement estimates the length of catheter required for placement of the catheter tip in the superior vena cava.

from the proposed insertion site to the sternal notch. Fig. 4-1 depicts such an estimation being obtained from a proposed arm vein insertion.

Before its insertion, the outside of the PA catheter should be wiped off with sterile solution and all open lumens thoroughly flushed. The balloon of the flotation catheter should be inflated with the recommended volume of air (written on the shaft of the catheter) and immersed in sterile water to check for possible leaks as indicated by the presence of small bubbles in the water.

If a thermodilution PA catheter is used, the thermistor wires should be checked before insertion by adjoining the cardiac output (CO) cable to the appropriate thermistor hub of the catheter (Fig. 4-2). The CO computer will flash "Faulty cath" if the thermistor wires are damaged. In this case, a new PA catheter should be used.

If an SvO_2 PA catheter is being inserted, calibration of the fiberoptics should be performed by inserting the catheter tip into the provided calibration receptable according to the manufacturer's directions. This is performed under sterile conditions.

The distal lumen of the PA catheter should be connected to a transducer via fluid-filled tubing so hemodynamic waveforms can be monitored during insertion and advancement of the PA catheter.

Percutaneous Catheterization

In 1953 Dr. Sven-Ivar Seldinger, a Stockholm radiologist, described the procedure for percutaneous arterial insertion of a catheter using a guidewire. This simple but revolutionary technique has stood the test of time and now is the preferred method of catheter insertion into either an artery or a vein.

Percutaneous insertion of central venous catheters has become widely accepted, not only because of speed of placement, but also because of the reduced risk of infection. In addition, percutaneous venous catheterization often preserves the integrity of the vessel, thus permitting future access.

The basic tools of the Seldinger technique of catheterization consist of an introducing needle, a guidewire, and a catheter. While any type of needle could be used

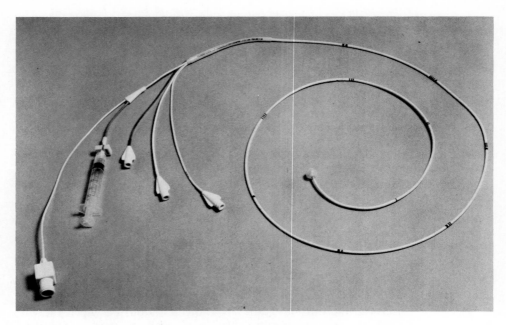

Fig. 4-2. Swan-Ganz flow-directed, balloon-tipped thermodilution catheter for PA and RA pressure monitoring and cardiac output measurement. Syringe is used for inflating the balloon with air. (Courtesy American Edwards Laboratories, Santa Ana, Calif.)

for the Seldinger technique, thin-walled needles are preferred, because the lumen can accommodate a guidewire without substantially increasing the outside diameter. Consequently, virtually all percutaneous puncture needles today have thin walls.

Fig. 4-3 illustrates the basic steps involved in percutaneous catheterization. Fig. 4-4 illustrates the same technique for percutaneous insertion of a sheath.

Procedure

Arm vein. Cannulation of a vein in the antecubital fossa has long been the most popular technique for inserting central catheters and has the lowest major complication rate. In some institutions it still remains the first choice, although catheterization of the central veins directly has become more common since the advent of balloon flotation PA catheters. When fluoroscopy is not used, improper positioning of central venous catheters from an arm vein occurs much more frequently than clinically suspected, with reported incidences of from 36% to 52%. In addition, arm movement can cause catheter tip movement of several centimeters, increasing the risk of phlebitis. For pacemakers, this movement may result in electrode dislodgment or RV perforation.

A central venous line can usually be inserted through the median vein or the basilic vein distal to the antecubital fossa. The cephalic vein is an equally large vein, but its sharp angle at the shoulder makes it more difficult to navigate.

ANATOMY. Venous blood from the arm drains through two main intercommunicating veins—the basilic and the cephalic veins. The basilic vein is deeper and ascends along the ulnar surface of the forearm (Fig. 4-5). It is joined by the median cubital vein in front of the elbow and continues up along the medial side of the

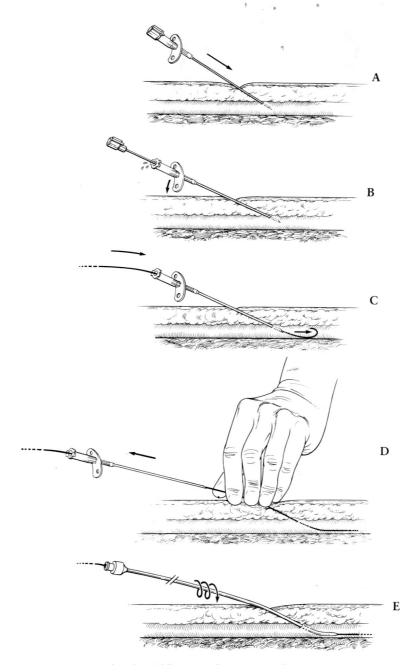

Fig. 4-3. Basic procedure for the Seldinger technique. **A,** The vessel is punctured with the needle at a 30- to-40 degree angle. **B,** The stylet is removed and free blood flow is observed; the angle of the needle is then reduced. **C,** The flexible tip of the guidewire is passed through the needle into the vessel. **D,** The needle is removed over the wire while firm pressure is applied at the site. **E,** The tip of the catheter is passed over the wire and advanced into the vessel with a rotating motion.

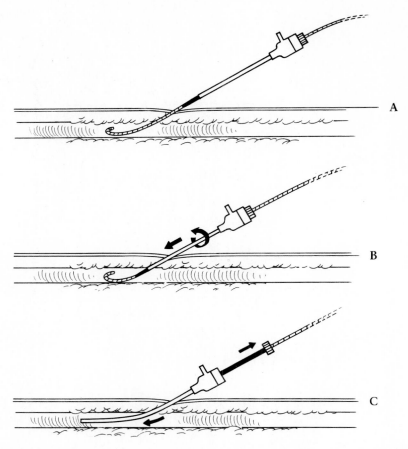

Fig. 4-4. Seldinger technique with use of a catheter introducer. **A,** The dilator and sheath are advanced over the guidewire until 6 to 10 cm of wire protrudes from the hub. **B,** The dilator and sheath are advanced through the skin into the vessel using a rotating motion. **C,** The guidewire and dilator are removed as a unit, leaving the sheath in place within the vessel.

brachial artery to the lower border of the teres major, where it becomes the axillary vein. The cephalic vein ascends on the radial aspect of the forearm. It communicates with the basilic vein through the median cubital vein just in front of the elbow and ascends laterally until it curves sharply as it pierces the clavipectoral fascia, crosses the axillary artery, and passes beneath the clavicle to join the axillary vein, or occasionally the external jugular vein. Because of this anatomy, the cephalic vein is more difficult to catheterize, making the basilic vein preferable.

EQUIPMENT. The basic equipment for venous cannulation consists of the basic percutaneous catheterization tray, a needle, and a catheter (central venous or PA) that is sufficiently long to reach the central vein. A small catheter can be inserted through a needle into the superior vena cava for CVP monitoring. However, it is more common today to insert PA catheters to monitor both central venous pressure (CVP) and pulmonary artery pressure (PAP) or pulmonary artery wedge pressure (PAWP). The PA catheter is inserted over a guidewire or through a catheter sheath by means of the Seldinger technique.

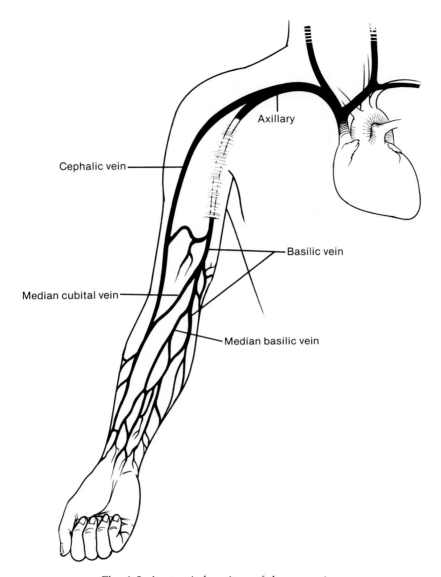

Cephalic vein

Axillary

Basilic vein

Median cubital vein

Median basilic vein

Fig. 4-5. Anatomic locations of the arm veins.

PATIENT PREPARATION. The patient is first prepared as described on p. 57. Additional specific preparation is conducted as follows:

1. Locate the vein. This may be easier if you temporarily apply a tourniquet above the antecubital fossa and the patient makes a fist to distend the veins.
2. Abduct the selected arm 30- to 45-degree from the body and secure it on a flat, padded arm board.
3. For placement of a central venous catheter without fluoroscopy, estimate the length of catheter needed as described on p. 57.

PROCEDURE. This discussion will be limited to insertion of a PA catheter into an antecubital vein via the Seldinger technique.

1. Apply a venous tourniquet to the upper arm.

2. While retaining traction on the skin distal to the insertion with one hand, puncture the vein with the needle held bevel side upward at a 15- to 20-degree angle.
3. With the appearance of the backflow of blood in the needle, insert the guidewire into the vein approximately 2 to 4 cm beyond the tip of the needle.
4. Release the tourniquet and slowly continue to advance the guidewire several centimeters.
5. Withdraw the needle from the vein while firmly holding the guidewire in place in the vessel.
6. Wipe the guidewire with a sterile moist gauze pad.
7. Insert the catheter of choice or a catheter introducer sheath over the guidewire into the vein.
8. Remove the guidewire. If a catheter introducer set is used, remove the inner dilator along with the guidewire, flush the sheath's side arm, and temporarily close the stopcock. Insert the catheter of choice into the sheath.
9. Aspirate and flush the catheter and connect both the catheter and side arm of the sheath to a heparinized flushing solution.
10. Position the catheter in the proper location.
11. Suture the catheter to the skin with 3-0 silk. (If a catheter sheath is used, suture the sheath and catheter separately to the skin.)
12. Apply an iodophor ointment and a sterile dressing to the insertion site and tape securely.
13. Immobilize the arm with an arm board.
14. Perform chest x-ray examination to verify the position of the catheter (if fluoroscopy is not used).

Special precautions

MEETING RESISTANCE. Do not force the catheter to advance. Withdraw the catheter 2 to 3 cm, rotate it slightly, and readvance it. Other maneuvers that may facilitate catheter passage include further abduction of the arm, having the patient move his or her shoulder anteriorly or posteriorly, having the patient inspire deeply, having the patient turn his or her head to the side of the venipuncture to prevent the catheter from entering the internal jugular vein, and partial inflation of the balloon of the catheter, if available.

ENSURING VISIBILITY. Do not attempt placement of a central venous catheter into a vein that cannot be made visible or palpable by means of a tourniquet, warm compresses, or placement of the arm in a dependent position with opening and closing of the hand. Choose another site in such a case.

Internal jugular vein. Catheterization of the internal jugular vein in the adult was first described by Hemosura in 1966. Since that time the internal jugular vein has been commonly used for percutaneous insertion of central venous, PA, and pacing catheters because its anatomic location provides a straight path to the right side of the heart, its landmarks are more definite and constant, and the complication rate is lower than with the subclavian approach.

ANATOMY. The internal jugular vein emerges from the base of the skull to enter the carotid sheath, which also contains the carotid artery and the vagus nerve. Initially, the internal jugular vein is posterior and lateral to the more superficial carotid artery. However, near the terminal portion of the vein, above its juncture with the subclavian vein, the internal jugular vein becomes lateral and slightly anterior to the carotid artery.

The lower portion of the internal jugular vein lies within the triangle formed by the sternal and clavicular heads of the sternocleidomastoid muscle (Fig. 4-6). It is within this triangle that the internal jugular vein is best cannulated. Behind the sternal end of the clavicle, the internal jugular vein unites with the subclavian vein to form the innominate vein.

EQUIPMENT. The basic percutaneous equipment tray is required, as well as the catheter of choice (central venous, PA, or pacing).

PATIENT PREPARATION. The patient should first be prepared as described on p. 57. Additional specific patient preparation consists of the following:

1. If the patient is obese or muscular with a short neck, place a small pillow or rolled towel under the shoulders to extend the neck.
2. Locate the carotid artery by palpation.
3. Identify the internal jugular vein and mark it if necessary.
4. Turn the patient's head to the contralateral side.

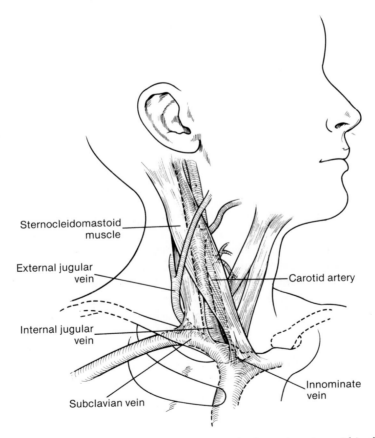

Fig. 4-6. Anatomy of the internal jugular vein showing its lower location within the triangle formed by the sternocleidomastoid muscle and the clavicle.

5. Place the patient in a 15- to 25-degree Trendelenburg position to distend the veins and prevent air embolism.

PROCEDURE. The literature describes at least 13 different variations of two basic approaches to percutaneous internal jugular vein cannulation. A high entry can be approached via a posterior (or lateral) route, an anterior (or medial) route, or a central route. Likewise, a low internal jugular puncture can be approached from a lateral or central route. In addition, either the right or left internal jugular vein can be cannulated. Most physicians prefer the right internal jugular vein because it is larger, forms a straight line to the superior vena cava and RA, the dome of the right lung and pleura lies lower than on the left side, and the large thoracic duct is not endangered. However, when right internal jugular vein cannulation fails and there is no hematoma, successful cannulation can usually be carried out on the left side.

Discussion here will be limited to cannulation of the internal jugular vein via the central approach described by Daily et al.

1. Identify the internal jugular vein by drawing a triangle from marks placed on the medial aspect of the clavicle, the medial aspect of the sternal head, and the lateral aspect of the clavicular head of the sternocleidomastoid muscle (Fig. 4-7). The center of the triangle is directly over the center of the internal jugular vein. (Having the awake patient lift his or her head slightly off the bed makes this triangle more visible and palpable.)

2. With a #11 blade, make a small (2 to 3 mm) stab wound at the insertion site (or do this after guidewire insertion).

3. Administer a local anesthetic and locate the internal jugular vein via a small (22- or 25-gauge) needle 3 to 4 cm above the medial aspect of the clavicle and 1 to 2 cm within the lateral border of the sternocleidomastoid muscle.

4. Attach a 3 or 5 ml syringe containing 2 or 3 ml of sterile saline or 1% lidocaine to the 18-gauge vascular needle. (The smaller syringe is easier to handle.)

5. Align the needle with the syringe (see Fig. 4-7) parallel to the medial border of the clavicular head of the sternocleidomastoid muscle. Direct the needle caudally at a 30-degree angle to the frontal plane directly over the internal jugular vein and aiming toward the ipsilateral nipple. (If the needle is positioned with its bevel side directed medially, the bevel aids in directing the guidewire medially into the central circulation.)

6. Puncture the skin and advance the needle while maintaining a slight negative pressure in the syringe until free flow of blood is obtained.

7. If the internal jugular vein is not entered initially, withdraw the needle while maintaining suction with the syringe and then redirect it 5- to 10-degree more laterally. If the vein has still not been entered, direct the needle more in line with the sagittal plane. Do not direct the needle medially across the sagittal plane lest the carotid artery be punctured. If possible, having the patient perform the Valsalva maneuver will distend the vein and improve the chance of successful cannulation.

8. After you observe free flow of venous blood in the syringe, instruct the patient to hold his breath and hum. During this time, quickly remove the syringe from the needle, place a thumb over the needle hub, and insert the soft, flexible tip

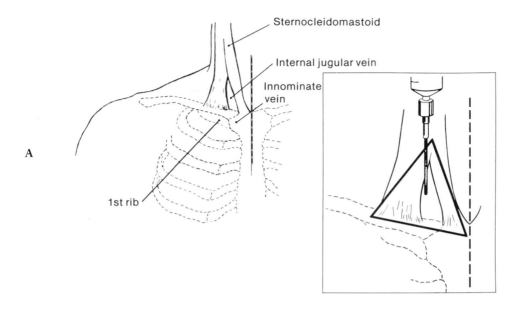

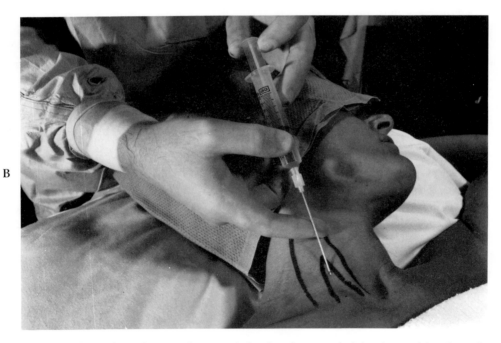

Fig. 4-7. Relationship of external anatomic landmarks to underlying internal jugular vein. **A,** Triangle drawn over clavicle and sternal and clavicular portions of sternocleidomastoid muscle is centered over internal jugular vein (inset). (From Daily PO, Griepp RB, and Shumway NE: Percutaneous internal jugular vein cannulation, Arch Surg 101:534-536, 1970. Copyright 1970, American Medical Association.) **B,** Alignment of the needle in the central portion of the triangle formed by the sternal and clavicular sections of the sternocleidomastoid muscle.

of the appropriate guidewire through the needle approximately 10 to 15 cm. Remove the needle and wipe the guidewire with a sterile, moist gauze pad. Instruct the patient to resume normal breathing.

9. Insert the catheter introducer set over the guidewire until 10 to 15 cm of wire extends beyond the hub of the sheath. Advance the dilator and sheath through the skin and subcutaneous tissue into the vein. If the introducer has a side arm, this should be closed to the patient.
10. Remove the dilator and the guidewire together from the sheath.
11. Aspirate and flush the sheath side arm with saline and temporarily close the stopcock toward the patient or connect it to a heparin IV infusion.
12. Insert the catheter of choice through the sheath and position it in the heart.
13. Aspirate and flush the catheter and sheath side arm and connect them to a heparinized IV infusion or pressure tubing.
14. Suture the sheath and catheter to the skin.
15. Apply an iodophor ointment and sterile dressing to the insertion site and tape it securely.
16. Return the patient to a flat position and remove the pillow or roll from the shoulders.
17. Perform chest x-ray examination to verify catheter position (if fluoroscopy was not used).

Subclavian vein. Cannulation of the subclavian vein for venous catheterization has grown in popularity since 1962, when Wilson et al described their successful experience with subclavian insertion of central venous catheters. Percutaneous catheterization of the subclavian vein has become a common approach to insertion of central venous, PA, and pacing catheters. This approach has been very popular for long-term placement of TPN catheters because it is easier to secure the catheter and there is less interference with the patient's mobility. The subclavian vein is also the easiest vein to cannulate in patients with profound circulatory collapse.

ANATOMY. The subclavian vein begins at the lateral border of the first rib as the continuation of the axillary vein, and it ends at the medial border of the anterior scalene muscle. It joins the internal jugular vein behind the sternoclavicular joint to form the innominate vein (Fig. 4-8). The vein is separated from its artery by the anterior scalene muscle, which is approximately 10 to 15 mm thick. The vein crosses the first rib and lies anteroinferior to the artery (posterior to the middle third of the clavicle). The apical pleura lies approximately 5 mm posterior to the junction of the jugular and subclavian veins. The subclavian vein is a large vein with an inside diameter of 1.5 to 2.0 cm or more.

EQUIPMENT. The equipment required is the same as that for the internal jugular vein approach (p. 65).

PATIENT PREPARATION. The patient should first be prepared as described on pp. 56 to 58. Additional preparation consists of the following:
1. Place a rolled towel under the patient's back between the scapulae.
2. Turn the patient's head to the contralateral side.
3. Place the patient in a 15- to 25-degree Trendelenburg position.

PROCEDURE. The subclavian vein can be approached from either the superior or inferior direction. Overall success and complication rates of both methods are very similar. However, the supraclavicular approach offers several practical advantages:

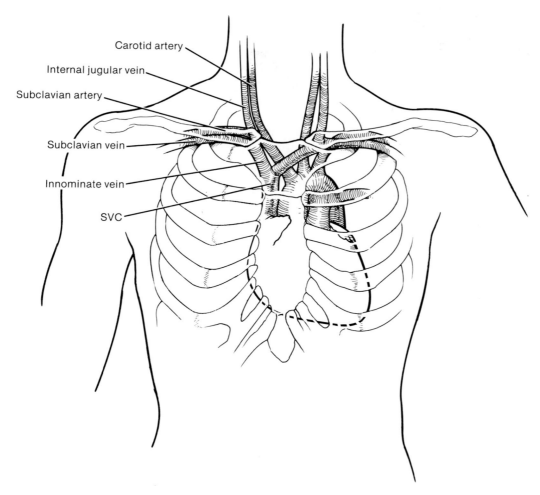

Carotid artery

Internal jugular vein

Subclavian artery

Subclavian vein

Innominate vein

SVC

Fig. 4-8. Anatomic location of the subclavian vein and surrounding structures. The subclavian vein joins the internal jugular vein to become the innominate vein at about the manubrioclavicular junction. The innominate vein becomes the superior vena cava (SVC) at about the level of the midmanubrium.

there is a shorter distance between the vein and the skin (0.5 to 4 cm); it is a more direct path to the superior vena cava; it is more easily performed during CPR with minimal or no interruption of chest compression; and the rate of correct catheter tip location is greater than with the infraclavicular approach.

Practical advantages notwithstanding, the infraclavicular approach to percutaneous subclavian catheterization remains the most popular method, and discussion here will be limited to this technique. Either the right or left subclavian vein may be cannulated, although the left subclavian vein may be preferred for catheter insertion because it gently curves into the innominate vein and no sharp bends of the catheter are required. However, the pleural dome is not as high on the right side as on the left side.

1. Identify the junction of the middle and medial thirds of the clavicle where the

first rib proceeds beneath the clavicle. Needle insertion should be approximately 1 or 2 cm lateral and inferior to this location. A frequent error is use of a more lateral insertion site at the midclavicle area. Another means of identification is to palpate the inferior surface of the clavicle and locate a tubercle on the clavicle approximately one third to one half the length of the clavicle from the sternoclavicular joint. This tubercle marks the site of needle entry.

2. Make a small (3 mm) skin nick at the insertion site using a #11 blade, sharp side upward (or do this after guidewire insertion).

3. Depress the area 1 to 2 cm beneath the junction of the distal and middle thirds of the clavicle with the thumb of the nondominant hand and place the index finger of the same hand approximately 2 cm above the sternal notch.

4. Administer a local anesthetic and locate the vein via a small (21- or 25-gauge) needle directed toward the index finger above the notch and at a 20- or 30-degree angle with the thorax. (Direct the bevel of the needle inferiomedially to encourage guidewire passage into the innominate vein.)

5. Insert the needle under the clavicle at the point identified in step 1 (Fig. 4-9).

6. Advance the needle, "walking" it down until it slips beneath the clavicle while maintaining gentle negative pressure within the syringe.

7. When the vein is entered, remove the smaller needle and attach the 18-gauge needle to a syringe containing 5 to 10 ml of heparin or lidocaine and repeat steps 3 to 6 while maintaining negative pressure in the syringe.

8. When the vein is entered with the cannulating needle, ask the patient to hold his or her breath or hum, while you quickly remove the syringe from the 18-gauge needle and immediately cap the needle hub with your thumb or index finger.

9. Insert the flexible tip of the guidewire 10 to 15 cm through the needle and remove the needle, maintaining gentle pressure on the puncture site. Instruct the patient to resume breathing.

10. With the sheath's side arm closed to the patient, advance the catheter introducer set (dilator and sheath) over the guidewire into the vein, using a slight twisting motion (the side arm is closed to the patient).

11. Remove the guidewire and dilator together from the sheath.

12. Aspirate and flush the side arm of the sheath and close its stopcock to the patient.

13. Insert the catheter of choice. Having the patient bring his or her ear to the shoulder on the side of the insertion site creates a sharp angle between the jugular and subclavian veins and helps prevent misdirection of the catheter into the internal jugular vein during advancement.

14. Advance and position the catheter in the heart.

15. Aspirate and flush the catheter and the side arm of the sheath and connect the side arm of the sheath and the hub of the catheter to a heparin IV infusion and pressure tubing.

16. Suture the sheath and catheter to the skin near the insertion site.

17. Apply an iodophor ointment and sterile dressing to the insertion site and tape it securely.

18. Return the patient to a flat position and remove the roll from his or her back.

19. Obtain a chest x-ray film to verify catheter position if fluoroscopy is not used.

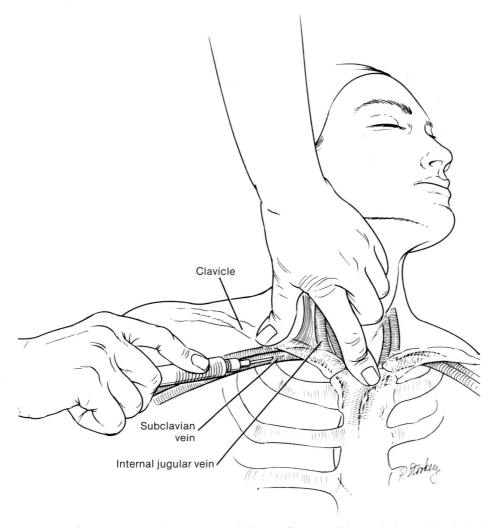

Clavicle

Subclavian
vein

Internal jugular vein

Fig. 4-9. Puncture of the subclavian vein with the needle inserted beneath the middle third of the clavicle at a 20- to 30-degree angle aiming medially.

Special precautions

PREVENTION OF GUIDEWIRE MISDIRECTION INTO THE JUGULAR VEIN. If guidewire passage is not entirely smooth, the wire may have entered the jugular vein. The patient may complain of an unpleasant sensation in the area of the ipsilateral ear. The guidewire location should be confirmed with fluoroscopy and the wire repositioned before the catheter is advanced over it. A caudal direction of the bevel of the needle and having the patient bring his or her ear down to the shoulder on the insertion side during guidewire passage are steps that may prevent guidewire misdirection into the jugular vein.

PASSAGE OF THE NEEDLE UNDER THE CLAVICLE. If it proves difficult to depress the needle sufficiently to pass under the clavicle into the vein, the needle may be bent smoothly over its entire length to form a gentle arc. The needle should then be inserted at a 45-degree angle under the clavicle, and following its 30-degree arc, it will usually enter the vein.

REDUCING THE RISK OF PNEUMOTHORAX. The operator can reduce the risk of pneumothorax by avoiding too lateral or too deep a needle insertion. Multiple attempts at cannulation should be avoided. Generally, if three attempts prove unsuccessful, another site should be chosen. Patients with chronic obstructive pulmonary disease with overinflated stiff lungs, especially those receiving ventilatory support, are at a higher risk for pulmonary complications resulting from attempted subclavian cannulation. Thus, subclavian vein cannulation is best avoided in these patients. If cannulation is attempted but unsuccessful, a chest radiograph should be obtained to rule out pneumothorax before contralateral insertion.

CORRECT AIM OF THE NEEDLE IN THE ELDERLY. In elderly patients the subclavian vein may be more inferior, requiring aiming of the needle toward the inferior margin of the sternal notch. These patients may also have a bony prominence beneath the medial portion of the calvicle, making cannulation difficult.

PREVENTION OF PUNCTURE OF THE SUBCLAVIAN ARTERY. The operator can avoid puncture of the subclavian artery by keeping the puncture site away from the most lateral course of the vein and not angulating the needle too far posteriorly. If the subclavian artery is punctured, the needle should be removed and firm pressure applied over the puncture site for 10 minutes.

Surgical Cutdown Technique

Although percutaneous catheterization provides more rapid access into the vascular system, surgical cutdown may be necessary in some emergency situations. This procedure was first described in 1940 as an alternate access procedure in patients in shock with collapsed veins, or in patients with very small veins. This technique continues to be useful in hypovolemic patients and children.

The basic equipment necessary for arterial or venous cutdown is listed on this page. Additional equipment includes sterile heparinized IV solution for maintenance of catheter patency and appropriate transducer components for hemodynamic pressure monitoring.

Brachial or basilic vein cutdown

1. Make a transverse incision through the skin and superficial fascia directly over the selected vessel with a #15 blade. The incision should be wide enough to permit adequate exposure of the vessel.
2. Separate the tissues by gentle, blunt, longitudinal dissection with a curved forceps.
3. Identify the selected vessel and bring it to the surface by placing the forceps tips underneath it.
4. Tag the vessel both proximally and distally using 3-0 or 4-0 silk (6 to 10 cm long) for the vein and umbilical or silicone rubber (Silastic) tape for the artery. For arterial cutdown, the Silastic tapes are usually double-wrapped around the proximal and distal portions of the vessel. The ends of each tape are then secured with a small straight forceps.
5. Occlude blood flow through the vessel. (Retract the upper tie around the artery or tie the lower tie in the vein).

6. While pinching the top portion of the vessel with a forceps, make a small incision (approximately one-third the diameter) into the vessel using a #11 blade sharp side up.

7. Insert the selected catheter into the vessel. A small vein introducer hook may facilitate venous entry.

8. Temporarily release tension on the upper suture around the vein and advance the catheter to the desired position. If necessary, apply tension to the proximal and distal ties to control any bleeding.

9. For long-term indwelling catheters in a vein, tie and cut off the upper tie around the catheter and vein, taking care not to occlude the catheter. For long-term use of catheters in an artery, remove the proximal and distal ties and compress the artery for several minutes.

10. Irrigate the wound with sterile saline and carefully observe for any bleeding.

11. Close the skin with three or four interrupted sutures of 4-0 silk.

12. Suture the catheter to the skin at the insertion site.

13. Clean the incision with sterile saline, and apply povidone-iodine ointment and a sterile dressing.

An alternate method of venous catheter insertion involves a modified cutdown in which the vein is located and exposed through a surgical incision and the vein then directly punctured with the needle. The venous catheter is then inserted via the Seldinger technique over a guidewire. This direct approach is helpful in patients with very small or inaccessible veins and eliminates the necessity to ligate the vein.

Basic equipment for vascular cutdown

Antiseptic solution
Drapes, towels, and towel clips
Bowl of sterile saline with heparin
4 × 4-inch gauze pads
Lidocaine 1% without epinephrine
25- and 21-gauge needles, 1½ and 2 inches long
5 and 10 ml syringes
#11 and #15 scalpels
Curved mosquito forceps
Plain forceps
Self-retracting retractors
Small rakes
Fine-toothed forceps (for arterial cutdown)
Two pieces of umbilical tape and/or Silastic tape (for arterial cutdown)
4-0 Silk suture
6-0 Monofilament suture
Iris scissors
Small plastic introducer
Needle holder
Heparin
Catheter of choice

The CVP catheter should be inserted into the vein and advanced until its tip lies in the SVC, just above the RA (Fig. 4-10). The catheter should be aspirated and flushed and connected to fluid-filled tubing and monitoring system (either a water manometer or transducer). Placement should be checked via a chest x-ray.

The PA catheter should be connected to a fluid-filled transducer system before insertion to provide continuous pressure monitoring during advancement. When the catheter tip reaches the SVC, the balloon of the catheter should be partially inflated to promote flotation into the RA (Fig. 4-11, *A* and *B*). When the tip of the catheter reaches the RA, as indicated by an RA waveform with marked respiratory variation (Fig. 4-12), inflate the balloon with approximately 1 ml of air. The catheter should then float into the RV (Fig. 4-11, *C*) and an RV waveform will be displayed on the monitor (see Fig. 4-12). (Watch the ECG closely for signs of ventricular irritability when the catheter is in the RV.) Advance the catheter as quickly and smoothly as possible until the catheter resists advancement and a PA waveform is present on the monitor (see Fig. 4-12). Deflate the balloon, obtain a PA pressure recording and slightly advance the catheter (Fig. 4-13). Slowly inflate the balloon until a PAW waveform appears on the screen (see Fig. 4-12). *Inflate only for a brief period of time and only enough to change the waveform from PA to PAW.* If there is a discrepancy between the PAW and PAed pressures, repeat the measurements several times to verify. Ensure that the balloon is completely deflated after each inflation by removing the inflating syringe. Actively withdrawing the air back into the syringe is not recommended because it can damage the balloon.

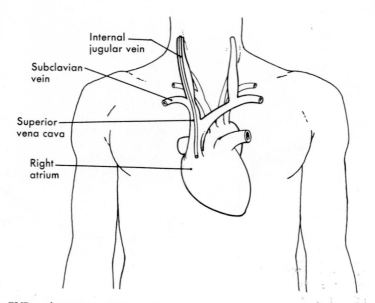

Fig. 4-10. CVP catheter in position with the tip in the superior vena cava just above the junction of the right atrium.

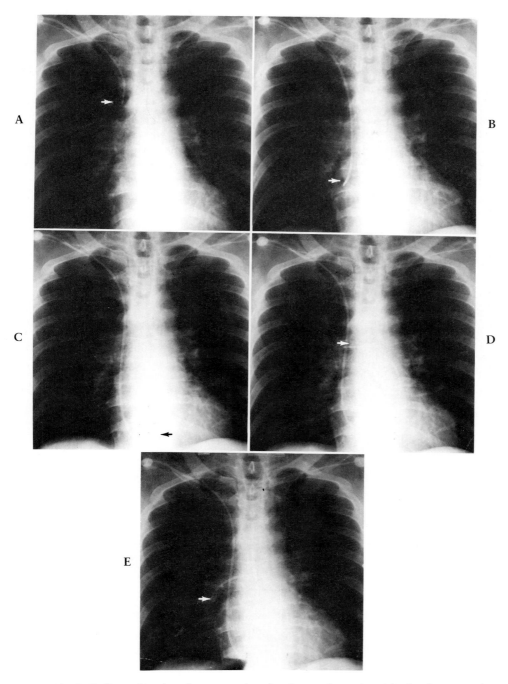

Fig. 4-11. A, Balloon-tipped catheter entering the thorax from the right basilic vein; the catheter tip is in the superior vena cava. **B,** Catheter tip is in the midright atrium. **C,** Catheter tip is in the right ventricle. **D,** Catheter tip is in the pulmonary artery. **E,** Catheter tip is advanced to a PAW position.

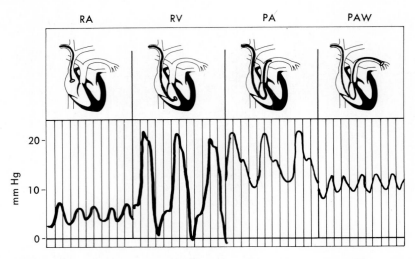

Fig. 4-12. Flow-directed, balloon-tipped catheter locations with corresponding pressure tracings. (From Schroeder JS, and Daily EK: Hemodynamic monitoring. Tampa Tracings slide series, Tarpon Springs, Fla, 1976, Tampa Tracings.)

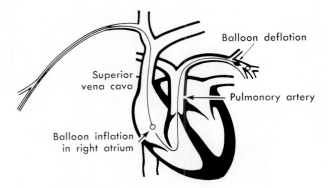

Fig. 4-13. Flow-directed, balloon-tipped catheter showing inflation of balloon in the right atrium and consequent "floating" of the catheter through the right ventricle and out to a distal PA branch. The balloon is deflated, advanced slightly, and reinflated slightly to obtain a PAW pressure.

Complications

Complications common to all venous cannulation techniques include hematoma, thrombosis, phlebitis, sepsis, cellulitis, and air embolism. Other complications are specific to the site of insertion and are presented in Table 4-2, along with rates of successful insertion, central venous catheter malposition, and overall complications. Experience and meticulous attention to technique are the best safeguards against these complications. Even then, life-threatening complications may occur.

Venous air embolism. Venous air embolism is a rare but catastrophic complication of central venous catheter placement, with a mortality of approximately 50%. Lethal air embolism occurs with central injection of 200 to 300 cc of air at a rate

Table 4-2. Insertion success rate, central venous catheter malposition, overall complication rate, and specific complications associated with various venous insertion sites

Site	Insertion success rate (%)	Catheter malposition rate (%) (without fluoroscopy)	Complication rate (%)	Specific complications and rate (%)
Basilic	58-98	25-52	3-5	Thrombophlebitis (3-5) Thrombosis (<1-5) Phlebitis/cellulitis (1-20)
Internal jugular	80-94	0-6 (Right) 0-20 (Left)	<1-13	Carotid artery puncture (1-15) Myocardial perforation of pacing catheter (1-10) Pneumothorax (<1) Hemothorax (<1) Air embolism (<1) Catheter embolism (<1) Nerve damage (rare) Thrombosis (rare) Horner's syndrome (rare)
Subclavian vein	85-98	20-33	<1-17	Pneumothorax (<1-10) Subclavian artery puncture (1-20) Sepsis (<1-2) Hemothorax (1) Hydrothorax (1) Air embolism (<1) Thrombophlebitis (<1) Thrombosis (rare) Catheter embolism (rare) Brachial plexus injury (rare) Phrenic nerve injury (rare) Sternoclavicular osteomyelitis (rare)
Femoral vein	89-95	—	4-20	Evidence of thrombus (15-20) Infection (3-20) Femoral artery puncture (4-10)
External jugular vein	61-99	6	0-4	Hematoma (<5) Air embolism (rare) Thrombosis (rare)

of 70 to 150 cc/sec, although as little as 20 cc of air may cause harm to a critically ill patient. The rate of air entry depends on both the inside diameter and the length of the tubing inserted. Air can enter a vein, particularly a large vein such as the internal jugular or subclavian, by one of three methods: (1) through a disconnection of or leak in the catheter, the infusion tubing, or the connecting sites; (2) through the needle or sheath at the time of insertion into the vein; or (2) along the formed track of a removed catheter that had been in place for a prolonged period, especially in a thin person with little subcutaneous tissue. This complication is more likely to occur when the patient is in an upright position, takes a deep breath, or is in a state of hypovolemia with low central venous pressure.

Massive air embolism can cause obstruction of the right ventricular outflow tract and interfere with gas exchange, presenting with manifestations that are similar to that of pulmonary thromboembolism. The diagnosis of venous air embolism is primarily clinical; the condition should be suspected whenever sudden cardiovascular collapse occurs in patients with a central venous catheter in place. Two-dimensional ecohocardiography has been shown to be of value in the diagnosis of venous air embolism. High-resolution computed tomographic (CT) scanning and magnetic resonance imaging (MRI) are helpful in the diagnosis of arterial air emboli of the central nervous system. The clinical manifestations and methods of prevention and treatment of venous air embolism are listed on page 79.

ARTERIAL ACCESS

Catheterization of the arterial system is indicated for pressure measurements, angiography, cardiac output determination, and counterpulsation. In addition, continuous intra-arterial pressure monitoring and multiple arterial blood sampling are frequently necessary in patients with unstable ischemic heart disease (with or without myocardial infarction), adult respiratory distress syndrome, severe arterial hypertension undergoing afterload-reducing therapy, hypotension or shock, and in patients who have undergone cardiac surgery.

Arterial Cannulation Sites

The arterial system can be cannulated either percutaneously or via a cutdown at several sites. If necessary the arterial system can also be entered via cannulation of arterial grafts. To reduce complications and obtain the most accurate hemodynamic data, catheters are preferably placed in the large-diameter arteries. In order of size this would be the femoral, axillary, brachial, and radial arteries. However, in clinical practice, cannulation of the axillary artery is infrequently used. Femoral and brachial arteries have traditionally been cannulated primarily in the cardiac catheterization laboratory on a short-term basis for pressure measurements and arteriography. This practice may be changing as more clinicians become aware of the benefits and familiar with the skills of femoral artery cannulation. Because of the poor collateral supply, cannulation of the brachial artery for long-term pressure monitoring is discouraged.

Table 4-3 lists some advantages and disadvantages of each arterial insertion site.

Patient preparation

MODIFIED ALLEN TEST. Before cannulation of the radial artery it is imperative to assess the adequacy of collateral blood flow to the hand. This can be done via a Doppler flow probe, a finger pulse monitor, or performance of the Allen test. A modified Allen test is performed in the manner described below.

1. Elevate the patient's arm well above the heart level.
2. Clench the fist of the elevated arm, either passively or actively.
3. Place the thumb of one hand over the ulnar artery and the thumb of the other

---

Manifestations, prevention, and treatment of air embolism

Manifestations
    Acute respiratory distress, apnea, occasional wheezing
    Sudden hypotension and syncope
    Profound hypoxia, cyanosis
    Audible machinery ("mill wheel") murmur
    Elevated CVP (or JVP)
    Neurologic deficits (hemiplegia, aphasia) in presence of right-to-left shunt
    Cardiac arrest with asystole or VF
Prevention
    Use meticulous technique, occluding needle and catheter hub as necessary
    Elevate venous pressure (Trendelenburg position; volume expansion, if venous
        pressure is low)
    Use sheaths with pneumatic valve and check competency of valve before using
    Use Luer-Lok connections
    Securely seal all central catheters and connections
    Restrain uncooperative, agitated, or confused patients
    Do not allow containers of IV solutions to completely empty
Treatment
    Immediately place patient in left lateral Trendelenburg position
    Have the patient perform the Valsalva maneuver, if possible
    Administer 100% oxygen and ventilatory support
    Aspirate air via CVP or PA catheter
    Hyperbaric oxygen treatment (DAN)*
    CPR if necessary

---

*Dividing accident network

hand over the radial artery and firmly compress both arteries for approximately 5 seconds.

4. While maintaining arterial compression, lower the arm and relax the hand, which will be very white.

5. Release the pressure only on the ulnar side of the artery.

6. Observe and time the appearance of a pink flush over the palm, including the thumb and fingers. The entire hand should regain color in less than 15 seconds; if so, the test is negative. Ulnar filling is deemed slow if flushing does not occur before 7 to 15 seconds and suggests that part of the hand depends on radial circulation for perfusion. This would be a positive Allen test and is an absolute contraindication for placement of a cannula in the radial artery; such placement would seriously compromise perfusion to the hand. The Allen test should be repeated, releasing compression on the radial artery only to evaluate radial adequacy. If either artery demonstrates a delay in color return, the radial artery should not be cannulated.

The Allen test may be difficult to perform in dark-skinned persons or in uncooperative patients. Under these circumstances the use of a Doppler flow probe, and more particularly the finger-pulse transducer, provides accurate assessment of the adequacy of ulnar collateral blood flow to the hand.

Table 4-3. Advantages and disadvantages associated with percutaneous cannulation of specific arterial sites

Site	Advantages	Disadvantages
Radial artery	Readily accessible Good collateral circulation Superifical location Collateral circulation can be assessed before the procedure	High risk of occlusion because of small size High rate of catheter malfunction In shock states with low blood pressure and peripheral vasoconstriction this site may not reflect central aortic pressure
Brachial artery	Accessible in most patients with peripheral vascular disease	Higher complication rate Deeper location makes control of bleeding more difficult Closely surrounded by major tendons, veins, and nerves
Axillary artery	Arm position permits biplane angiography and oblique views Less patient immobilization Left axillary artery insertion associated with successful selective catheter placement Decreased risk of occlusion because of large size Extensive collateral circulation	Increased risk of nerve damage Risk of hematoma or pseudoaneurysm
Femoral artery	Large vessel easy to cannulate with decreased risk of occlusion Easier to cannulate in presence of vasoconstriction or hypotension Accurate central pressures even in shock states Long catheter life Easy to compress after catheter removal	Reduced patient mobility Insertion site not as easily located in obese patients Risk of hematoma in very obese patients in whom direct compression may be difficult

7. General patient preparation as described on p. 57.
8. Immobilize the patient's nondominant hand (if possible) palm side up on a padded arm board, providing approximately 60-degree extension of the wrist.
9. Secure a peripheral IV line or heparin lock.

Percutaneous Cannulation

Percutaneous insertion of arterial catheters is the preferred method of cannulation because of its ease and speed of insertion, reduced infection rate, and fewer equipment requirements.

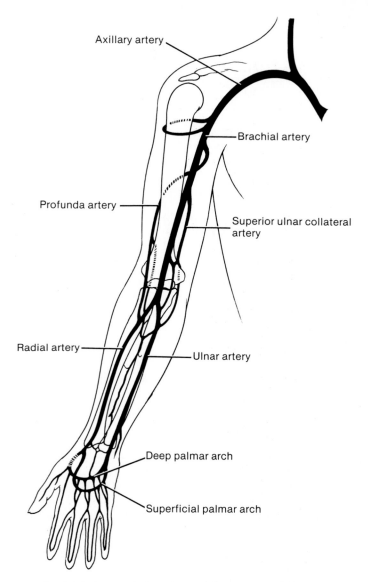

Axillary artery

Brachial artery

Profunda artery

Superior ulnar collateral
artery

Radial artery

Ulnar artery

Deep palmar arch

Superficial palmar arch

Fig. 4-14. Anatomic locations of the arteries of the arm.

Radial artery

Percutaneous cannulation of the radial artery is traditionally the most common means of arterial access in the critical care or emergency setting.

Anatomy. The radial artery is a small, superficially located terminal branch of the brachial artery (Fig. 4-14). It arises in the antecubital fossa and passes downward to the wrist along the radial side of the forearm. Its pulsations can be readily palpated at the wrist before the flexor carpi radialis tendon of the lateral anterior border of the radius.

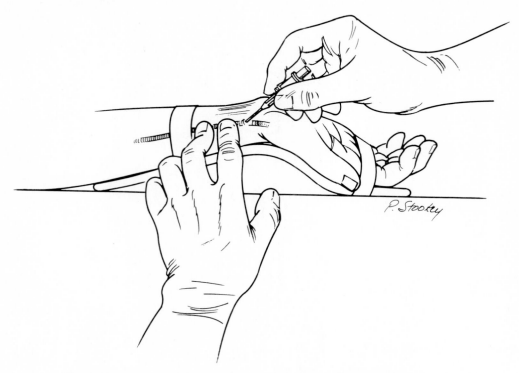

Fig. 4-15. Puncture of the radial artery with the needle at a 30-degree angle.

The radial artery anastamoses with the ulnar artery in the hand, forming the deep palmar arch, the dorsal arch, and the superficial palmar arch.

Procedure

1. Palpate the radial artery to determine its exact location and direction.
2. Make a shallow 1 to 2 mm skin incision over the radial artery with a #11 scalpel.
3. Align a 20-gauge needle with stylet at a 20-degree angle over the radial artery approximately 3 to 4 cm proximal to the styloid process of the radius.
4. While palpating the pulse with one hand, insert the needle into and through the radial artery (Fig. 4-15).
5. Remove the inner stylet and slowly withdraw the needle until it is located in the artery; proper location is indicated by bright red blood pulsating from the needle hub.
6. Insert the soft flexible tip of an 0.018-inch (0.46 mm) guidewire 10 to 15 cm into the artery. While securely holding the wire in place, remove the needle. Wipe the guidewire with a moistened gauze pad. Insert a short (5 cm) 3 Fr catheter over the guidewire into the artery; remove the guidewire. Alternately, and more commonly, a catheter-over-needle is inserted into the radial artery for long-term monitoring. If a catheter-over-needle is being used, remove the stylet and slowly withdraw the catheter and needle until bright red blood pulsates from the needle hub. Advance the Teflon catheter into the artery while simultaneously withdrawing the needle.

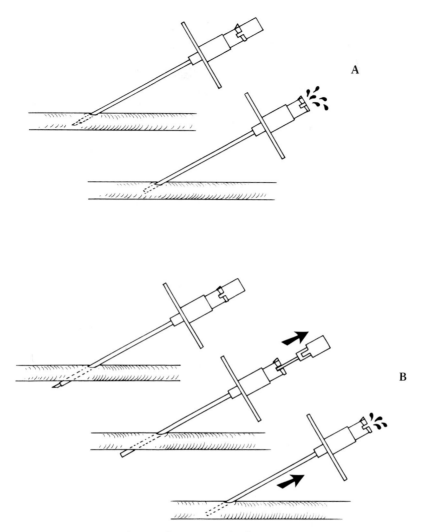

Fig. 4-16. Methods of arterial cannulation via (**A**) direct puncture or (**B**) transfixation in which both walls are punctured, after which the inner stylet is removed and the cannula is slowly withdrawn until blood flow appears at the hub.

7. Aspirate, discard the aspirate, and gently flush the catheter. Attach the heparinized IV solution and stopcock to the catheter.
8. Suture the hub of the catheter to the skin with 3-0 silk.
9. Cleanse the area and apply an iodophor ointment and a sterile dressing secured with tape.

Special precautions

DIMINISHED RADIAL PULSE. Occasionally the radial artery pulse will diminish or disappear after infiltration with lidocaine. This is usually temporary. However, return of the pulse can sometimes be hastened by gentle massage of the surrounding tissues.

PULSATILE BLOOD CESSATION. If cessation of pulsatile blood occurs at any time during catheter advancement, slowly withdraw the catheter until blood flow resumes. Withdraw the catheter 1 to 2 mm more, then readvance the catheter. If no blood flow reappears during the second catheter withdrawal, remove the catheter entirely and apply compression for 5 minutes before repuncturing the artery. If there never was evidence of blood flow, the artery was probably never punctured; in this case compression is not necessary before repuncturing the artery.

METHODS OF CANNULATION (FIG. 4-16). Cannulation can be successfully performed by either direct threading or fixation, as described in step 5. Transfixation of the vessel by deliberate puncture of both the anterior and posterior wall of the artery is a commonly used method in the smaller arteries. Reports indicate no significant difference in the complication rates of these methods.

CIRCULATORY ASSESSMENT OF THE HAND. Circulation in the hand should be assessed every 4 hours and the catheter removed immediately upon any signs of circulatory compromise.

PREVENTION OF BLEEDING. Bleeding from the puncture site can be prevented by applying firm pressure for 5 to 10 minutes after catheter removal. The puncture site should then be observed for several minutes to assure the adequacy of hemostasis. This should be followed by application of a light pressure dressing and frequent evaluations of the radial pulse and blood flow to the hand.

Table 4-4. Insertion success rate and specific complications associated with percutaneous cannulation of arterial insertion sites

Site	Insertion success rate (%)	Specific complications and reported rates (%)
Radial artery	85	Thrombosis 2.5-60 Hematoma 0-30 Emboli 0-23 Infection 0-14 Diminished pulse 1-15 Distal ischemia 1-7 Sepsis 0-5 Bleeding 1 Distal necrosis <1 Pseudoaneurysm <1
Femoral artery	99	Hematoma 1-5 Thrombosis 1-4 Distal ischemia 3 Emboli <2 Sepsis 0-4
Brachial artery	Varied data	Diminished pulse 0-45 Ischemia 0-1.5
Axillary artery	70-90	Brachial plexus injury <1-9 Hematoma 1-6 Neuropathy 0-3 Pseudoaneurysm <1 Sepsis <1

A loose connection from the arterial line can quickly cause hemorrhage. For this reason, only Luer-Lok connections should be used. All connections should be secured tightly and all connectors should be readily visible so that leaks can be immediately detected.

Complications

RADIAL ARTERY THROMBOSIS. The most significant determinants of radial artery thrombosis seem to be catheter size, shape, and composition and the length of time the catheter is left in the artery. For these reasons it is strongly recommended that the radial artery be cannulated with a nontapered Teflon catheter no larger than 20 gauge and that the catheter be removed as soon as clinically possible. Short-term cannulation for less than 4 hours can be safely performed with little risk of thrombosis. The risk of arterial occlusion is also higher if the artery is punctured more than once during attempted cannulation. Despite the high rate of thrombotic complications with radial artery catheters, permanent damage occurs infrequently, with resolution of symptoms usually within 48 hours to 7 days of catheter removal. Therapeutic maneuvers that may improve distal blood flow include heparin infusion, administration of lidocaine, performance of a sympathetic nerve block, or thrombectomy via a Fogarty catheter. Careful attention to technique, use of a small, preferably nontapered Teflon catheter for short periods of time, and meticulous nursing care can markedly reduce the risk of serious complications. Other complications and their reported rate of occurrence are listed in Table 4-4.

REFERENCES

Abrams HL: Angiography, Boston, 1983, Little, Brown & Co.

Asimacopoulos PJ, Bagley FH, and McDermott WF: A modified technique for subclavian puncture, Surg Gynecol Obstet 150:241, 1980.

Bedford RF, and Wollman H: Complications of percutaneous radial artery cannulation in objective prospective study in man, Anesthesiology 38:228-236, 1973.

Bernard RW, and Stahl WM: Subclavian vein catheterizations: a prospective study. I. Non-infectious complications, Ann Surg 173:184, 1971.

Blitt CD, Wright WA, Petty WC, and Webster TA: Central venous catheterization via the external jugular vein: a technique employing the J-wire, JAMA 229:817, 1974.

Brinkman AJ, and Costley DO: Internal jugular venipuncture, JAMA 223:182, 1973.

Brown M, Gordon LH, Brown OW, and Brown EM: Intravascular monitoring via the axillary artery, Anesth Intensive Care 13:38-40, 1984.

Bryan-Brown CW et al: The axillary artery catheter, Heart Lung 12:492-497, 1983.

Campeau L: Percutaneous brachial catheterization (letter), Cathet Cardiovasc Diagn 11:443-444, 1985.

Civetta JM, Gabel JC, and Gemer M: Internal-jugular-vein puncture with a margin of safety, Anesthesiology 36:622, 1972.

Cooper MW: A simple method for insertion of multiple catheters through a single venipuncture site, Cathet Cardiovasc Diagn 8:305, 1982.

Daily PO, Griepp RB, and Shumway NE: Percutaneous internal jugular vein cannulation, Arch Surg 101:534, 1970.

Davis FM: Methods of radial artery cannulation and subsequent arterial occlusion, Anesthesiology 56:331, 1982.

Dronen S, Thompson B, Nowak R, and Tomlanovich M: Subclavian vein catheterization during cardiopulmonary resuscitation: a prospective comparison of supraclavicular and infraclavicular percutaneous approaches, JAMA 247:3227, 1984.

Eisenberg RL, Mani RL, and McDonald EJ, Jr: The complication rate of catheter angiography by direct puncture through aortofemoral grafts, AJR 126:814-816, 1976.

English ICW, Frew RM, and Pigott JFG: Percutaneous cannulation of the internal jugular vein, Thorax 24:496, 1969

Feliciano DV, et al: Major complications of percutaneous subclavian vein catheters, Am J Surg 138:869, 1979.

Fergusson DJG, and Kamada RO: Percutaneous entry of the brachial artery for left heart catheterization using a sheath, Cathet Cardiovasc Diagn 7:111-114, 1981.

Folland ED et al: Brachial artery catheterization employing a side arm sheath, Cathet Cardiovasc Diagn 10:55-61, 1984.

Goldfarb G, and Lebrec D: Percutaneous cannulation of the internal jugular vein in patients with coagulopathies: an experience based on 1000 attempts, Anesthesiology 56:321, 1982.

Gottdiener JS et al: Detection of venous air embolism by 2D echocardiography: evidence for entry of air into intracardiac shunt, Circulation 72(suppl III):III-352, 1985

Gurman GM, and Krierman S: Cannulation of big arteries in critically ill patients, Crit Care Med 13:217-220, 1985.

Hales S: Statistical essays: Hemostaticks, vol 2, ed 3, London, 1738, W Innys & R Manby.

Hemosura B: Measurment of pressure during intravenous therapy, JAMA 195:181, 1966.

Huyghens L et al: Cardiothoracic complications of centrally inserted catheters, Acute Care 11:53-56, 1985.

Jacob AS, and Schweiger MJ: A method for inserting two catheters, pulmonary arterial and temporary pacing, through a single puncture into a subclavian vein, Cathet Cardiovasc Diagn 9:611, 1983.

Jernigan WR, and Gardner WC: Use of the internal jugular vein for placement of central venous catheter, Surg Gynecol Obstet 130:520, 1970.

Johnston AOB, and Clark RG: Malpositioning of central venous catheters, Lancet 2:1395, 1972.

Jones RM, Hill AB, Nahrwold ML, and Bolles RE: The effect of the method of radial artery cannulation on post cannulation blood flow and thrombus formation, Anesthesiology 55:76-78, 1981.

Kaiser CW et al: Choice of route for central venous cannulation: subclavian or internal jugular vein: a prospective randomized study, J Surg Oncol 17:345, 1981.

Kashuk JL, and Penn I: Air embolism after central venous catheterization, Surg Gynecol Obstet 159:249, 1984

Kearns PJ, Haulk AA, and McDonald TW: Homonymous hemaniopia due to cerebral air embolism from central venous catheters, West J Med 140:615, 1984.

Kelly J, Braverman B, Land PC, and Ivankovich AD: Comparison of Allen test, Doppler and finger-pulse transducer to assess patency of ulnar artery, Anesthesiology 59(supp.):A178, 1983.

Langston CS: The aberrant central venous catheter and its complications, Diagn Radiol 100:55, 1971.

Legler D, and Nugent M: Doppler localization of

the internal jugular vein facilitates its cannulation (abstract), Anesthesiology, 1983, p. A179.

Linos DA, Mucha P, and Van Heerden JA: Subclavian vein, a golden route, Mayo Clin Proc 55:315, 1980.

Mani RL, and Costin BS: Catheter angiography through aortofemoral grafts: prevention of catheter separation during withdrawal, AJR 128:328-329, 1977.

Maouad J, Herbert JL, Fernandez F, and Gay J: Percutaneous brachial approach using the femoral artery sheath for left heart catheterization and selective coronary angiography, Cathet Cardiovasc Diagn 11:539-546, 1985.

Mostert JW, Kenny GM, and Murphy GP: Safe placement of central venous catheter into internal jugular vein, Arch Surg 101:431, 1970.

O'Reilly MV: The technique of subclavian vein cannulation, Can Med Assoc J 108:63, 1973.

Pepine CJ, Von Gunten C, and Hill JA: Percutaneous bracial catheterization using a modified sheath and new catheter system, Cathet Cardiovasc Diagn 10:637-642, 1984.

Rao TLK, Wong AY, and Salem MR: A new approach to percutaneous catheterization of the internal jugular vein, Anesthesiology 46:362, 1977.

Rapoport S et al: Pseudoaneurysm: a complication of faulty technique in femoral arterial puncture, Radiology 154:529-530, 1985.

Russell JA et al: Prospective evaluation of radial and femoral artery catheterization sites in critically ill adults, Crit Care Med 11:936-939, 1983.

Schatzki SC: Catheter angiography through prosthetic vascular grafts using a Teflon sheath, Radiology 148:565, 1983.

Schwartz AJ, Jobes DR, and Gruchow E: Carotid artery puncture with internal jugular cannulation using the Seldinger technique: incidence, recognition, treatment, and prevention, Anesthesiology 51:S160, 1979.

Schwartz AJ, Jobes DR, and Levy WJ: Intrathoracic vascular catheterization via the external jugular vein, Anesthesiology 56:400, 1982.

Seneff MG: Central venous catheterization: a comprehensive review (II). J Intens Care Med 2:218-232, 1987.

Shenoy PN, Leaman DM, and Field JM: Safety of short-term percutaneous arterial cannulation, Anesth Analg 58:256-258, 1979.

Simon RR, and Brenner BE: Procedures and techniques in emergency medicine, Baltimore, 1984, Williams & Wilkins Co.

Skowronski GA, and Pearson IY: A technique for insertion of two intravascular catheters via a single puncture, Crit Care Med 10:404, 1982.

Smith DC: Catheterization of prosthetic vascular grafts: acceptable technique (editorial), AJR 143:1117-1118, 1984.

Soderstrom CA et al: Superiority of the femoral artery for monitoring: a prospective study, Am J Surg 144:309-312, 1982.

Swanson RS, Uhlig PN, Gross PL, and McCabe CJ: Emergency intravenous access through the femoral vein, Ann Emerg Med 13:244, 1983.

Sznajder JI et al: Central vein catheterization: failure and complication rates by three percutaneous approaches, Arch Intern Med 146:259-261, 1986.

Thomas F et al: The risk of infection related to radial vs. femoral sites for arterial catheterization, Crit Care Med 11:807-81, 1983.

Valeix B, et al: Selective coronary arteriography by percutaneous transaxillary approach, Cathet Cardiovasc Diagn 10:403-409, 1984.

Weinshelbaum A, and Carson SN: Separation of angiographic catheter during arteriography through vascular graft, AJR 134:583-584, 1980.

Weiss BM, and Gattiker RI: Complications during and following radial artery cannulation: a prospective study, Intens Care Med 12:424-428, 1986.

Zajko AB et al: Percutaneous puncture of venous bypass grafts for transluminal angioplasty, AJR 137:799-801, 1981.

Chapter 5

Central Venous and Pulmonary Artery Pressure Monitoring

Central venous catheters have been widely used in the coronary care unit for over 20 years for administration of fluids, blood sampling for routine laboratory analysis, venous oxygen saturation determination, and central venous pressure (CVP) measurement. It was previously thought the CVP reflected changes in left ventricular (LV) function that would allow accurate assessment of the patient's hemodynamic status, response to therapy, or both. It has now been documented through further clinical experience that severe left-sided hemodynamic abnormalities may occur rapidly after myocardial infarction without significant changes in superior vena cava (SVC) pressures. However, CVP measurement does provide useful information about right ventricular function and cardiovascular status, and is frequently used to monitor the volemic state of patients who do not require pulmonary arterial (PA) pressure monitoring.

As a more immediate, accurate reflection of LV function, the PA pressure has become an important parameter for optimal monitoring of LV function. The development of a flow-directed, balloon-tipped catheter for PA pressure and mixed venous oxygen saturation monitoring has significantly contributed to the expansion of vascular monitoring in the coronary care and intensive care units.

CENTRAL VENOUS PRESSURE MONITORING
Physiologic Review

The CVP is a reflection of the right atrial (RA) pressure and thus provides useful information about both the preload of the right side of the heart and the adequacy of venous return.

True preload of the right ventricle is really the end-diastolic myocardial fiber length. However, the clinical measurement of preload of the right side of the heart is the pressure during filling of the right ventricle (end-diastolic pressure). Except in tricuspid stenosis, the pressure in the RA *is* the preload or filling pressure of the

RV. Thus RAP or CVP is clinically valuable in assessing preload of the right side of the heart.

Venous return, or the amount of blood returning to the heart, is determined by the difference between mean systemic pressure and the RA pressure. The greater the difference between the two pressures, the greater the volume of blood returning to the heart. Decreases in RAP or CVP at a constant mean arterial pressure (MAP) result in increased venous return until the CVP falls below zero, at which point the veins leading into the thorax tend to collapse. Likewise, increases in RAP or CVP above 7 mm Hg at a constant MAP result in reduced venous return and hence cardiac output.

The CVP reflects RA pressure, which primarily reflects changes in RV diastolic pressure. Although the CVP will eventually reflect left-sided heart failure or other abnormalities, the timing and sequence of the pressure changes in the superior vena cava are less predictable. There is less value in monitoring the CVP in a patient with rapidly changing cardiovascular status, because the CVP may be the last parameter to show a change.

Clinical Application

The CVP is most valuable in monitoring blood volume, adequacy of central venous return, and RV function. It is particularly helpful after surgery, during active bleeding, or in assessing dehydration, when it may be difficult to determine the true blood volume of the patient. The CVP actually reflects the pressure in the great veins as blood returns to the heart (Fig. 5-1). If blood return decreases, the pressure may decrease also. In general, a low pressure (less than 5 cm H$_2$O) would indicate that additional fluid or blood can be given safely without overloading the

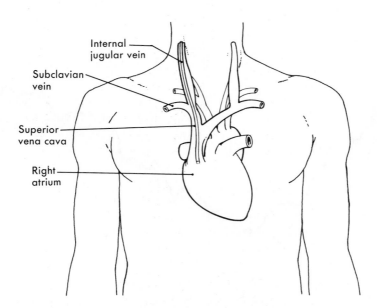

Fig. 5-1. CVP catheter properly positioned in the SVC just above the RA junction. The catheter has been inserted through the right internal jugular vein.

Table 5-1. Patient data for Case 2

	5 AM	6 AM	8 AM	Noon	6 PM
CVP (cm H$_2$O)	?	0	2	8	6
Blood pressure	90/60	85/60	100/65	115/75	112/83
Urinary output (ml/hr)	30	22	54	125	115
Blood administration (units)	3	—	2	3	—

intravascular space of the heart. This additional volume of blood or fluid causes increases in the central venous return and the CVP. The increase in these filling pressure contributes to the increase in cardiac output and systemic pressures, according to Starling's Law.

The CVP is also useful in differentiating right ventricular failure from left ventricular failure. With failure of the RV, usually following RV infarction, the CVP is high because of decreased compliance of the RV, requiring higher filling pressures. The pulmonary artery wedge (PAW) pressure, however, is characteristically lower because of reduced volume filling the left side of the heart. The reverse hemodynamic picture frequently occurs with LV failure, where the PAW pressure is elevated and the CVP may be normal or low.

When PA pressure monitoring is not possible, the CVP may be used to monitor the patient with chronic right and left heart failure. In these patients the CVP *tends* to follow the PAW pressure, rising with increased LV failure and falling with certain treatments, such as diuresis.

Case 1

A 54-year-old man was admitted to the coronary care unit with an anteroseptal myocardial infarction. On hospital day 2, he had recurrence of chest pain, suggesting an extension of the infarction. Shortly thereafter, he complained of increasing shortness of breath, but the CVP remained stable at 8 cm H$_2$O. A floating balloon-tipped catheter was advanced to the pulmonary artery, showing a PA systolic pressure of 35, a PA diastolic pressure of 21, and a mean PAW pressure of 23 mm Hg.

In the absence of severe pulmonary emphysema, pulmonary vascular disease, or mitral valve disease, we can conclude that the patient was indeed in LV failure, with an elevated LVEDP leading to rises in the LA, PAW, and PA pressures, as measured. The elevated PAW pressure caused additional fluid to shift into the patient's pulmonary alveolar space, accounting for his complaint of shortness of breath.

Case 2

A 22-year-old man was brought to the emergency room with a pneumothorax and hemothorax following an automobile accident. Bleeding from the chest tube continued. After he had received 3 units of whole blood, his hematocrit reading was 38% despite a continuing decrease in arterial blood pressure and a decreasing urinary output. Was he developing hemorrhagic shock caused by blood volume depletion?

A CVP catheter was advanced to the superior vena cava through the right antecubital basilic vein. A fluid-filled manometer showed a pressure of 0 cm H$_2$O when the manometer zero level was held at midchest level. He was given 5 additional units of whole blood before the CVP showed a rise to 8 cm H$_2$O. Thus the additional fluid was given safely and resulted in a return of his cardiac output and systemic pressures to normal. Table 5-1 shows data charted on this patient.

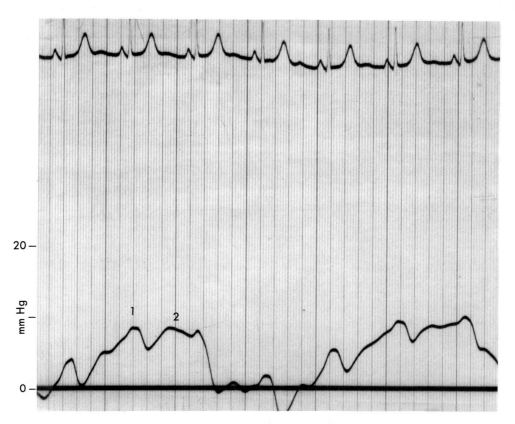

Fig. 5-2. CVP waveform showing *a* (*1*), and *v* (*2*) waves and normal respiratory variation.

CVP MEASUREMENT

The CVP Waveform

Fig. 5-2 depicts a normal central venous waveform obtained using a calibrated pressure transducer. Its morphology is identical to an RA waveform consisting of three positive waves, an *a* wave, a *c* wave, and a *v* wave. The *a* wave is followed by a fall in pressure termed the *x* descent; the *v* wave is followed by the *y* descent. (See p. 98 for a discussion of the components of the CVP or RA waveform.) The normal CVP ranges from 0 to 7 mm Hg (0 to 10 cm H_2O) with a normal average reported to be approximately 3 mm Hg (4 cm H_2O).

Pressure in the central veins is affected by changes in intrathoracic pressure. For this reason, the CVP falls during spontaneous inhalation and rises during spontaneous exhalation. To minimize the effects of these respiratory changes, the CVP should be measured at end-expiration whether the pressure is measured via a H_2O manometer or a transducer. This is true also if the patient is breathing spontaneously or with mechanical ventilation.

Methods of Measuring CVP

The CVP can be measured with a water manometer (the original technique), or with a calibrated transducer. The increased use of disposable pressure transducers

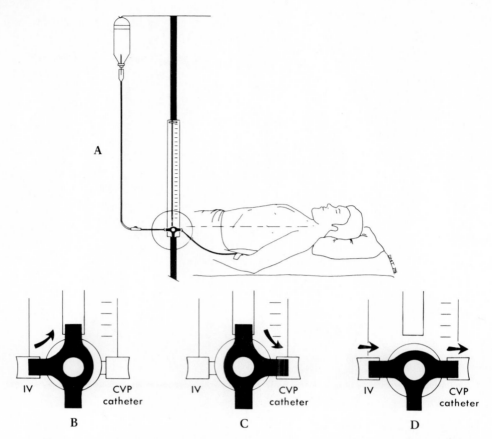

Fig. 5-3. Procedure for measuring CVP with manometer. **A,** Manometer and IV tubing in place. **B,** Turn the stopcock so that the manometer fills with fluid above the level of the expected pressure. **C,** Turn the stopcock so that the IV is off and the manometer flows to the patient. Obtain a reading after the fluid level stabilizes. **D,** Turn the stopcock to resume the IV flow to the patient.

in the critical care arena has made the latter technique more commonly used today. When the CVP is measured with a water manometer, its measurement is in centimeters of water (cm H_2O). When measured with the use of a pressure transducer, its measurement is in millimeters of mercury (mm Hg). These differences in units of measurement may cause some confusion, which can be avoided if the manometrically measured CVP is converted to mm Hg.

An easy way to make the conversion is to remember that mercury is 13.6 times heavier than water. Therefore 1 mm Hg equals 13.6 mm H_2O which equals 1.36 cm H_2O. The saline manometer pressures are more commonly reported in centimeters of water. Centimeters of water can be converted to millimeters of mercury by dividing the centimeters of water by 1.36:

$$5 \text{ cm } H_2O = \frac{5 \text{cm } H_2O}{1.36} = 3.7 \text{ mm Hg}$$

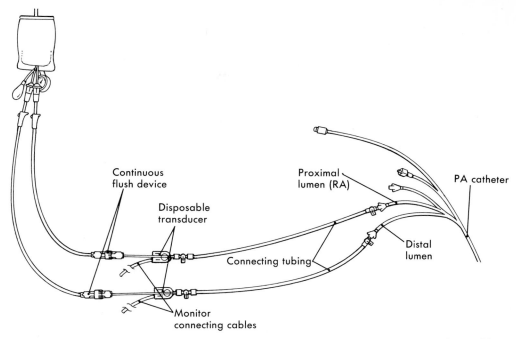

Fig. 5-4. An appropriate setup for monitoring of PA and RA pressures using disposable transducers and one IV solution bag.

Perhaps an easier formula for conversion is 1 cm H_2O equals 0.74 mm Hg. Using this formula, centimeters of water are converted to millimeters of mercury by multiplying by 0.74:

$$5 \text{ cm } H_2O = 5 \text{ cm } H_2O \times 0.74 \text{ mm Hg} = 3.7 \text{ mm Hg}$$

Use of a water manometer. Use of a plastic disposable or glass manometer with a three-way stopcock is an easy method for measuring CVP and involves the following steps:

1. Place the patient flat before setting the zero level of the manometer and for all subsequent CVP measurements. Place the zero level of the manometer at mid-chest level, which is the approximate level of the right atrium. The manometer may be secured to an IV pole. If the patient cannot tolerate lying flat, a mark can be made on the skin at midchest level; the zero level of the manometer is then always held at this mark for serial CVP measurements.
2. Connect the IV tubing to one side of the three-way stopcock; connect the manometer to the upper part; and connect the CVP catheter to the other side, using extension tubing if necessary. Different brands of the disposable or metal stopcocks have varying methods of showing the direction of flow. CVP measurement setups that are already properly connected are available commercially. See the package directions for specific instructions.
3. Check the catheter for patency by allowing the IV fluid to drip rapidly before taking the CVP measurement.

4. To obtain a CVP reading, turn the stopcock so that the manometer fills with fluid above the level of the expected pressure (Fig. 5-3). Do *not* allow the manometer to overflow; overflowing may result in contamination.

5. Turn the stopcock so that the IV tubing is closed and the fluid in the manometer flows into the patient (see Fig. 5-3). The fluid column will then equalize to the hydrostatic pressure level at the tip of the catheter.

6. The fluid level in the manometer should fall rapidly and fluctuate with respiration. It will drop with inspiration as the intrathoracic pressure decreases and will rise with expiration. A reading may be taken when the fluid level stops falling and at end expiration.

7. Turn the stopcock to resume the IV flow (see Fig. 5-3) after the measurement is obtained.

8. Record the pressure on the appropriate vital sign sheet.

Use of a transducer. With the widespread use of hemodynamic monitoring via the PA catheter, use of a transducer to measure the CVP or RAP has become the more common practice today. In addition to providing a more accurate measurement of the mean CVP or RAP, it permits observation and analysis of the actual waveform (see Fig. 5-2). Fluid-filled tubing and the transducer are attached to the proximal port of the PA catheter (Fig. 5-4) following the steps outlined on pp. 132-133. Transduced pressures can also be obtained from single-lumen CVP catheters in the same manner.

As with PA and PAW pressure monitoring, the reference port of the transducer system should be positioned to approximate the RA level.

Risks and Complications

The risks and complications associated with CVP catheterization are basically those of PA catheterization (see the discussion on p. 134). Of noteworthy difference, however, is the increased risk of cardiac perforation and tamponade with the use of CVP catheters. Most commonly, perforation by the catheter tip occurs in the RA, although perforations of the RV and SVC have also been reported. Perforation and tamponade may occur acutely after catheter insertion or from hours to days after insertion. When late tamponade occurs it is usually because of endocardial damage and gradual erosion from catheter adherence. Such perforations are more likely to occur when CVP catheters are inserted through an arm vein, where subsequent movement of the extremity can cause the catheter to advance against the vessel or myocardial wall. The clinical signs of tamponade may occur slowly or dramatically and can often be misleading because of the similarity to other, more common, problems. However, since tamponade is associated with such high mortality, it is essential for the critical care nurse to be aware of its likelihood and diligently observe for any evidence of the development of tamponade. Cardic tamponade should be suspected in any patient with a CVP catheter who develops unexplained hypotension. If the diagnosis of tamponade is confirmed, infusion through the CVP catheter should be immediately discontinued and aspiration of fluid attempted through the catheter to try to remove fluid from the pericardial sac. The CVP catheter should then be removed and pericardiocentesis performed.

Precautions to minimize cardiac perforation with CVP catheters include the following:

1. Place the CVP catheter tip just above (approximately 2 cm) the SVC/RA junction at the time of insertion (see Fig. 5-1).
2. Verify the position of the CVP catheter tip with a chest x-ray.
3. Suture the catheter securely to the skin.
4. Avoid CVP catheter insertion through the arm veins.
5. Use soft catheters without beveled edges.
6. Frequently (at least once per shift) check the ability to aspirate blood back from the catheter.

Table 5-2 identifies some other causes of problems commonly encountered with CVP catheters as well as appropriate preventions and interventions.

Table 5-2. Problems encountered with CVP catheters

Problem	Cause	Prevention	Treatment
Pain and inflammation above insertion site	Mechanical irritation of catheter leading to sterile thrombophlebitis	Prepare skin properly. Use sterile technique during insertion and dressing change.	Remove catheter (mandatory if infection is at insertion site).
	Bacterial infection ascending along catheter at insertion site	Insert catheter smoothly. Change dressing, stopcocks, and connecting tubing daily. Rotate insertion site every 48 to 72 hr.	Apply warm compresses. Give pain medication as necessary.
Poor infusion of IV fluid	Partial clotting at catheter tip	Use continuous drip. May help to use 1 unit heparin/1 ml IV fluid. Occasionally hand flush or use rapid drip. Flush with large volume after blood withdrawal.	Attach syringe to catheter and attempt to aspirate clot. Irrigate gently; *do not* forcibly flush catheter without consulting physician; remove catheter and reinsert at another site if it cannot be irrigated easily.
	External kinking of catheter	Coil and tape catheter carefully after insertion.	Remove dressing and check for possible kinking of catheter. Straighten catheter, retape, and apply new sterile dressing.
	Catheter tip against myocardium	Position catheter just above RA. Check chest x-ray after insertion.	Check for free backflow of blood from catheter. Reposition catheter.
Catheter tip missing when catheter is removed	Catheter cut or sheared	Never pull back catheter and readvance through needle.	Locate by palpation if in arm or by chest x-ray film; may require venous cutdown if proximal end is in arm or cardiac catheterization if proximal end is in thorax.

PA AND PAW PRESSURE MONITORING
Physiologic Review

The development of the flow-directed, balloon-tipped catheter presented the opportunity to indirectly acquire important diagnostic and therapeutic information regarding LV function. As the major pumping chamber of the heart, the left ventricle's performance correlates closely with overall cardiac function and indicates the severity of cardiac dysfunction. The LV end-distolic volume or preload (LVEDP) is one of the primary determinants of LV performance, since it affects the myocardial fiber stretch during diastole when the LV passively fills. The pressure developed in the LV during this period is exponentially related to the volume (Fig. 5-5). For this reason, an elevated LVEDP usually signifies an increase in volume, whereas a low LVEDP signifies a decrease in volume. However, the diastolic pressure-volume relationship of the LV can be altered by changes in ventricular compliance and LV geometry and by certain therapeutic interventions. Changes in ventricular compliance occur when the heart is prevented from expanding normally during ventricular filling. This can be because of pericardial restriction or disease, PEEP, or myocardial disease, especially associated with ischemia.

Fig. 5-5 illustrates the altered pressure-volume curve seen in a patient with decreased ventricular compliance resulting from myocardial infarction. A higher filling pressure is required for the same amount of volume filling the ventricle. For this reason, a patient with a stiff, diseased left ventricle requires a higher filling pressure (in the range of 15 to 20 mm Hg) to maintain adequate stroke volume.

In the patient with normal lungs and a normal mitral valve, the PA end-diastolic pressure closely reflects the LVEDP as an index of LV function or dysfunction. At the end of diastole, just before the next systole, the mitral valve is still open and the left ventricle is filled with blood. At this point there is an equilibration of pressures between the left ventricle and the left atrium (in the absence of mitral valve disease). Since there are no valves in the pulmonary venous system, the pressure equilibrates between the pulmonary veins, pulmonary capillaries, and the pulmonary artery at end-diastole. Therefore, at this point, the PA end-diastolic pressure is equal to the LVEDP. Fig. 5-6 illustrates this correlation.

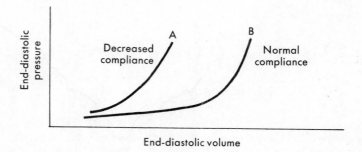

Fig. 5-5. Relationship between ventricular end-diastolic volume and end-diastolic pressure. With normal ventricular compliance, relatively large increases in end-diastolic volume are accompanied, up to a point, by relatively small increases in end-diastolic pressure *(curve B)*. In the noncompliant ventricle, small increases in end-diastolic volume are associated with marked increases in end-diastolic pressure. *Curve A* illustrates the effects of decreased compliance.

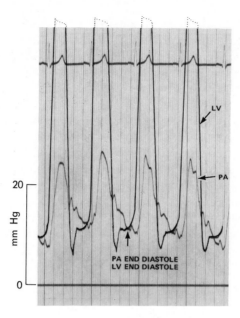

Fig. 5-6. Simultaneous LV and PA pressure tracing. Note the close correlation between LV and PA end-diastole. PA systolic pressure = 29 mm Hg; diastolic pressure = 12 mm Hg. LV systolic pressure is off scale; diastolic pressure = 12 mm Hg. The dark vertical time lines are 1 sec apart; the light lines mark every 0.2 sec.

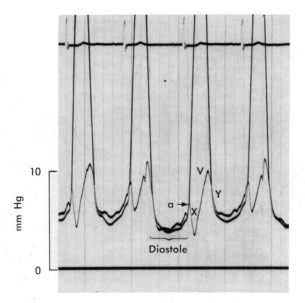

Fig. 5-7. Simultaneous recording of LV and PAW pressures. Note the normal *a* and *v* waves with *x* and *y* descents. During diastole, the PAW pressure is barely 1 mm higher than the LV pressure when the mitral valve is open and blood is flowing from the left atrium to the left ventricle.

The PAW pressure is obtained by inflating the balloon of the catheter to occlude a branch of the pulmonary artery. This occlusion causes a cessation of forward blood flow in that branch of the pulmonary artery so that the catheter lumen at the tip "sees" only the pressure ahead in the more distal pulmonary capillary and pulmonary venous system. This pressure is a direct retrograde reflection of the LA pressure. Like the pulmonary diastolic pressure, the PAW pressure provides information about pressure events during LV diastole, that is, when the mitral valve is open (Fig. 5-7). Since the PAW pressure is the pressure in the pulmonary capillary, it is also a critical determinant affecting the movement of fluid from the vascular bed to the interstitial and alveolar spaces of the lung. Mild pulmonary congestion is usually evident when the PAW pressure is elevated to 18 to 20 mm Hg. Acute pulmonary edema can occur with PAW pressure >30 mm Hg. The PA diastolic and PAW pressures are essentially equal (within a few mm Hg) when the pulmonary vascular resistance (PVR) is normal. Situations that increase PVR, such as pulmonary embolism, hypoxia, or chronic lung disease, also increase the PA pressure, whereas the PAW pressure may remain normal. In these situations the PA pressure reflects the high PVR and not the LVEDP. To properly evaluate the LVEDP in these instances, the PAW pressure must be monitored. Generally, however, the PA diastolic pressure is most suitable and safer to monitor.

RIGHT-SIDED HEART PRESSURE WAVEFORMS

The morphology and characteristics of the waveforms produced by the chambers and vessels of the right side of the heart are related to the underlying physiologic and electrophysiologic cardiac events. Pressure waveform changes (increases as well as decreases) are reflections of physiologic changes in myocardial fiber tension (myocardial fibers are either contracting or relaxing) or changes in blood volume (blood is either entering or exiting a chamber). Since cardiac electrical stimulation precedes mechanical activity, the ECG defines the timing of the corresponding mechanical response. A sound understanding of normal hemodynamic waveforms is essential in differentiation of abnormal waveforms from a variety of causes.

RA Pressure
Physiology and morphology

The pressure changes produced by the right atrium are small and usually consist of three distinct positive waves—*a, c,* and *v*—followed by negative waves—*x, x¹,* and *y* descents (Fig. 5-8). The *a* wave is a small pressure rise that is produced by the action of atrial systole. The decline in pressure that immediately follows the *a* wave is termed the *x* descent and reflects atrial relaxation (immediately following systole). The *c* wave may appear as a distinct wave, as a notch on the *a* wave, or may be absent altogether. It reflects a slight increase in pressure in the right atrium produced by closure of the tricuspid valve leaflets. The negative wave immediately following the *c* wave is termed the *x¹* descent. It is produced by a downward pulling of the septum during ventricular systole. (If the *c* wave appears only as notch on the *a* wave, the single descent following the *ac* wave is termed the *x* descent.)

The *v* wave is an increase in atrial pressure produced by right atrial filling dur-

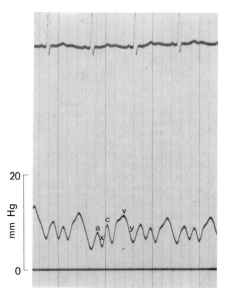

Fig. 5-8. RA pressure waveform showing *a*, *c*, and *v* waves with *x* and *y* descents. Note that the recorded waveforms are delayed from the corresponding electrical event in the P-QRS-T. This delay occurs because of the delay in recording pressure events through a long catheter.

ing concomitant right ventricular systole, which causes the leaflets of the closed tricuspid valve to actually bulge back into the right atrium. The *y* descent immediately follows the *v* wave and is produced by the opening of the tricuspid valve and emptying of the right atrium into the right ventricle.

Since the pressure rises produced during both the atrial systolic (*a* wave) and diastolic (*v* wave) events are nearly the same (usually within 3 to 4 mm Hg of each other), we generally take an average or a mean of the pressure rises. The normal resting mean right atrial pressure is 2 to 6 mm Hg.

ECG correlation

The *a* wave, which represents mechanical atrial systole, immediately succeeds electrical atrial depolarization, that is, after the P wave of the ECG. Because of the time required for the mechanical event to reach the sensing device (the transducer) and depending on the length of tubing used, there is a varying degree of delay between the recorded electrical event and the mechanical event. At any rate, the *a* wave of the atrial pressure generally is seen 80 to 100 msec after the P wave or at some time within the PR interval of the ECG.

The *c* wave, reflecting closure of the tricuspid valve, corresponds to the RST junction of the ECG. Its timing following the *a* wave approximates the PR interval.

The *v* wave, occuring during ventricular systole, would naturally succeed electrical ventricular depolarization and can be looked for any time in the TP interval.

Atrial fibrillation is characterized by the absence of uniform atrial depolarization and consequently results in absent P waves in the ECG and absent *a* waves in the right atrial pressure waveform (Fig. 5-9). For every QRS complex, there will be

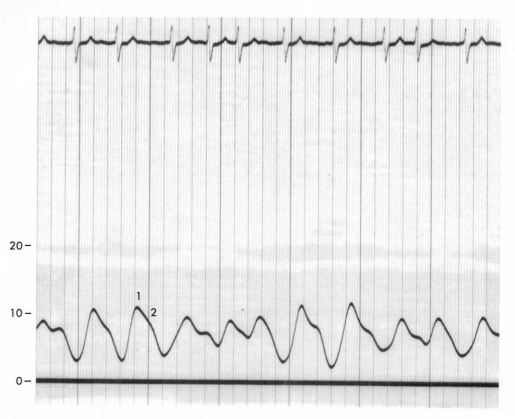

Fig. 5-9. Normal RA waveform with absent *a* waves in a patient with atrial fibrillation. (1 = *v* wave; 2 = *y* descent.) Note the effect of varying R-R intervals on the extent of the *y* descent reflecting changes in RV filling (and RA emptying).

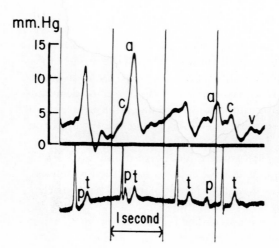

Fig. 5-10. RA pressure waveform in a patient with A-V dissociation showing the presence of cannon *a* waves as the atria contracts against a closed tricuspid valve. Note the change in the RA waveform with normal *a* and *v* waves when the patient converts to normal sinus rhythmn.

(From Kory, RC, Tsagaris, TJ, and Bustamente, RA: A primer of cardiac catheterization, Springfield, Ill, 1965, Charles C Thomas, Publisher.

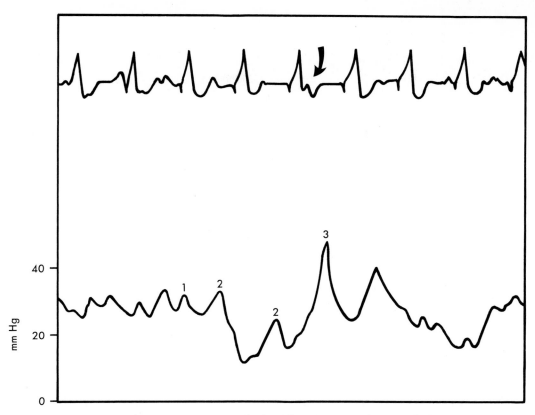

Fig. 5-11. RA waveform in a patient with A-V dissociation and a paced rhythm. *1* = *a* wave; *2* = *v* wave; *3* = cannon *a* wave following the retrograde P wave (*arrow*) as the atria contract against a closed tricuspid valve.

one distinct pressure rise, the *v* wave. Frequently, however, it is possible to see small flutter or fibrillatory waves throughout the pressure tracing.

In *junctional rhythm* or during certain beats of *AV dissocation* where the atria contract against a closed tricuspid valve, giant *a* or cannon *a* waves are seen in the right atrial pressure tracing (Fig. 5-10). Cannon *a* waves can also be seen following a premature ventricular contraction (PVC). Close scrutiny of the atrial waveform is often very helpful in determining the atrial activity associated with paroxysmal supraventricular tachycardia (PSVT) in which retrograde P waves may be disguised within the QRS complex. Reviewing the atrial waveform at a faster paper speed (50 mm/sec) facilitates correlation of the electrical and mechanical events of the heart.

Patients with a ventricular pacemaker may have absent *a* waves, occasional, random *a* waves, or even cannon *a* waves at times, depending on the underlying rhythm (Fig. 5-11). This is the result of absent or dissociated atrial activity that does not relate to the QRS.

Abnormal findings

Elevated RA pressures occur in the following cases:
1. Right ventricular failure

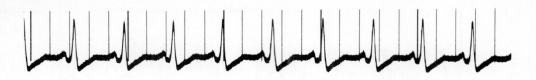

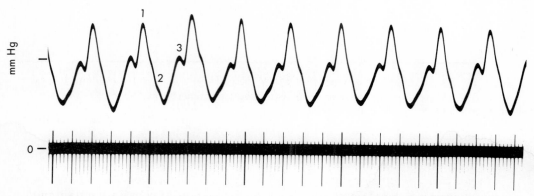

Fig. 5-12. Elevated RA pressure with exaggerated *a* wave (*1*) in a patient with RV failure and increased resistance to ventricular filling. (*2* = *x* descent; *3* = *v* wave.)

2. Tricuspid stenosis and regurgitation
3. Cardiac tamponade
4. Constrictive pericarditis
5. Pulmonary hypertension (primary or secondary)
6. Chronic left ventricular failure
7. Volume overload

The *a* wave of the RA pressure tracing is exaggerated and elevated in any condition that increases the resistance to right ventricular filling. These include tricuspid stenosis, RV failure, pulmonary hypertension, and pulmonic stenosis (Fig. 5-12).

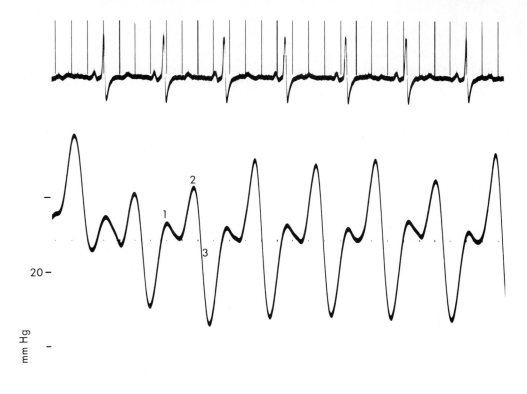

Fig. 5-13. Elevated RA pressure with exaggerated *v* wave (2) and rapid *y* descent (3) in a patient with tricuspid regurgitation as a result of acute RV failure. The *a* wave (1) of approximately 26 mm Hg reflects an elevated RVedp and RV failure.

The *v* wave of the RA pressure tracing is exaggerated and elevated in tricuspid regurgitation because of a reflux of blood into the right atrium during ventricular systole through the insufficiently closed tricuspid valve (Fig. 5-13). Clinically, tricuspid regurgitation most commonly occurs secondary to acute RV failure and dilatation. Flotation of the PA catheter into the RV and out to the PA is often very difficult in such situations.

In cardiac tamponade both the *a* and *v* waves are equally elevated and reflect the elevated diastolic filling pressures in all chambers of the heart. The contour of the RA pressure tracing is distinct, however, showing a predominant *x* descent with a very short or absent *y* descent *(Xy)* (Fig. 5-14). The mean value of the RA pressure is elevated and approximates the PAW mean value as well as the PA end-diastolic value (Fig. 5-15). Generally, the normal respiratory response is observed, with a decline in RA pressure during spontaneous inhalation and an elevation during exhalation.

In constrictive pericardial disease the *a* and *v* waves of the RA pressure tracing

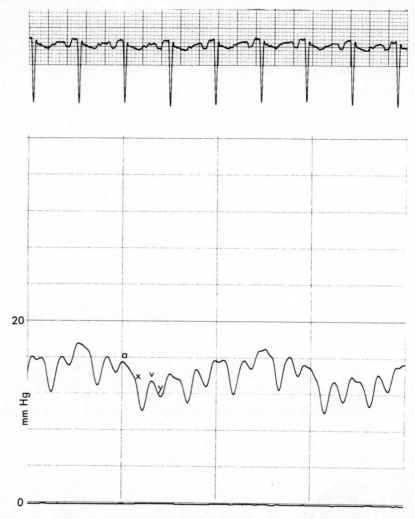

Fig. 5-14. Elevated RA pressure with characteristic waveform appearance associated with cardiac tamponade, that is, a normal x descent with a very brief y descent (Xy). Both a and v waves are equally elevated with a mean pressure of approximately 15 mm Hg.

are also elevated, but the contour of the waveform differs from cardic tamponade, showing either a predominant y descent or equally dominant x and y descents (Fig. 5-16). Additionally, Kussmaul's sign (a rise rather than a fall in right atrial pressure during inspiration) can be seen in constrictive disease but rarely, if ever, in cardiac tamponade. Kussmaul's signs and elevation of the RA waveform with an xY or xy pattern can also be seen in patients with acute right ventricular infarction in which an acutely dilated RV is restricted by the noncompliant pericardium. As in tamponade, the value of the elevated RAP in patients with constrictive pericarditis or RV infarction usually equals the PAEDP and PAW pressure. Very low RA pressures occur with hypovolemia from any cause (Fig. 5-17).

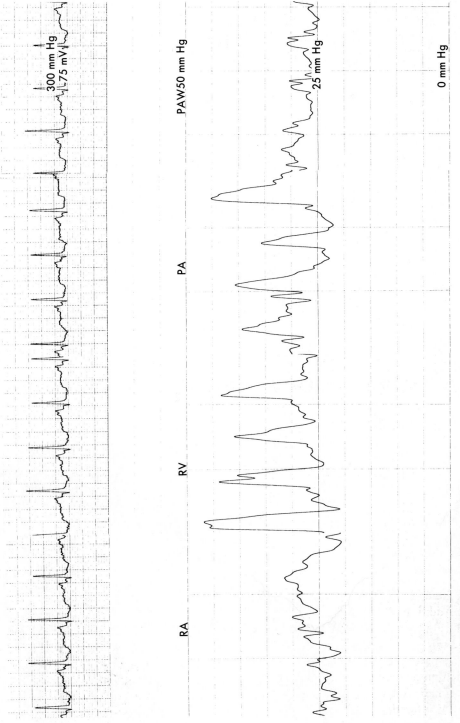

Fig. 5-15. Near equalization of RA mean, RV diastolic, PA diastolic, and PAW mean pressures in a patient with cardiac tamponade. The slightly lower RA mean value may be a result of hypovolemia.

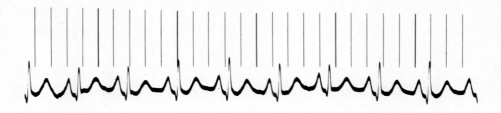

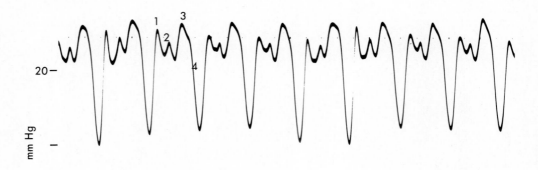

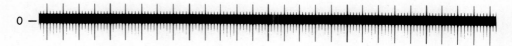

Fig. 5-16. Elevated RA pressure with characteristic waveform appearance associated with constrictive pericarditis, that is, a normal or brief *x* descent with an exaggerated *y* descent. The exaggerated *y* descent is a result of rapid ventricular filling (atrial emptying) during early diastole followed by an abrupt rise in pressure as the size of the heart is increased and compressed by the inelastic, constricted pericardium. The *a* and *v* waves are both equally elevated with a mean RA pressure of approximately 19 mm Hg. (1 = *a* wave; 2 = *c* wave; 3 = *v* wave; 4 = *y* descent.)

RV Pressure

Physiology and morphology

The pressure changes in the right ventricle reflect the dynamic, pumping action of that chamber. In general, the phases are systole and diastole; however, these are broken down further into seven specific events that constitute ventricular dynamics (Fig. 5-18).

Systolic events	Diastolic events
1. Isovolumetric contraction	4. Isovolumetric relaxation
2. Rapid ejection	5. Early diastole
3. Reduced ejection	6. Atrial systole (kick)
	7. End-diastole

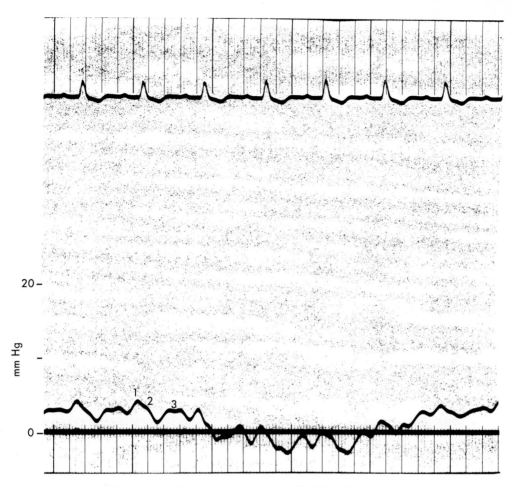

Fig. 5-17. A low RA pressure of approximately 3 mm Hg. Note the negative pressure during spontaneous inspiration. (1 = *a* wave; 2 = *x* descent; 3 = *v* wave.)

Isovolumetric contraction refers to the increase in tension or pressure as a result of ventricular muscle contraction without any change in ventricular volume. ("Iso" means equal; "volumetric" refers to volume.) This is because both the tricuspid and pulmonic valves are closed during this time. The continued rise in ventricular pressure, however, forces the pulmonic valve open, and *rapid ejection* of blood into the pulmonary artery occurs. *Reduced ejection* is characterized by a drop in ventricular pressure, even though some blood is still being pumped into the PA.

Diastole occurs when the ventricular pressure has dropped lower than the PA pressure, causing the pulmonic valve to close. This sharp decline in pressure results from *isovolumetric relaxation*. The ventricular muscle fibers are relaxing and losing tension while both pulmonic and tricuspid valves are closed, obviating any changes in ventricular volume. When the ventricular diastolic pressure falls below the RA pressure, the tricuspid valve opens, resulting in passive filling of the right

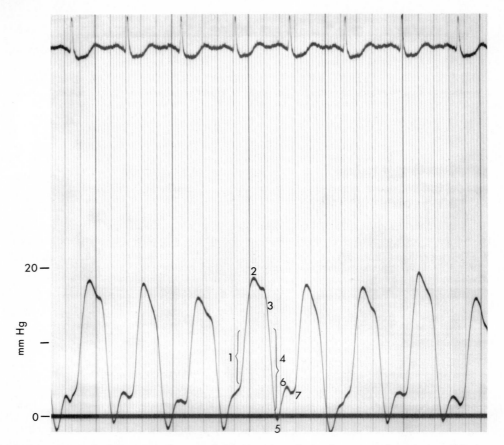

Fig. 5-18. Normal RV pressure waveform (1 = isovolumetric contraction; 2 = rapid ejection; 3 = reduced ejection; 4 = isovolumetric relaxation; 5 = early diastole; 6 = atrial systole; 7 = end-diastole).

ventricle. This period is termed *early diastole* or the rapid filling phase. This is soon followed by atrial systole, which forces an additional volume (anywhere from 10% to 15%) of blood into the ventricle. It is evidenced by an increase in pressure, termed the *atrial kick* or simply the *a* wave.

The period immediately succeeding the *a* wave, just before the systolic pressure rise occurs, is termed *end-diastole*. The pressure during this period reflects end-diastolic volume. It is the ventricular end-diastolic volume that determines the extent of fiber shortening and the subsequent stroke volume according to the Starling law. The normal RV systolic pressure is only 20 to 30 mm Hg, about one sixth of the pressure generated by the LV. The RV end-diastolic pressure is normally <5 mm Hg.

ECG correlation

The systolic ejection phase of the RV waveform corresponds to ventricular depolarization, or more generally the QT interval of the ECG. The diastolic period occurs, generally, in the TQ period of the ECG.

Abnormal findings

Elevation of the right ventricular systolic pressure occurs with pulmonary hypertension (whatever the cause), VSD, or pulmonic stenosis. Normally the RV and PA systolic pressures are essentially equal. In pulmonic stenosis the RV systolic pressure is much greater than the PA systolic pressure because of the resistance to ejection met at the narrowed pulmonic valve.

The RV diastolic pressure is elevated in right ventricular failure, constrictive pericarditis, or cardiac tamponade. Left-sided heart failure of long standing may also be reflected back as an increase in RVEDP.

Right ventricular pressure is usually not directly monitored at the bedside. However, it is indirectly monitored through evaluation of the PA systolic pressure, which equals RV systolic pressure, and the RA mean pressure, which approximates the RV end-diastolic pressure (if tricuspid or pulmonic valvular disease is not present). Knowledge of the events producing the RV pressure waveform is useful, since the same physiologic events produce the left ventricular pressure. Accurate identification of RV pressure waveform is essential for safe, accurate hemodynamic monitoring. The presence of an RV pressure waveform on the oscilloscope (Fig. 5-19) requires withdrawal of the catheter to the RA or inflation of the balloon for flotation of the catheter out to the PA.

PA Pressure
Physiology and morphology

The pulmonary artery (PA) pressure is divided into two phases: systole and diastole. Systole begins with the opening of the pulmonic valve, resulting in rapid ejection of blood into the pulmonary artery. On the PA pressure tracing this is seen as a sharp rise in pressure, followed by a decline in pressure as the volume decreases (Fig. 5-20). When the RV pressure falls below the level of the PA pressure, the pulmonic valve snaps shut. This sudden closure of the valve leaflets produces a small notch on the downslope of the PA pressure and is termed the *dicrotic notch.* The systolic value referred to is the peak systolic pressure reached. Normal PA systolic pressure is 20 to 30 mm Hg (the same as the RV systolic pressure).

Diastole follows closure of the pulmonic valve. During this time, runoff to the pulmonary system occurs without any further blood flow from the right ventricle until the next systole. The PA diastolic value referred to is the end-diastolic pressure just before the next systole. This value corresponds closely to the LV end-diastolic pressure (LVEDP) in the absence of pulmonary disease or mitral valve disease. Normal PA end-diastolic pressure is 8 to 12 mm Hg.

ECG correlation

The systolic phase of the PA pressure should correspond closely to ventricular depolarization. However, catheter length and the amount of tubing used can delay this somewhat. Generally, it occurs in the QT interval of the ECG.

In atrial fibrillation the value of the PA pressure varies greatly (Fig. 5-21), depending on the RR intervals and length of time for ventricular filling. The shorter the RR interval, the shorter the ventricular filling time, the less stroke volume ejected, and the less pressure rise in the PA. The contour of the PA pressure tracing remains normal, however.

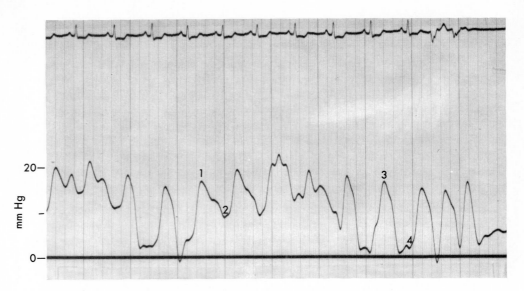

Fig. 5-19. Pressure tracing obtained from the distal lumen of the PA catheter with the catheter tip moving back and forth across the pulmonic valve producing PA and RV pressure waveforms. It is not in a safe location for monitoring purposes (note the occurrence of PVC's). It would also be impossible to obtain a PAW pressure with the catheter tip in this location. Frequently, inflation of the balloon will float the catheter tip distally to the PA, although it may not float distally enough to obtain a PAW pressure. (1 = PA systole; 2 = PA end-diastole; 3 = RV systole; 4 = RV end-diastole.)

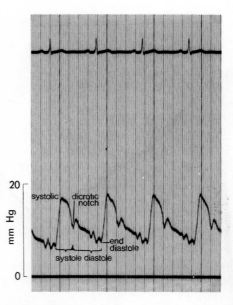

Fig. 5-20. PA pressure waveform showing phases of systole, dicrotic notch (pulmonic valve closure), and end diastole. Normally, PA end diastole closely represents LVEDP.

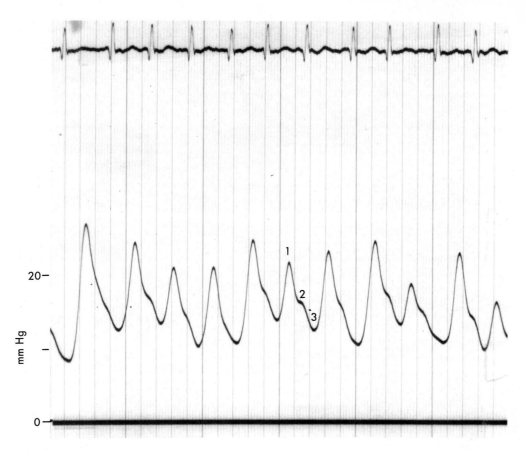

Fig. 5-21. PA pressure waveform in a patient with atrial fibrillation showing the varying systolic pressures associated with varying R-R intervals and length of time for diastolic filling. (1 = PA systole; 2 = dicrotic notch; 3 = PA end-diastole.)

Abnormal findings

Certain pathologic conditions alter the PA pressure. Elevation of PA pressure occurs with the following:

1. Increased pulmonary blood flow, as in a left-to-right shunt caused by an atrial or ventricular septal defect
2. Increased PVR, as in pulmonary diseases, pulmonary hypertension or pulmonary embolus(i)
3. Increased pulmonary venous pressure, as in mitral stenosis and LV failure

Because of the increased risks associated with PAW pressure measurements, such as pulmonary infarction or even pulmonary rupture, monitoring the PA diastolic (PAd) pressure is commonly used as a reflection of LVEDP. Normally, the PAd and PAW pressures are nearly the same (within 2 to 4 mm Hg) (Fig. 5-22). Situations where this is not true, thus obviating the use of PAd pressure monitoring as a reflection of LVEDP, are the following:

1. Pulmonary disease (chronic obstructive pulmonary disease, adult respiratory distress syndrome)

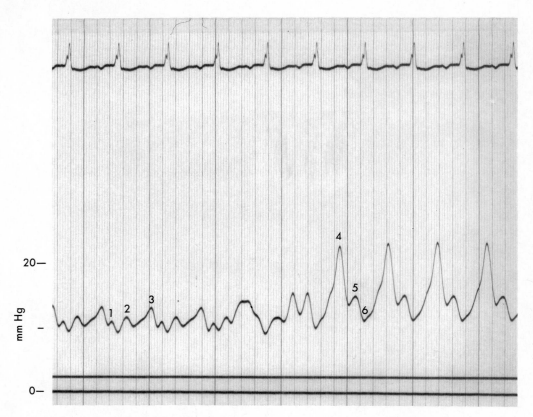

Fig. 5-22. Normal PAW to PA pressure waveforms associated with deflation of the balloon of the PA catheter. Note the mean PAW pressure of approximately 12 mm Hg is closely related to the PA end-diastolic pressure of 11 mm Hg. Once this correlation has been established, the PAEDP can be reliably used to monitor left heart filling pressures (LVEDP) and, thereby, avoid frequent balloon inflations. (1 = PAW *a* wave; 2 = PAW *c* wave; 3 = PAW *v* wave; 4 = PA systolic, 5 = PA dicrotic notch; 6 = PA end-diastolic pressure.)

2. Pulmonary embolus
3. Heart rates greater than 130 beats/min

Elevations of the PVR, from whatever cause, elevate the PA pressure. However, inflation of the balloon of the catheter stops the flow of blood in that branch of the PA. Thus the effects of increased resistance are no longer met, and the pressure obtained is a retrograde pressure from the LA. For this reason, PAW pressure usually equals LA pressure, even in situations such as pulmonary disease and pulmonary embolus (Fig. 5-23).

Tachycardias (>130 beats/min) abbreviate the duration of diastole and therefore falsely elevate the PAEDP and invalidate the usual relationship between the PAEDP and PAW or LVEDP (Fig. 5-24).

In addition to pathologic abnormalities, mechanical abnormalities frequently alter the PA pressure both in contour and value. "Fling" or "whip" in the PA pressure tracing (Fig. 5-25), consisting of exaggerated oscillations, can occur with excessive catheter coiling in either the RA or RV or when the catheter tip is located

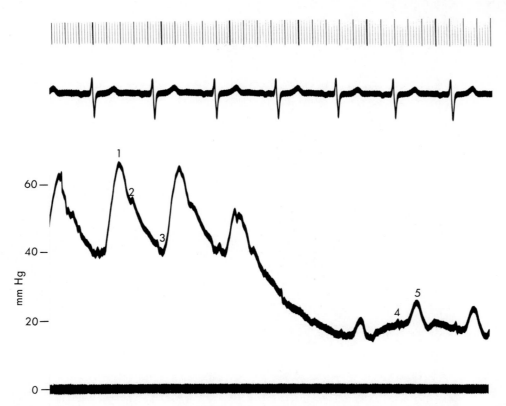

Fig. 5-23. Elevated PA pressure (65/40) with a normal to mildly elevated PAW pressure (mean = 19 mm Hg). The wide disparity between the PAEDP and PAW mean pressures is because of chronic pulmonary disease and does not reflect the left heart filling pressures. Monitoring of left heart filling pressures in such situations requires balloon inflation and measurement of the PAW pressure. (1 = PA sysole; 2 = dicrotic notch; 3 = PA end-diastole; 4 = PAW *a* wave; 5 = *v* wave.)

near the pulmonic valve, where blood flow is turbulent. Patients with pulmonary hypertension and dilated pulmonary arteries frequently exhibit fling in the PA pressure tracing. In these situations accurate measurement of the PA pressure is difficult, and manipulation and repositioning of the catheter are necessary.

Damping of the PA pressure, resulting from a variety of causes, changes both the contour and the value of the PA waveform in a characteristic manner (Fig. 5-26). The entire waveform loses any sharp definition and becomes rather rounded out in appearance. Frequently the upstroke of the systolic pressure is slow and the dicrotic notch is absent or poorly defined. The value of the PA pressure is decreased considerably and as such is an inaccurate pressure. Most often fibrin at the tip of the catheter is the culprit when pressures become damped. Careful aspiration followed by gentle flushing usually corrects this problem, but occasionally catheter replacement is necessary. Placement of the tip of the catheter against the wall of the vessel also produces damped pressures and requires repositioning of the catheter. The presence of an air bubble(s) anywhere within the system also dampens the pressure waveform. Kinks in either the catheter itself or the extension tubing produce a dampened, lowered pressure waveform.

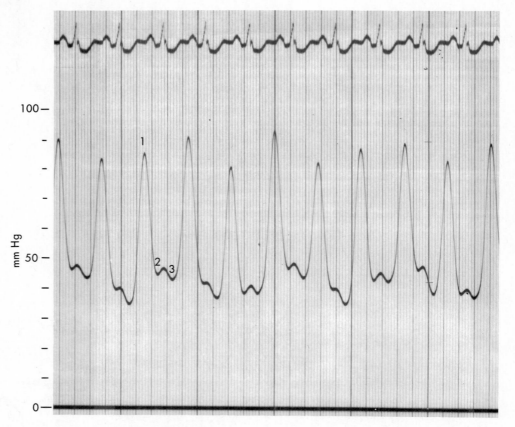

Fig. 5-24. Markedly elevated PA pressure in a patient with sinus tachycardia and pulmonary hypertension. Note the abbriviated diastolic phase as a result of the rapid heart rate. (1 = systole; 2 = dicrotic notch; 3 = end-diastole.)

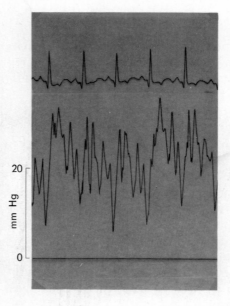

Fig. 5-25. PA pressure waveform demonstrating catheter fling caused by excessive catheter movement, making it impossible to accurately measure the pressure.

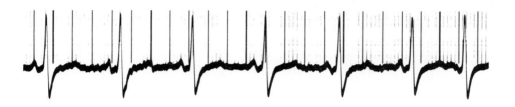

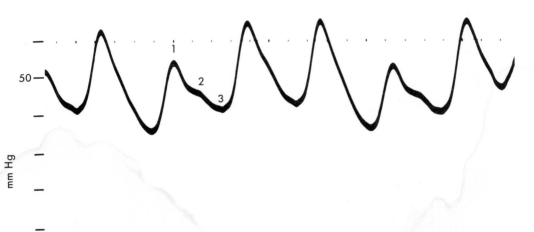

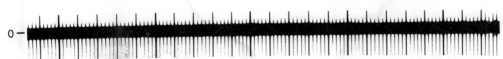

Fig. 5-26. Elevated PA pressure showing a damped waveform with poor definition and possible inaccurate measurement. (1 = PA systole; 2 = dicrotic notch; 3 = PA end-diastole.)

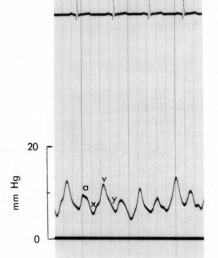

Fig. 5-27. Normal PAW pressure waveform showing *a* and *v* waves and *x* and *y* descents.

PAW Pressure
Physiology and morphology

When proper position in a small branch of the PA is achieved, inflation of the balloon of the PA catheter actually occludes flow in that segment of the pulmonary artery. The pressure obtained with balloon inflation is termed the PAW. This pressure reflects left atrial (LA) pressure and has similar contour and characteristics as the right atrial pressure (*a*, *c*, and *v* waves) since the pressure is produced by the same physiologic events (Fig. 5-27). The *a* wave of the PAW pressure is produced by LA systole and is followed by the *x* descent, reflecting left atrial relaxation following systole. The *c* wave that is produced by closure of the mitral valve frequently gets lost in retrograde transmission and often is not observed in the PAW pressure waveform although it can sometimes be seen. The *v* wave is produced by filling of the LA and bulging back of the mitral valve during ventricular systole. The decline succeeding the *v* wave is the *y* descent, which represents opening of the mitral valve with a decrease in LA pressure and volume during passive emptying into the LV.

Although the contour of the PAW pressure is the same as the RA pressure, the value of the PAW pressure is normally higher. As with the RA pressure, we generally record the mean of the PAW pressure, since the *a* and *v* waves are normally of approximately the same value. The normal resting PAW mean pressure is 4 to 12 mm Hg. If, however, either the *a* or the *v* wave is particularly dominant or elevated, it is not accurate to average the pressure rises. In those instances the value of both the *a* wave and the *v* wave should be noted.

ECG correlation

Timing of the electrical and mechanical events is the same as with the RA pressure; that is, the *a* wave follows the P wave of the ECG, and the *v* wave follows the

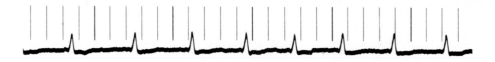

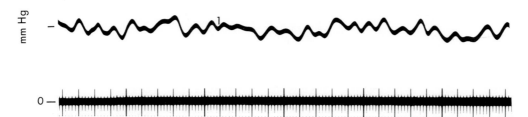

20—

mm Hg

0—

Fig. 5-28. Normal PAW pressure in a patient with atrial fibrillation and absent *a* waves. Numerous small waves in this pressure tracing are likely a result of the fibrillatory activity of the atrium. (1 = *v* wave.)

T wave of the ECG. However, a greater time delay between electrical and mechanical events is frequently noted with the PAW pressure as it is a retrograde measurement of LA pressure.

The effects of arrhythmias on the PAW pressure are the same as those discussed with the RA pressure. In atrial fibrillation there are no *a* waves in the PAW pressure waveform, and only a *v* wave follows each QRS complex (Fig. 5-28). Junctional rhythm or AV dissociation can produce giant or cannon *a* waves.

Abnormal findings

Elevated PAW pressures occur in the following conditions:
1. LV failure
2. Mitral stenosis or regurgitation
3. Cardiac tamponade
4. Constrictive pericarditis
5. Volume overload

The *a* wave of the PAW pressure is exaggerated and elevated in any condition that increases the resistance to LV filling (Fig. 5-29). Elevation of the PAW *a* wave

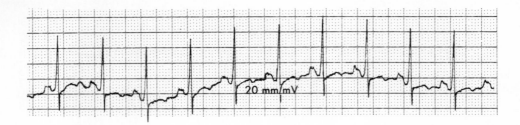

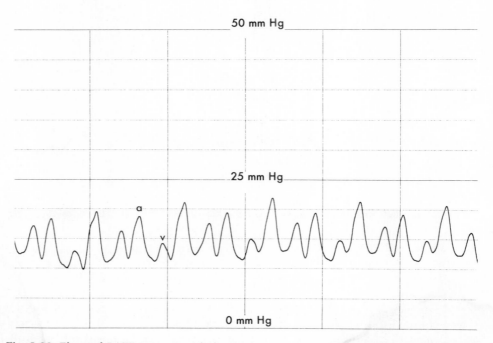

Fig. 5-29. Elevated PAW pressure with dominant *a* wave as a result of LV hypertrophy with decreased compliance during LV filling.

with LV failure reflects the increased filling pressure required with elevated LV diastolic pressures. In pure mitral stenosis the PAW *a* wave is dominant and elevated as a result of the resistance met at the narrowed mitral orifice. It represents the increased force of contraction required to eject blood through the stenotic valve. The *y* descent of the PAW pressure is usually prolonged in mitral stenosis, indicating increased resistance to passive filling of the LV.

The *v* wave of the PAW pressure is exaggerated and elevated with mitral insufficiency because of regurgitation of blood back into the LA during ventricular systole (Fig. 5-30). Mitral regurgitation can occur in varying degrees of severity and from a variety of causes. A mildly elevated and dominant *v* wave is commonly seen with LV failure and dilatation. Rheumatic fever or bacterial endocarditis can cause destruction to the valve leaflets and produce chronic mitral regurgitation. Acute

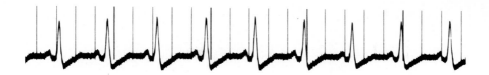

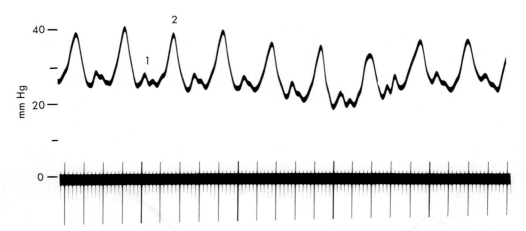

Fig. 5-30. Elevated PAW pressure with a dominant and elevated v wave (2) as a result of mitral regurgitation. The a wave (1) is also elevated indicating LV failure. In this case, the mitral regurgiation is likely functional 2° LV failure and dilatation.

mitral regurgitation, with giant v waves can occur with ruptured papillary muscle following myocardial infarction (Fig. 5-31).

Such large v waves significantly elevate the pulmonary venous pressure, resulting in acute pulmonary edema. Often a giant v wave can be transmitted onto the PA waveform, producing a bifid appearance to the PA pressure wave (Fig. 5-32). Occasionally, the v wave may even be higher than the PA systolic pressure resulting in a PA waveform as seen in Fig. 5-33. Such an occurrence results in retrograde flow of blood and early closure of the pulmonic wave. However, not *all* elevations of the v wave of the PAW pressure are because of mitral regurgitation. Increases in

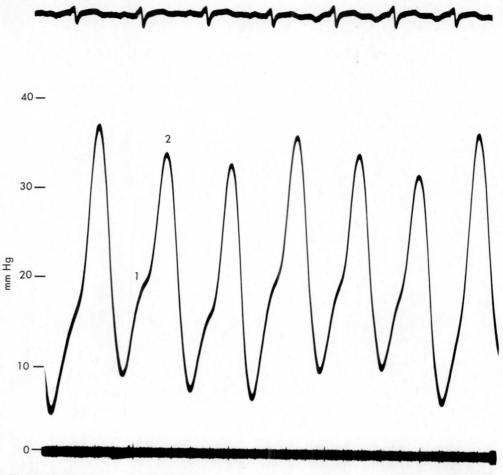

Fig. 5-31. PAW pressure waveform with a dominant and elevated v wave (2) as a result of acute mitral regurgitation associated with papillary muscle dysfunction from an acute MI. The almost obscured a wave, (1) is only minimally elevated.

the v wave can also occur as a result of decreased compliance of the left atrium. Abnormal elevations of the v wave of the PAW pressure may cause the PAW waveform to resemble a PA waveform (Fig. 5-34). This is particularly likely in patients with atrial fibrillation in whom the PAW waveforms consist solely of a large v wave. Such an error could result in permanent wedging of the PA catheter with the associated risks of pulmonary infarction or rupture. Close inspection of the timing of the PAW waveform in relation to the ECG (best done at fast paper speed) usually reveals the v wave following the T wave, whereas the upstroke of the PA systolic pressure usually occurs earlier, and corresponds to the QRS of the ECG.

If some doubt still exists as to whether the pressure is actually a PAW pressure or a damped PA pressure, obtaining a small blood sample while the balloon is inflated may confirm the location. If the catheter is indeed wedged, occluding for-

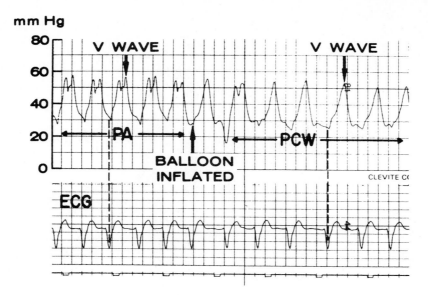

Fig. 5-32. Elevated PA and PAW pressures showing a large *v* wave of the PAW reflected in the PA pressure giving it a bifid appearance (double-peaked). Careful examination of the mechanical events with the ECG reveals the PA systolic pressure occurring earlier in the cardiac cycle than the PAW *v* wave. (From Buchbinder N, and Ganz W: Hemodynamic monitoring: invasive techniques, Anesthesiology 45: 146, 1976.)

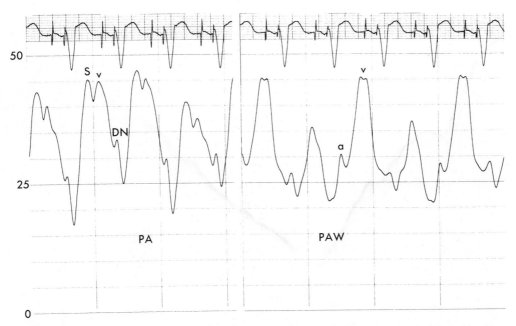

Fig. 5-33. PA pressure with retrograde reflection of the *v* wave from the LA. In this case, the *v* wave is higher that the systolic (S) PA pressure. (DN = dicrotic notch.) The PAW pressure on the right reveals an elevated *v* wave of approximately 45 mm Hg.

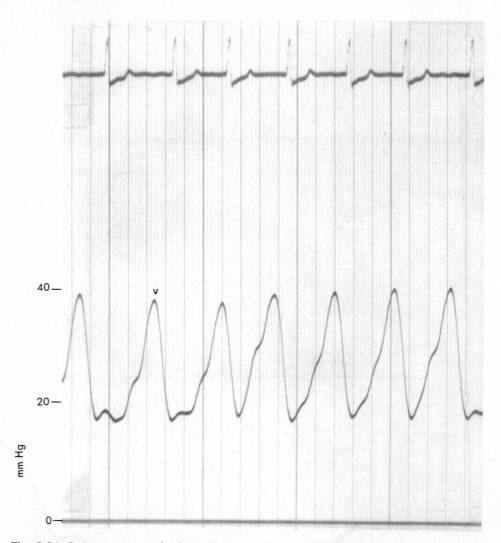

Fig. 5-34. Paw pressure with elevated *v* wave because of mitral regurgitation. Absent *a* waves in this waveform are a result of the underlying atrial fibrillation. The appearance of this PAW waveform somewhat resembles a PA waveform. Differentiation can be done by obtaining a blood sample from the distal lumen of the catheter. (See discussion in text.)

ward blood flow, the blood sample obtained will be from the postcapillary vasculature and therefore should be arterialized blood. If the catheter is not wedged, the blood sample obtained will be darker venous blood. These observations are generally made visually, because often not enough blood can be drawn from a wedged catheter for the laboratory to determine oxygen saturation. After the blood sample is withdrawn from the PAW, it is essential to deflate the balloon before flushing the catheter to ensure that flushing is done in the PA and not in the PAW position.

In cardiac tamponade, constrictive pericardial disease, and hypervolemia the PAW *a* and *v* waves are both elevated. In cardiac tamponade the *x* descent is

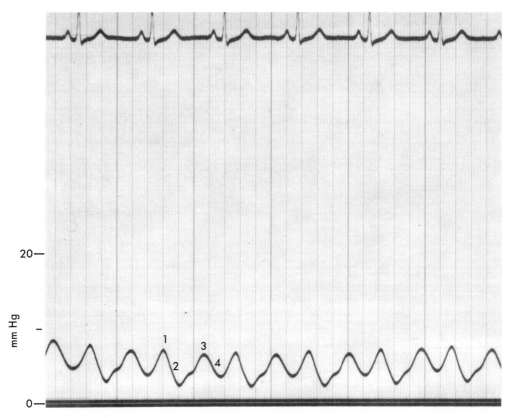

Fig. 5-35. PAW pressure waveform of normal configuration but low value with a mean of approximately 4 mm Hg. (1 = *a* wave; 2 = *x* descent; 3 = *v* wave; 4 = *y* descent.)

prominent, whereas in constrictive pericarditis either the *y* descent is prominent or the *x* and *y* descents are equal, giving an M pattern to the PAW pressure waveform (see Fig. 5-15).

Hypovolemia produces a low PAW pressure (Fig. 5-35). In the normal heart, PAW pressures less than 4 or 5 mm Hg indicate hypovolemia, whereas in the compromised heart, hypovolemia may be present despite higher PAW pressures.

Mechanical abnormalities of the PAW pressure produce changes in both the value and the contour of the PAW pressure waveform. *Overwedging,* which is caused by overinflation or eccentric inflation of the balloon of the catheter or an exceedingly distal location of the catheter tip, may produce an artifactually elevated, damped, and inaccurate PAW pressure (Fig. 5-36). In addition, there is usually a linear increase or decrease in the pressure waveform. (It resembles a line at an approximately 10- to 20-degree angle). Slow, careful, and accurate balloon inflation or, if the catheter is too distally positioned, withdrawal to a more proximal PA location may alleviate this problem.

Damping of the PAW pressure produces the same type of rounded-out appearance as with the PA pressure with lack of defined *a* and *v* waves (Fig. 5-37). The balloon should be deflated before the catheter is aspirated and then gently flushed. Never flush in the PAW position.

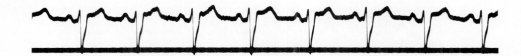

20—

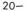

mm Hg

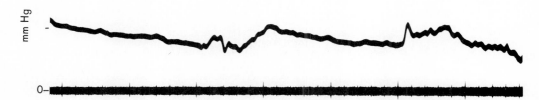

0—

Fig. 5-36. PAW pressure lacking the normal characteristics as a result of overwedging. Over-wedging can occur when the balloon of the catheter is inflated with an excessive amount of air for the size of the vessel in which the catheter is positioned. Careful monitoring of the pressure waveform during balloon inflation, with immediate cessation of inflation when a PAW waveform is obtained can prevent this problem.

Occasionally a mixed PA/PAW pressure is obtained because of incomplete wedging of the catheter tip (Fig. 5-38). Sometimes the changes are directly related to respirations, with a PA pressure observed during expiration and a PAW pressure observed during inspiration. In this circumstance, slight advancement of the catheter is necessary to obtain an accurate PAW pressure.

The PAW mean pressure should be lower than the PA mean pressure, and a noticeable fall in pressure should occur as the balloon in balloon-tipped catheters is inflated (see Fig. 5-22). Similarly, there should be an abrupt rise in pressure as the balloon is deflated. The PAW pressure, like all hemodynamic pressures, should be measured at the end of expiration. Since the digital display presents an average of the sweep, it is necessary to measure the pressure marking the end-expiratory phase of the respiratory cycle on a calibrated oscilloscope or graph paper.

Frequently, direct left atrial (LA) pressures are measured via a small catheter placed in the LA at the time of open heart surgery. Since the PAW pressure is an indirect measurement of LA pressure, both the contour and the value of the LA pressure are the same as the PAW pressure (Fig. 5-39). The LA *a* wave, produced by left atrial systole, is followed by the *x* descent, a decline in pressure as a result of reduced LA volume. The *c* wave is produced by closure of the mitral valve leaflets and may or may not be evident in the LA waveform. The *v* wave results from filling of the LA and bulging back of the mitral valve during ventricular systole.

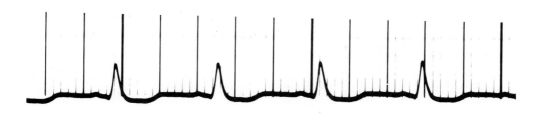

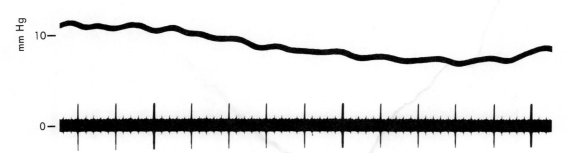

Fig. 5-37. Excessively damped PAW pressure lacking the normal characteristics and contour. After deflation to ensure the catheter is no longer wedged, the catheter should be aspirated and flushed.

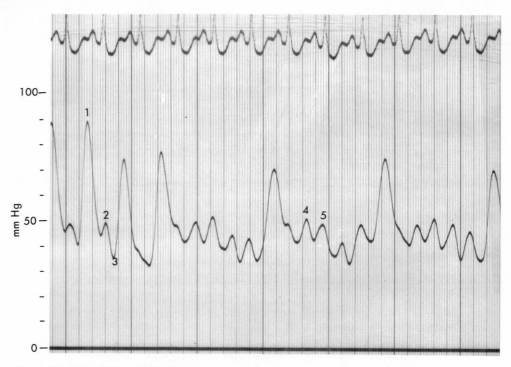

Fig. 5-38. Mixed PA and PAW pressure waveforms as a result of forward migration of the PA catheter tip. The change from PA to PAW appears to be cyclical and regular indicating that the changes follow the respiratory pattern. Slight withdrawal of the catheter tip should eliminate this problem.

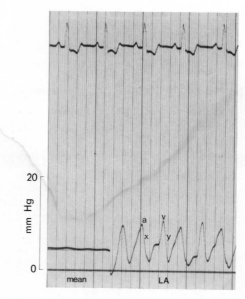

Fig. 5-39. LA pressure waveform demonstrating similarity to PAW waveform. This pressure is normal.

This is followed by the *y* descent, reflecting a decrease in LA volume during passive filling of the LV. The delay between electrical and mechanical events that one sees in the PAW pressure is less apparent with the direct LA pressure; for example, the LA *a* wave more immediately follows the P wave of the ECG.

Normal values of the LA pressure are a mean pressure of 4 to 12 mm Hg.

PAW interpretation

Although the PAW pressure is commonly used as a reflection of the LVEDP, its limitations must be appreciated. Situations in which the PAW pressure *does not* equal or approximate the LVEDP include:

1. Mitral stenosis
2. Left atrial myxoma
3. Pulmonary venous obstruction
4. Decreased ventricular compliance
5. Increased pleural pressure
6. Placement of the catheter tip in a nondependent zone of the lung

The first three pathological disorders cause an increase in the LA pressure and, therefore, the PAW pressure. However, the diastolic filling pressure of the left ventricle may be normal or even low as a result of reduced volume. Indirect assessment of LVEDP is not possible in these situations.

Decreases in ventricular compliance from any cause require higher filling pressures for the same filling volume. The pressure-volume curve depicted in Fig. 5-5 illustrates this increase in pressure as compliance decreases. In such cases, it is possible for normal or higher PAW pressures to accompany relative hypovolemia. Nonetheless, it is the pressure in the pulmonary capillary, not the volume in the ventricle, that is responsible for the transudation of fluid out of the vascular space.

Increases in juxtacardiac and pleural pressures are transmitted to cardiac chambers and vessels. PAW pressures obtained in patients with increased pleural pressure reflect the elevated juxtacardiac pressure rather than a high LVEDP. (See Chapter 13 for further discussion of this.)

When the tip of the PA catheter lies in nondependent lung zone I or II and the balloon of the catheter is inflated to measure the PAW pressure, the flow is interrupted causing the vasculature beyond the catheter tip to collapse. The recorded PAW pressure in such cases reflects the alveolar or airway pressure rather than the LVEDP. (This concept is discussed in greater detail in Chapter 13) Fig. 5-40 schematically illustrates the possible causes responsible for an elevation of the recorded PAW pressure.

The possibility of such conditions affecting the PAW pressure measurement must be assessed before clinically interpreting an elevated PAW pressure. An elevated PAW pressure does not always mean the LVED pressure or volume is elevated. It could be a result of increased surrounding pleural pressure, or a noncompliant ventricle, or interruption of the fluid column between the catheter tip and the LA.

RESPIRATORY EFFECTS ON HEMODYNAMIC PRESSURES

Since the heart lies between the lungs within the chest, an intimate relationship exists between cardiac and the surrounding airway, esophageal, and pleural pres-

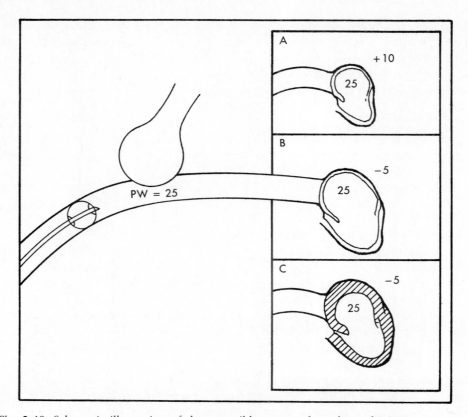

Fig. 5-40. Schematic illustration of three possible causes of an elevated PAW pressure: **A,** The PAW, LA and LVed pressures are elevated as a result of increased pleural pressure (+10), although the end-diastolic ventricular volume (preload) is normal, or reduced. **B,** The LV, LA and PAW pressures are all elevated as a result of increased LV preload and ventricular dilatation with normal compliance and normal pleural pressure. In this situation, the PAW pressure accurately reflects the LVedp and volume. **C,** Elevated LV, LA and PAW pressures with normal pleural pressure surrounding a noncompliant ventricle. In this case, the elevated PAW pressures with normal pleural pressure surrounding a noncompliant ventricle. In this case, the elevated PAW pressure reflects the decrease in ventricular compliance and not the preload or end-diastolic volume of the ventricle, which is actually reduced. All three possible causes of elevated PAW pressures must be considered, when applicable, for accurate assessment of LV preload. (From Wiedemann HP, Matthay MA, and Matthay RA: Cardiovascular-pulmonary monitoring in the intensive care unit (Part I), Chest 85: 537-549, 1984.)

sures. The cardiac as well as vascular structures within the thorax are constantly subjected to continually changing surrounding pressures of −2 to −7 mm Hg and even higher in certain disease states. Normally, however, the intrathoracic pressure changes are fairly small and constant from one respiratory cycle to another. For this reason, it is common practice to reference intravascular pressures to atmospheric pressure rather than surrounding pleural pressure. However, referencing intracardiac or intravascular pressures to atmospheric pressure may not be appropriate when intrathoracic pressures are increased. In these situations, it is more accurate to measure *transmural* intracardiac or intravascular pressures. Transmural pressures are determined by subtracting the intrapleural pressure from the mea-

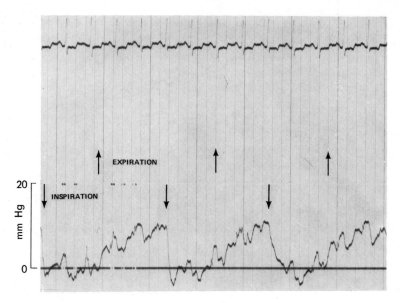

Fig. 5-41. CVP or RA pressure tracing showing pressure variation during respiration. At maximal inspiration there is actually a negative pressure in the thorax and right atrium in comparison with rest of the body and atmospheric pressure.

sured hemodynamic pressure. Intrapleural pressure can be measured with esophageal catheters, but this method is difficult in the critically ill patient. More commonly, the intrapleural pressure is estimated, as discussed in Chapter 13.

During spontaneous *inspiration*, lung volume increases and the pressure in the intrathoracic cavity becomes negative relative to atmospheric pressure. This decrease in intrathoracic pressure is transmitted to the structures in the thoracic cavity, causing a decrease in intravascular and intracardiac pressures during inspiration (Fig. 5-41). Consequently, it is normal to observe falls in RA, PA, PAW, LA, and arterial pressures during normal, spontaneous inspiration. However, if true transmural pressures were measured (that is, the pressure within the heart chamber or vessel relative to the surrounding pleural pressure rather than the pressure in the atmosphere), the pressures would reflect the changes in volume that occur during the respiratory cycle. During inspiration, decreased intrapleural pressure causes venous return to increase, resulting in an increase in RA volume and therefore transmural RA pressure (relative to pleural pressure). Similarly, there is an increase in RV volume and end-diastolic pressure relative to pleural pressure. As a result of this increase in RV preload, pulmonary arterial outflow and therefore transmural PA pressure actually increase slightly during spontaneous inspiration.

The effects of inspiration on the left side of the heart are not as consistently explained as those of the right side of the heart. The inspiratory effect of increasing RV volume or preload causes an increase in RV size. Several studies have demonstrated that increasing RV size through the mechanism of ventricular interdependence may lead to decreased LV size, stiffening of the LV, and alterations in the LV pressure-volume curve. Decreases in LV filling pressures have been attributed to decreased pulmonary venous return as a result of pooling of blood in the lungs during inspiration. This distribution of blood in the pulmonary vasculature is thought to be caused by increased compliance of the pulmonary vasculature during inspiration and results in decreased LV filling. Recent evidence reveals increases in effective or transmural LV filling pressure during inspiration in some patients. This probably reflects the imposed alterations in the LV pressure-volume curve during inspiration as a result of decreased compliance of the LV.

The net result of these inspiratory effects on LV performance is a decrease in stroke volume. This decrease in stroke volume is caused not only by changes in LV preload but by increases in afterload that occur with decreased pleural pressure. Because stroke volume decreases during spontaneous inspiration, arterial pulse pressure falls.

During expiration, intrathoracic pressure increases, resulting in increased pulmonary venous return to the LA with increased filling of the LV and increased stroke volume. Therefore both intravascular and intracardiac pressures rise during spontaneous expiration.

Because the PA and PAW pressure can vary markedly as a result of intrathoracic pressure changes during respiration, all pressures should be measured at end-expiration, when intrathoracic pressure comes closest to atmospheric pressure.

PA and PAW Pressure Measurement

A pressure transducer, monitoring equipment, and an oscilloscope allow pressure monitoring during catheter insertion at the bedside. This technique permits location of the catheter tip position without fluoroscopy by means of the pressure measurement and the pressure waveform on the oscilloscope. The various types of transducers and monitoring equipment are described in Chapter 3.

Flotation catheters are now available to meet virtually every need in hemodynamic monitoring (Fig. 5-42). In addition to thermistors, which allow measurement of cardiac output by the thermodilution technique, these catheters come equipped with pacing wires and an additional RA port for the infusion of fluids or drugs or measurement of RV ejection.

The accuracy, reliability, and reduced cost of disposable pressure transducers have resulted in their widespread use in bedside hemodynamic monitoring. These preassembled, sterile devices have eliminated some of the contamination problems associated with the use of nondisposable transducers.

Before pressure measurements are obtained, the reference port of the transducer must be set level to the patient's phlebostatic axis or midchest height, approximately the level of the RA (Fig. 5-43). The transducer is then connected to the monitor, which has been warming up at least 15 minutes. With the reference stopcock open to room air, the zero dial on the monitor is set, and the calibration is checked. (Disposable transducers do not require calibration checks with a mercury manometer. However, the calibration of the monitor system should be checked during the initial setup.)

The catheter is connected to the transducer by short stiff extension tubing and stopcocks (Fig. 5-44). The connecting tubing should be just long enough to connect the catheter to the transducer. Excessive tubing lengths cause distortion of the pressure waveforms. Ideally, the transducer should be connected directly

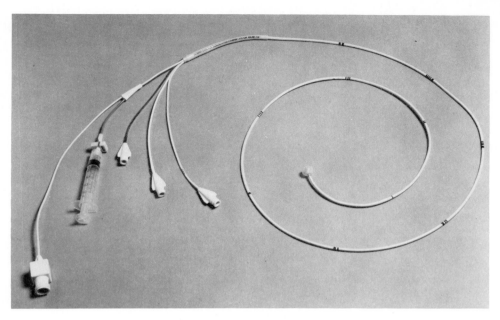

Fig. 5-42. Swan-Ganz flow-directed, balloon-tipped thermodilution catheter for PA and RA pressure monitoring and cardiac output measurement. Syringe is used for inflating the ballon with air. (Courtesy American Edwards Laboratories, Santa Ana, Calif.)

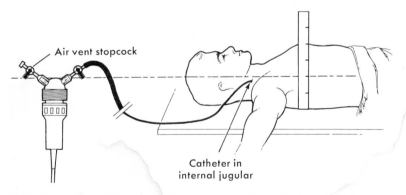

Fig. 5-43. The patient's midchest position is measured, marked, and used as an anatomic reference point for placement of the transducer.

to the catheter via a stopcock. The connector tubing must be flushed with IV fluid before it is connected to the catheter. To prevent a thrombus from forming at the catheter tip, 1 unit heparin/1 ml IV fluid is added and a continuous flush device is used.

Equipment

Hemodynamic monitoring of RA, PA, and PAW pressures requires the following equipment:

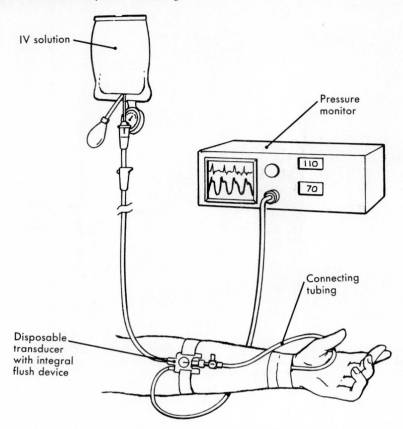

Fig. 5-44. Setup showing connections between catheter, continuous flush device, disposable transducer, IV solution, and pressure monitor.

1. Catheter of choice (CVP or PA catheter)
2. Catheter/sheath introducer
3. Sterile catheter sleeve
4. Pressure transducer (disposable or reusable)
5. Sterile transducer dome (if reusable transducer is used)
6. Electronic monitor and oscilloscope
7. Heparinized infusion fluid in a plastic IV bag
8. Pressure tubing
9. IV tubing with pediatric drip chamber
10. Three-way stopcocks
11. Continuous flush device
12. Pressurized IV cuff or pump
13. Fluoroscope (optional)
14. Paper recorder
15. Cardiopulmonary resuscitation equipment

Setting up equipment

1. Plug transducer cable into the monitor.
2. Select appropriate scale on the monitor (venous or arterial).

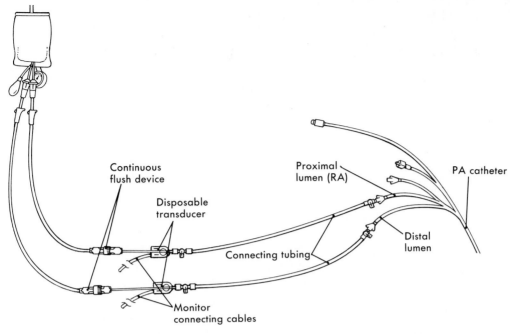

Fig. 5-45. Use of one IV solution bag for monitoring of 2 different pressure lines.

3. Activate monitor power switch to "on."
4. Add heparin to IV solution in a collapsible bag via the medication port. Label solution bag.
5. Remove all air from the IV bag via a 22-gauge needle inserted into the medication port.
6. Remove protective cap from the drip chamber and insert into outlet port of IV bag. If desired, a second drip chamber can be inserted into the medication port of the IV bag, thus using only one IV bag for two monitoring lines (Fig. 5-45). A single drip chamber distally divided into three monitoring lines is also available, allowing the use of one IV bag for three monitoring lines.
7. Open the IV roller clamp and lightly squeeze the drip chamber. Do not fill the drip chamber more than 0.5 cm, because the fluid level increases when pressure is applied to the bag.
8. Close the IV roller clamp, insert the IV bag into a pressure administration cuff, and hang the pressure cuff.
9. Replace all vented caps with dead-ender caps on the sideports of all stopcocks.
10. Attach the IV set to the designated female end of the continuous flush device (if not preassembled).
11. Attach a venting stopcock to one port of the transducer dome.
12. Attach a Luer-Lok stopcock to the remaining port of the transducer dome.
13. Attach the female end of the continuous flush device to the Luer-Lok stopcock on the transducer dome.
14. Open the transducer venting stopcock to air.
15. Open the IV roller clamp, pull the fast flush device, and allow the IV solution

to completely fill the tubing, the stopcocks, the flushing device, and the transducer dome. (It may be necessary to rotate the dome while fast flushing to purge all air bubbles from the dome.)

16. Close the transducer venting stopcock.
17. Remove dead-ender cap at patient end of the connecting tubing; attach a Luer-Lok stopcock (if not preassembled) and close off its sideport.
18. Pull fast flush device and slowly flush entire monitoring line (using gravity pressure only), taking special care to ensure that no air is trapped in any stopcocks.
19. Pressurize cuff to 300 mm Hg. (Make sure the drip chamber does not completely fill.)
20. Hold the catheter hub end in a downward position and allow blood to completely fill the hub.
21. While pulling the fast flush device, attach the IV line to the hub of the catheter, securing tightly.
22. Check drip rate to ensure flow of 1 to 5 ml/hr.
23. Check all connecting sites and label tubing (arterial, proximal, or distal) near the continuous flush device and near the drip chamber.
24. Place transducer reference at patient's midchest level and secure in this position (either on IV pole holder or directly on patient's arm or chest).
25. Open the transducer reference stopcock to air.
26. Turn zero control knob on monitor to obtain a zero reading.
27. Push calibration knob and check monitor calibration; adjust if necessary.
28. Close the transducer venting stopcock to air.

Many manufacturers now provide completely preassembled kits containing the disposable transducer with attached stopcocks, flush device, and IV tubing. These kits only require exchanging dead-ender caps for the vented caps during the setup.

Measurement of two pressures with a single transducer

To minimize equipment use, a single transducer can be used to monitor both RA and PA pressures. Although this method eliminates the ability to monitor both pressures simultaneously, a simple turning of two stopcocks makes either pressure tracing available. Fig. 5-46 illustrates an appropriate setup. Caution must be exercised to make sure the distal (PA) pressure is *continuously* monitored with occasional, brief monitoring of the proximal (RA) pressure. This allows continuous assessment of catheter tip location and the ability to immediately intervene if forward migration of the catheter tip occurs. A single transducer setup should never be used for PA and peripheral arterial catheters, since both pressures require continuous monitoring.

PROBLEMS AND COMPLICATIONS ENCOUNTERED WITH BALLOON-TIPPED CATHETERS

Although the relative ease of catheter insertion and the information obtained make PA pressure monitoring a valuable diagnostic tool, it is not without hazard. Reported overall complications rates for PA catheters are as high as 75%. However, this high rate relates to the frequent occurrence of transient and clin-

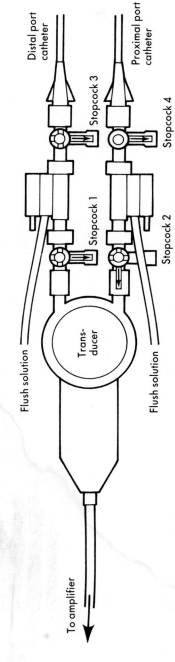

Fig. 5-46. Setup showing the use of a single quartz transducer for continous PA pressure monitoring and intermittent RA pressure monitoring. Stopcocks 1 and 3 are open, allowing monitoring of the PA pressure while stopcock 2 is closed to the transducer. Stopcock 4 is open between the flush solution and the proximal port of the catheter.

ically benign arrhythmias. The majority of complications that occur with PA catheterization are minor, although fatalities may be associated with major complications. Potentially life-threatening complications have been reported to occur in approximately 4% of patients who have undergone PA catheterizations.

Cardiac Arrhythmias

Either atrial or ventricular arrhythmias frequently occur during right heart catheter insertion and are usually transient and benign, subsiding with completion of catheter passage out to the PA. Transient PVCs and nonsustained ventricular tachycardia are the most common arrhythmias, but occasionally sustained ventricular tachycardia develops, requiring drug therapy or prompt cardioversion or both. Rarely, ventricular fibrillation may occur and is treated by immediate defibrillation. The occurrence of ventricular arrhythmias is highly correlated with the presence of shock, acute myocardial ischemia or infarction, hypokalemia, hypocalcemia, hypoxemia, acidosis, and prolonged catheter insertion times.

The prophylactic use of lidocaine to control cardiac arrhythmias has been reported. This is not routinely used, but may be of some value in selected high-risk cases.

Bundle Branch Block

Right bundle branch block may occur during manipulation of the catheter in the right ventricle. This is generally not a problem unless the patient has preexisting left bundle branch block (LBBB), resulting in complete AV block. In patients with preexisting LBBB, it may be prudent to insert a PA catheter with pacing electrodes to prevent ventricular asystole. If a pacing catheter is not inserted, transvenous or transcutaneous pacing equipment should be readily available.

The best prevention of the development of any cardiac arrhythmia or conduction abnormality is rapid placement of the catheter tip in the PA with minimal manipulation in the right ventricle or right atrium. In addition, the balloon should be fully inflated before entering the right ventricle to prevent catheter tip–induced arrhythmias.

Thrombus Formation

Although thrombus formation may occur with any intravascular catheter, the polyvinylchloride material of the PA catheter has been shown to be highly thrombogenic, with formation of a fibrin sleeve around the catheter within 60 to 130 minutes of catheter insertion. Small thrombi with erosion of the endothelium of the vein, endocardium, or valves along the course of the catheter have been found on autopsy. This same study revealed a significant increase of blood vessel thrombosis (from 41% to 79%) after 2 days of catheterization despite anticoagulation.

Thrombus can also develop at the insertion site. In venographic autopsy examination, Chastre et al found thrombosis of the internal jugular veins (the catheter insertion site) in 66% of patients despite lack of clinical evidence of thrombosis. The presence of a PA catheter has been shown to correlate with a continuing reduction in platelet count, likely caused by increased platelet consumption associated with aggregation along the catheter. The platelet count usually returns to normal within 2 to 4 days after catheter removal.

The incidence of thrombus formation is increased in patients with low cardiac output, disseminated intravascular coagulation, or congestive heart failure.

Reduction of the risk of thrombosis may occur with a continuous flush of heparinized saline or use of a catheter bonded with heparin. Use of a Teflon sheath with a side arm for continuous infusion may also reduce thrombus formation. Manual flushing of either the PA or arterial catheter should always be preceded by aspiration to remove any clots, if present. Flushing should then be performed gently with a small volume of fluid.

Pulmonary Infarction

Pulmonary infarction may occur as a result of embolization of thrombus from the catheter or as a result of catheter migration and prolonged wedging. Forward migration of the catheter occurs primarily during the first 24 hours as the catheter loop tightens with repeated RV contractions.

Prevention of this complication includes a review of a chest radiograph in the first 12 hours, continuous display of the pressure from the distal lumen of the catheter, wedging of the catheter only for a very brief time, monitoring of the PAEDP rather than PAW pressure (if a close correlation is established), and, perhaps, use of heparin-bonded catheters to reduce thrombolic occlusions. Chest radiographs should be repeated if catheter migration is suspected.

Infection

Infection secondary to PA catheterization can range from contamination to colonization to sepsis. Contamination, with a positive culture of the catheter tip, or colonization, with growth of the same organisms from both the catheter tip and another site (for example, sputum, urine), has been shown to occur in 5% to 35% of cases.

Colonization with bacteria (most commonly coagulase-negative staphylococci) has been shown to occur more frequently with polyvinylchloride PA catheters than with Teflon intravascular CVP catheters. Sepsis, in which the same pathogen is grown from the blood and the catheter tip, has been reported to occur in 1% to 8% of PA catheter placements. Septic endocarditis involving the right side of the heart is a rare complication of prolonged PA catheterization.

Prevention of infection includes meticulous aseptic technique during catheter insertion, daily care of the insertion site (including cleansing with a bactericidal agent and application of iodophor ointment and a new sterile dressing), and a short duration of catheter placement. Catheters left in place longer than 4 days are associated with a higher incidence of infection. To reduce the incidence of infection the Centers of Disease Control (CDC) recommends changing the IV solution, tubing, stopcocks, and transducer dome every 48 hours, using nonglucose IV solutions, and removing and replacing the catheter, if necessary, after 4 days. A recent bacteriologic evaluation of disposable pressure transducers showed no increase in contamination rates of disposable transducers changed every 4 days or every 2 days (3%). Advancement of PA catheters after initial placement should only be done if the proximal portion of the catheter has been maintained sterile inside a sleeve. In one study, short-term sterility was provided by catheter sleeves for 1 to 2 days if inserted under meticulous aseptic technique. All intravascular catheters should immediately be removed if colonization or sepsis develops, and appropriate antibiotic therapy instituted.

Pulmonary Artery Rupture

Rupture of the PA is a dramatic and usually fatal complication that occurs infrequently with the use of PA catheters. Because this complication is often associated with pulmonary hypertension, advanced age (>60 years), anticoagulation, and cardiopulmonary bypass surgery, PAWP measurements should be performed with caution in this subgroup of patients. In all patients, PAWP should be obtained with *continuous* visualization of the PAP during balloon inflation. Inflation should be discontinued immediately on visualizing a PAW waveform. Should the PAW wedge waveform become nonphasic, the balloon should immediately be deflated because this may represent overinflation or eccentric inflation, with the balloon extending around the catheter tip.

Although pulmonary hypertension, per se, may not render the arteries more fragile, the higher PAP tends to drive the catheter further distally into smaller vessels, thereby increasing the risk of perforation. Changes in the vessel wall that oc-

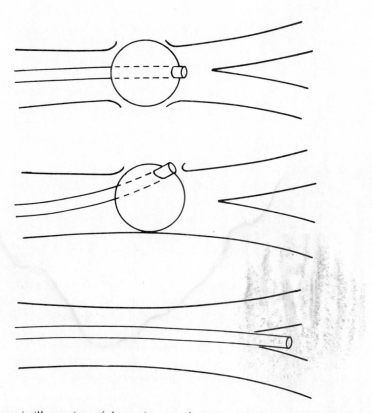

Fig. 5-47. Schematic illustration of the various mechanisms responsible for catheter-induced rupture of the PA: overinflation of the balloon, eccentric balloon inflation, and distal migration of the catheter tip.

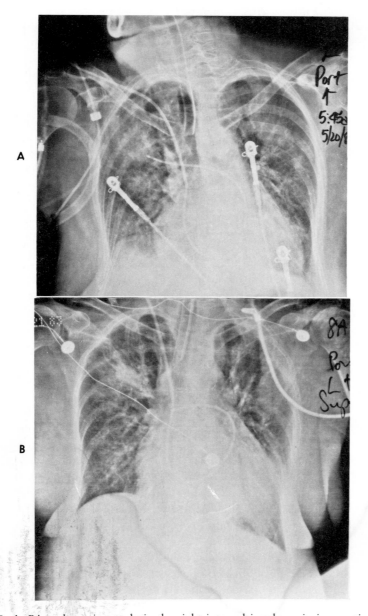

Fig. 5-48. A, PA catheter inserted via the right internal jugular vein in a patient with congestive heart failure and pulmonary edema. Note that the catheter tip has migrated distally into the upper lobe branch of the right PA with the beginning appearance of a wedge-shaped pulmonary infarction. **B,** Evolving right upper lobe pulmonary infarction is apparent in this same patient despite withdrawl of the catheter tip into the right PA.

cur in patients over the age of 60 years also result in lower rupturing pressures. The use of hypothermia, which stiffens the catheter, and manipulation of the heart during cardiac surgery also increase the risk of PA rupture. The four causes of PA rupture are distal migration of the catheter tip, overinflation of the balloon, eccentric inflation of the balloon, and manual flushing of a wedged catheter. Fig. 5-47 illustrates some of the mechanisms responsible for rupture of the PA.

To prevent this frequently fatal complication, the following procedures should be performed:

1. Monitor the distal lumen pressure continuously.
2. Radiographically confirm catheter tip location in the central PA.
3. Inflate the balloon slowly, using only that amount of air necessary to achieve a PAWP tracing, while constantly monitoring the pressure. Although the recommended balloon capacity of the 7 Fr catheter is 1.5 cc of air, an inflation volume of 0.8 to 1.0 cc of air is often sufficient.
4. Perform infrequent balloon inflations (monitor PAEDP, if possible).
5. Always deflate the balloon before performing a manual flush. If necessary, withdraw the tip of the catheter slightly to prevent forceful flushing in the wedge position.
6. Never inflate the balloon with an excessive volume of air (greater than the recommended volume of air). If a PAWP is obtained with less than the usual volume of air, check the catheter position for migration.
7. Never inflate the balloon with fluid. Carefully identify infusion ports before injections to avoid injecting fluid into the balloon lumen.

Fig. 5-48 illustrates the rupture of a branch of the PA caused by excessive balloon inflation. Although only 1.5 cc of air was injected, the distal location of the catheter tip in a small vessel caused pulmonary artery rupture during inflation.

If PA rupture is small, as indicated by a small amount of hemoptysis, the patient should be placed in a lateral recumbent position with the affected side down and closely monitored and observed. Anticoagulation should be stopped and reversed. Hemoptysis of 15 to 30 ml should prompt consideration of a "wedge" angiographic study to determine the amount and location of extravasation of dye. Massive hemoptysis can be controlled with insertion of a double-lumen endotracheal tube to prevent bleeding into the unaffected lung and aid ventilation. Prompt surgical repair may be necessary, along with pneumonectomy or lobectomy.

Cardiac Tamponade

Cardiac perforation resulting in cardiac tamponade can occur during manipulation of any catheter placed in the heart. This rare complication is associated with central venous (RA) catheters more commonly than PA catheters and may occur anywhere from minutes to days after catheterization. Clinical manifestations of cardiac tamponade in conjunction with low cardiac output and elevated RA and CVP pressures in patients with a right heart catheter should prompt suspicion of this complication.

Catheter Coiling or Knotting

Coiling or knotting of the PA catheter during catheter insertion is often associated with prolonged insertion time. This occurrence is considered a complication

Table 5-3. Problems encountered with PA catheters

Problem	Cause	Prevention	Treatment
Phlebitis or local infection at insertion site	Mechanical irritation or contamination	Prepare skin properly before insertion. Use sterile technique during insertion and dressing change. Insert smoothly and rapidly. Change dressings, stopcocks, and connecting tubing every 24 to 48 hr. Remove catheter or change insertion site every 4 days.	Remove catheter. Apply warm compresses. Give pain medication as necessary.
IV fluid infusing poorly Damped waveforms and inaccurate pressures	Partial clotting at catheter tip	Use continuous drip with 1 unit heparin/1 ml IV fluid. Hand flush occasionally. Flush with large volume after blood withdrawal. Use heparin-coated catheters.	Aspirate, then flush catheter with heparinized fluid (not in PAW position).
	Tip moving against wall	Obtain more stable catheter position.	Reposition catheter.
Abnormally low or negative pressures	Improper transducer reference level	Maintain transducer air-reference port at midchest level.	Remeasure level of transducer reference and reposition at midchest level.
	Incorrect zeroing and calibration of monitor	Zero and calibrate monitor properly.	Recheck zero and calibration of monitor.
Ventricular irritability	Looping of excess catheter in right ventricle	Suture catheter at insertion site; check chest x-ray.	Reposition catheter; remove loop.
	Migration of catheter from PA to RV	Position catheter tip in main right or left PA.	Inflate balloon to encourage catheter flotation out to PA.
	Irritation of the endocardium during catheter passage	Keep balloon inflated during advancement; advance gently.	Administer lidocaine if necessary; defibrillate if VF occurs.

(Continued.)

Table 5-3. Problems encountered with PA catheters—cont'd

Problem	Cause	Prevention	Treatment
Apparent wedging of catheter with balloon *deflated*	Forward migration of catheter tip caused by blood flow, excessive loop in RV, or inadequate suturing of catheter at insertion site.	Check catheter tip by fluoroscopy; position in main right or left PA. Check catheter position on x-ray film if fluoroscopy is not used. Suture catheter in place at insertion site.	Aspirate blood from catheter; if catheter is wedged, sample will be arterialized and obtained with difficulty or not at all. If wedged, slowly pull back catheter until PA waveform appears. If not wedged, gently aspirate and flush catheter with saline; catheter tip can partially clot, causing damping that resembles damped PAW waveform.
Pulmonary hemorrhage, infarction, or both	Distal migration of catheter tip Continuous or prolonged wedging of catheter Overinflation of balloon while catheter is wedged	Check chest x-ray immediately after insertion and 12 hr later; remove catheter loop in RA or RV. Leave balloon deflated with stopcock *open*. Suture catheter at skin to prevent inadvertent advancement. Position catheter in main right or left PA. Pull catheter back to pulmonary artery if it becomes wedged. Do no flush catheter when in wedge position. Inflate balloon slowly with only enough air to obtain a PAW waveform. Do no inflate 7 Fr catheter with more than 1 to 1.5 cc air. Do not inflate if resistance is met.	

Table 5-3. Problems encountered with PA catheters—cont'd

Problem	Cause	Prevention	Treatment
"Overwedging" or damped PAW	Overinflation of balloon Eccentric inflation of balloon	Watch waveform during inflation; inject only enough air to obtain PAW pressure. Do not inflate 7 Fr catheter with more than 1 to 1.5 cc air.	Deflate balloon; reinflate slowly with only enough air to obtain PAW pressure. Deflate balloon; reposition and slowly reinflate.
PA balloon rupture	Overinflation of balloon Frequent inflations of balloon Syringe deflation damaging wall of balloon	Inflate slowly with only enough air to obtain a PAW pressure. Monitor PAd pressure as reflection of PAW and LVEDP. Allow passive deflation of balloon through stopcock. Remove syringe after inflation.	Remove syringe to prevent further air injection. Monitor PAd pressure.
Infection	Nonsterile insertion techniques Fluid contamination through outlet ports of stopcocks	Use sterile techniques. Use sterile catheter sleeve. Use sterile dead-ender caps on all ports of stopcocks.	Remove catheter. Use antibiotics.
	Fluid contamination from transducer through membrane of disposable dome	Change IV solution, stopcock, and tubing every 24 to 48 hr. Do not use IV solution containing glucose. Check disposable domes for cracks. Sterilize nondisposable transducer before use. Change disposable domes or transducers every 48 hr. Change disposable dome after countershock. Do not use IV solution containing glucose.	

(Continued.)

Table 5-3. Problems encountered with PA catheters—cont'd

Problem	Cause	Prevention	Treatment
	Exposure of vessel to microorganisms	Use percutaneous insertion technique.	
	Prolonged catheter placement	Change catheter insertion site every 4 days.	
Heart block during insertion of catheter	Mechanical irritation of His bundle in patients with pre-existing left bundle branch block.	Insert catheter expeditiously with balloon inflated. Insert transvenous pacing catheter before PA catheter insertion.	Use temporary pacemaker or flotation catheter with pacing wire.

because it prevents correct catheter tip positioning and it can cause arrhythmias or endocardial trauma. Coiling can occur in either an enlarged RA or in the RV. If advancement of 15 cm of catheter does not result in a pressure change either from RA to RV or from RV to PA, the catheter should be slowly withdrawn and then readvanced to prevent knotting. Stiffening of the catheter by immersing it in or flushing it with iced saline or inserting a 0.025-inch (0.64 mm) guidewire may decrease the tendency for catheter coiling and enhance forward passage.

Knotting of the catheter can be handled in a variety of ways. Surgical removal may at times be necessary if intracardiac structures are involved in the knot.

Balloon Rupture

Balloon rupture after catheter insertion is usually a minor and infrequent complication that occurs as a result of improper technique. This may include overinflation of the balloon (more than 1.5 cc air for a 7 Fr catheter), inflation of the balloon with fluid instead of air, and active rather than passive deflation of the balloon. The balloon should only be passively deflated by removing the syringe and allowing the balloon to deflate. If the balloon air is actively withdrawn into the syringe, the latex of the balloon may be pulled into the side holes of the catheter, thus damaging the balloon.

Rupture of the balloon is indicated by a lack of feeling of resistance during inflation, failure of the bevel of the inflation syringe to spring back during passive inflation, and the inability to obtain a PA wedge waveform after inflation. The appearance of blood in the balloon lumen also indicates balloon rupture. Should this occur, the stopcock of the air lumen should be turned off, tape placed over the stopcock, and the message "do not inflate" inscribed on the tape. Table 5-3 summarizes the complications of PA monitoring along with causes, preventive measures, and appropriate interventions.

MAINTENANCE OF CATHETER PATENCY DURING PRESSURE RECORDING

Catheter patency is maintained by using continuous flush devices that use a pressure bag IV fluid system and deliver a maximum of 2 to 5 ml IV fluid/hr through the catheter while not altering the intravascular pressure being recorded. They also permit quick, high-flow flushes (30 to 40 ml/sec) without stopcock maneuvers. This system works well if there is pulsatile flow at the catheter tip. A low cardiac output in a critically ill patient tends to promote stasis and clotting, and catheters in these patients may require regular hand flushing even with the continuous flow device.

Care of Lines During Continuous Physiologic Monitoring

Dead-ender caps are applied to all open stopcock ports. New sterile dead-ender caps are applied each time the stopcock port is entered. Care is taken to make certain all blood is removed from tubing and stopcocks after withdrawing blood samples from the catheter. All connecting tubings, stopcocks, domes, and infusion solutions are changed at least every 48 hours. Since glucose is a medium in which bacterial organisms grow rapidly, it is recommended that IV solutions that do not contain glucose be used for continuous infusion. The dressing is changed every 24 hours, with fresh application of povidone-iodine (Betadine) ointment and inspection of the insertion site.

Table 5-4 lists several potential causes of inaccurate hemodynamic pressure measurements, as well as ways to possibly prevent and/or manage the problem.

Nursing Diagnoses

Nursing diagnoses as well as expected outcomes and interventions for patients undergoing invasive hemodynamic monitoring are located in Appendix D.

Table 5-4. Inaccurate pressure measurements

Problem	Cause	Prevention	Treatment
Damped pressure tracing or abnormally high reading	Catheter tip against vessel wall	Usually cannot be avoided.	Pull back or reposition catheter while observing waveform.
	Partial occlusion of tip by clot	Use continuous drip. May help to use 1 unit heparin/1 ml IV fluid. Occasionally hand flush rapidly and use rapid drip after blood withdrawal. Use heparin-bonded catheter.	Aspirate clot with syringe; flush with heparinized fluid.
	Pressure trapped by improper sequence of stopcock operation	Turn stopcocks in proper sequence when two pressures are measured on one transducer.	Thoroughly flush transducers with IV solution; rezero and turn stopcocks in proper sequence.

(Continued.)

Table 5-4. Inaccurate pressure measurements—cont'd

Problem	Cause	Prevention	Treatment
Inappropriate pressure waveform or measurement	Altered location of catheter tip (for example, in RV or PAW instead of in PA	Establish optimal position carefully when introducing catheter initially. Suture catheter at insertion site and tape catheter to patient's skin.	Review waveform on scope. Check position under fluoroscope and/or x-ray after reposition.
	Movement of catheter tip against wall of chamber	Usually cannot be avoided.	Reposition catheter.
Negative or inappropriately low pressure	Transducer reference level higher than midchest	Maintain transducer reference at midchest level.	Recheck transducer position.
	Loose connection	Use Luer-Lok stopcocks.	Check connections.
Damped pressure without improvement after catheter flush	Air bubbles in transducer	Set up carefully.	Check system; flush rapidly through transducers.
No pressure available	Transducer not open to catheter Amplifiers still on *cal, zero,* or *off*	Follow routine, systematic steps for pressure measurement.	Check system, stopcocks.
Noise or fling in pressure waveform	Excessive catheter movement, particularly in pulmonary artery	Avoid excessive catheter length in ventricle.	Try different catheter tip position. Purposely damp waveform with damping device.
	Excessive tubing length	Use shortest tubing possible (<3 to 4 feet).	Eliminate excess tubing.
	Excessive stopcocks	Minimize number of stopcocks.	Eliminate excess stopcocks.

REFERENCES

Abernathy WS: Complete heart block caused by the Swan-Ganz catheter, Chest 65:349, 1974.

Abbott N, Walrath JM, and Scanlon-Trump E: Infection related to physiologic monitoring: venous and arterial catheters, Heart Lung 12:28-34, 1983.

Alderman E, and Glantz S: Diastolic pressure-volume curves in man, Circulation 54:665-670, 1976.

Alpert JS: Hemodynamic monitoring: the basics, Primary Cardiol, pp. 113-126, May 1981.

Amin DK, Shah PK, and Swan HJC: The Swan-Ganz catheter: indications for insertion, J Crit Illness 1:54-61, 1986.

Ansley DM et al: The relationship between central venous pressure and pulmonary capillary wedge pressure during aortic surgery, Can J Anaesth 34:594-600, 1987.

Archer G, and Cobb LA: Long term pulmonary artery pressure monitoring in the management of the critically ill, Ann Surg 180:747-752, 1974.

Baciewicz BJ, and Gallucci A: Pulmonary artery catheter induced pulmonary artery rupture in patients undergoing cardiac surgery, Can Anaesth Soc J 32:258-264, 1985.

Baele P, Pedemonte O, Zech F, and Kestens-Servaye Y: Clinical use and bacteriologic studies of catheter contamination sleeves, Intens Care Med 10:297-300, 1984.

Baigrie RS, and Morgan CD: Hemodynamic monitoring: catheter insertion techniques, complications and trouble-shooting, Can Med Assoc J 121:885-892, 1979.

Band JD, and Maki DG: Safety of changing intravenous delivery systems at longer than 24-hour intervals, Ann Intern Med 91:173-178, 1979.

Barash PG et al: Catheter-induced pulmonary artery perforation: mechanisms, management and modifications, J Thorac Cardiovasc Surg 82:5-12, 1981.

Berryhill RE, Benumof JL, and Rauscher LA: Pulmonary vascular pressure reading at the end of exhalation, Anesthesiology, 49:365-368, 1978.

Bodai BI, and Holcroft JW: Use of the pulmonary arterial catheter in the critically ill patient, Heart Lung 11:406-416, 1982.

Bolton E: Procedural guidelines for the use of balloon-tipped, flow-directed catheters, Crit Care Nurse 1:33-40, 1981.

Boutros A, and Albert S: Effect of the dynamic response of transducer-tubing system on accuracy of direct blood pressure measurement in patients, Crit Care Med 11:124-127, 1983.

Boyd KD, Thomas J, Gola J, and Boyd AD: A prospective study of complications of pulmonary artery catheterization in 500 consecutive patients, Chest 84:245-249, 1983.

Brandstetter RD, and Gitter B: Thoughts on the Swan-Ganz catheter, Chest 89:5-6, 1986.

Brinkman AJ, and Costley DO: Internal jugular venipuncture, JAMA 223:182-183, 1973.

Buchbinder N, and Ganz W: Hemodynamic monitoring: invasive techniques, Anesthesiology 45:146-155, 1976.

Buxton AE et al: Failure of disposable domes to prevent septicemia acquired from contaminated pressure transducers, Chest 74:508-513, 1978.

Calvin MP et al: Pulmonary damage from a Swan-Ganz catheter, Br J Anaesth 47:1107-1109, 1975.

Campbell ML, and Greenberg CA: Reading pulmonary artery wedge pressure at end-expiration, Focus on Critical Care 15:60-63, 1988.

Centers for Disease Control: Guidelines for prevention of infections related to intra-vascular pressure-monitoring systems, Infect Control 3:68, 1982.

Centers for Disease Control: Nosocomial bacteremia from intravascular pressure monitoring systems. In National nosocomial infections study report, 1977 (6-month summaries), Atlanta, 1979, US Department of Health, Education, Welfare.

Cengiz M, Crapo RO, and Gardner R: The effect of ventilation on the accuracy of pulmonary artery and wedge pressure measurements, Crit Care Med 11:502-507, 1983.

Chabanier A, Dany F, Brutus P, and Vergnoux H: Iatrogenic cardiac tamponade after central venous catheter, Clin Cardiol 11:91-99, 1988.

Collier PE, Ryan JJ, and Diamond DL: Cardiac tamponade from central venous catheters. Reports of a case and review of the English literature, Angiology 35:595-600, 1984.

Conahan TJ et al: Valve competence in pulmonary artery catheter introducers, Anesthesiology 58:189-191, 1983.

Connors AF, Castele RJ, Farhat NZ, and Tomashefski JF: Complications of right heart catheterization, Chest 88:567-572, 1985.

Connors AF, Jr et al: Evaluation of right-heart catheterization in the critically ill patient without acute myocardial infarction, N Engl J Med 308:262-267, 1983.

Daily PO, Griepp RB, and Shumway NE: Percutaneous internal jugular vein cannulation, Arch Surg 101:534-536, 1970.

Damen J: Ventricular arrhythmias during insertion and removal of pulmonary artery catheters, Chest 88:190, 1985.

Deren MM, et al: Perforation of the pulmonary artery requiring pneumonectomy after use of a flow-directed (Swan-Ganz) catheter, Thorax 34:550-553, 1979.

Disposable pressure transducers, Health Devices 13:268-289, 1984.

Donowitz LG et al: *Serratia marcescens* bacteremia from contaminated pressure transducers, JAMA 242:1749-1751, 1979.

Duncan JW, and Powner DJ: Complications associated with the use of pulmonary artery catheters, Arizona Med 39:433-435, 1982.

Eaton RJ, Taxman RM, and Avioli LV: Cardiovascular evaluation of patients treated with PEEP, Arch Intern Med 143:1958-1961, 1983.

Edwards H, and King TC: Cardiac tamponade from central venous catheters, Arch Surg 117:965-967, 1982.

Elliott CG et al: Complications of pulmonary artery catheterization in the care of the critically ill patients, Chest 76:647-652, 1979.

Ellis DM: Interpretation of beat-to-beat blood pressure values in the presence of ventilatory changes, J Clin Monitoring 1:65-70, 1985.

Farber DL et al: Hemoptysis and pneumothorax after removal of persistently wedged pulmonary artery catheter, Crit Care Med 9:494-495, 1981.

Fisher ML et al: Assessing left ventricular filling pressure with flow-directed (Swan-Ganz) catheters, Chest 68:542-547, 1975.

Foote GA et al: Pulmonary complications of the flow-directed balloon-tipped catheter, N Engl J Med 290:927-931, 1974.

Forrester JS et al: Bedside diagnosis of latent cardiac complications in acutely ill patients, JAMA 222:59-63, 1972.

Forrester JS et al: Filling pressures in the right and left sides of the heart in acute myocardial infarction, N Engl J Med 285:190-193, 1971.

Frog M, Berggren L, Brodin M, and Wickbom G: Pericardial tamponade caused by central venous catheters, World J Surg 6:138-143, 1982.

Fromm RE, Guimond JG, Darby J, and Snyder JV: The craft of cardiopulmonary profile analysis. In Snyder JV and Pinsky MR: Oxygen Transport in the Critically Ill, Chicago, 1987, Year Book Medical Publishers, Inc.

Gardner RM: Direct blood pressure measurement: dynamic response requirements, Anesthesiology 54:227-236, 1981.

Geer RT: Interpretation of pulmonary-artery wedge pressure when PEEP is used, Anesthesiology 46:383-384, 1977.

Goldberg RJ: Risks and benefits of pulmonary artery catheterization, J Intensive Care Med 3:69-70, 1988.

Goldman RH et al: Measurement of central venous oxygen saturation in patients with myocardial infarction, Circulation 38:941-946, 1968.

Gomez-Arnau J et al: Retrograde dissection and rupture of pulmonary artery after catheter use in pulmonary hypertension, Crit Care Med 10:694-695, 1982.

Grace MP, and Greenbaum DM: Cardiac performance in response to PEEP in patients with cardiac dysfunction, Crit Care Med 10:358-360, 1982.

Greene JF et al: Septic endocarditis and indwelling pulmonary artery catheters, JAMA 233:891-892, 1975.

Hannan AT, Brown M, and Bigman O: Pulmonary artery catheter-induced hemorrhage, Chest 85:128-131, 1985.

Hardy JF, Morissette M, Taillefer J, and Vauclair R: Pathophysiology of rupture of the pulmonary artery by pulmonary artery balloon-tipped catheters, Anesth Analg 62:925-930, 1985.

Hardy JF, Morisette M, Taillefer J, and Vauclair R: The pathophysiology of pulmonary artery ruptures by pulmonary artery balloon tipped catheters, Anesthesiology 59:A127, 1983.

Hardy JF, and Taillefer J: Inflating characteristics of Swan-Ganz catheter balloons: clinical considerations, Anesth 62:363-364, 1983.

Heard SO et al: Influence of sterile protective sleeves on the sterility of pulmonary artery catheters, Crit Care Med 15:499-502, 1987.

Hoar PF et al: Heparin bonding reduces thrombogenicity of pulmonary artery catheters, N Engl J Med 305:993-995, 1981.

Horst HM, Obeid FN, Vij D, and Bivins B: The risks of pulmonary arterial catheterization, Surg Gynecol Obstet 159:229-232, 1984.

Iberti TJ, Benjamin E, Gruppi L, and Raskin JM: Ventricular arrhythmias during pulmonary artery catheterization in the intensive care unit, Am J Med 78:451-454, 1985.

Jesudian MCS, Fabian JA, and Chen J: An unusual complication of a pulmonary artery catheter, J Cardiovasc Surg 28:345-346, 1987.

Johnston WE et al: Influence of balloon inflation and deflation on pulmonary catheter tip location, Anesthesiology 65:A23, 1986.

Johnston WE et al: Short-term sterility of the pulmonary artery catheter inserted through an external plastic shield, Anesthesiology 61:461-464, 1984.

Kaplan JA, and Miller ED: Insertion of the Swan-Ganz catheter, Anesth Rev, pp. 22-25, Nov 1976.

Katz JD et al: Pulmonary artery flow-guided catheters in the perioperative period, JAMA 237:2832-2834, 1977.

Kaye W: Catheter- and infusion-related sepsis: the nature of the problem and its prevention, Heart Lung 11:221-228, 1982.

Kaye W: Invasive monitoring techniques: arterial cannulation, bedside pulmonary arery catheterization and arterial puncture, Heart Lung 12:395-427, 1983.

King EG: Influence of mechanical ventilation and pulmonary disease on pulmonary artery pressure monitoring, Can Med Assoc J 121:901-904, 1979.

Kronberg GM et al: Anatomic locations of the tips of pulmonary artery catheters in supine patients, Anesthesiology 51:467-469, 1979.

Lalli SM: The complete Swan-Ganz, RN 41:65-77, 1978.

Lange HW, Galliani CA, and Edwards JE: Local complications associated with indwelling Swan-Ganz catheters: autopsy study of 30 cases, Am J Cardiol 52:1108, 1983.

Lantiegne KC, and Civetta JM: A system for maintaining invasive pressure monitoring, Heart Lung 7:610-621, 1978.

Lapin ES, and Murray JA: Hemoptysis with flow-directed cardiac catheterization, JAMA 220:1246, 1972.

Luskin RL et al: Extended use of disposable pressure transducers, JAMA 255:916-920, 1986.

Maki DG, and Band JD: A comparative study of polyantibiotic and iodophor ointments in prevention of vascular catheter-related infection, Am J Med 70:739-744, 1981.

Marini JJ et al: Estimation of transmural cardiac pressures during ventilation with PEEP, J Appl Physiol 53:384-391, 1982.

Marini JJ, O'Quin R, Culver BH, and Butler J: Estimation of transmural cardiac pressures during ventilation with PEEP, J Appl Physiol 53:384-391, 1982.

Marini JJ: Pulmonary artery occlusion pressure: clinical physiology, measurement and interpretation, Am Rev Respir Dis 128:319-326, 1983.

McDonald DH, and Zaidan JR: Pressure-volume relationships of the pulmonary artery catheter balloon, Anesthesiology 59:240-243, 1983.

Meister SG et al: Potential artifact in measurement of left ventricular filling pressure with flow-directed catheters, Cathet Cardiovasc Diag 2:175-179, 1976.

Michel L et al: Infection of pulmonary artery catheters in critically ill patients, JAMA 245:1032-1036, 1981.

Michel L, March HM, and McMichan JC: Infection of pulmonary artery catheters in critically ill patients, JAMA 245:1032-1036, 1981.

Mitchell MM et al: Accurate, automated, continuously displayed pulmonary artery pressure measurement, Anesthesiology 67:294-300, 1987.

Muller BJ, and Gallucci A: Pulmonary artery catheter induced pulmonary artery rupture in patients undergoing cardiac surgery, Can Anaesth Soc J 32:258-264, 1985.

Myers ML, Austin TW, and Sibbald WJ: Pulmonary artery catheter infections: a prospective study, Ann Surg 201:237-241, 1985.

Nemens EJ, and Woods SL: Normal fluctuations in pulmonary artery and pulmonary capillary wedge pressures in acutely ill patients, Heart Lung 11:393-405, 1982.

Pace NL: A critique of flow-directed pulmonary arterial catheterization, Anesthesiology 47:455-465, 1977.

Page DW et al: Fatal hemorrhage from Swan-Ganz catheter, N Engl J Med 291:260, 1974.

Paulson DM et al: Pulmonary hemorrhage associated with balloon flotation catheters, J Thorac Cardiovasc Surg 80:453-458, 1980.

Pinilla JC et al: Study of the incidence of intravascular catheter infection and associated septicemia in critically ill patients, Crit Care Med 11:21-25, 1983.

Reeves JG: Cardiac physiology and monitoring, Can Anaesth Soc J: 32:S1-S11, 1985.

Robotham JL et al: Effects of respiration on cardiac performance, J Appl Physiol 44:703-709, 1978.

Rosenblum WE et al: Pulmonary artery dissection induced by a Swan-Ganz catheter, Cleve Clin Q 51:671-675, 1984.

Rowley KM, Clubb KS, Smith GJW, and Cabin HS: Right-sided infective endocarditis as a consequence of flow-directed pulmonary artery catheterization: clinopathologic study of 55 autopsied patients, N Engl J Med 311:1152-1156, 1984.

Roy R et al: Pulmonary wedge catheterization during positive end-expiratory pressure ventilation in the dog, Anesthesiology 46:385-390, 1977.

Russell RO, and Rackley CE: Hemodynamic monitoring in a coronary intensive care unit, Mt Kisco, NY, 1974, Futura Publishing Co, Inc.

Rutherford BD, McCann WD, and O'Donovan TP: The value of monitoring pulmonary artery pressure for early detection of left ventricular failure following myocardial infarction, Circulation 43:655-665, 1971.

Salmenpera M, Peltola K, and Rosenberg P: Does prophylactic lidocaine control cardiac arrhythmias associated with pulmonary artery catheterization? Anesthesiology 56:210-212, 1982.

Scharf SM et al: Effects of normal and loaded spontaneous inspiration on cardiovascular function, J Appl Physiol 47:582-590, 1979.

Scharf SM: Mechanical effects of respiratory system on cardiocirculatory function, Isr J Med Sci 17:715-720, 1981.

Shah KB, Rao TLK, Laughlin S, and El-Etr AA: A review of pulmonary artery catheterization in 6,245 patients, Anesthesiology 61:271-275, 1984.

Sharkey SW: Beyond the wedge: clinical physiology and the Swan-Ganz catheter, Amer J of Med 83:111-120, 1987.

Shasby MD et al: Swan-Ganz catheter location and left atrial pressure determine the accuracy of the wedge pressure when positive end-expiratory pressure is used, Chest 80:666-670, 1981.

Sheth NK et al: Colonization of bacteria on polyvinylchloride and Teflon intravascular catheters in hospitalized patients, J Clin Microbiol 18:1061-1063, 1983.

Shin B et al: Pitfalls of Swan-Ganz catheterization, Crit Care Med 5:125-127, 1977.

Shinn JA et al: Effect of intermittent positive pressure ventilation upon pulmonary artery and pulmonary capillary wedge pressures in acutely ill patients, Heart Lung 8:322-327, 1979.

Singh J et al: Catheter colonization and bacteria with pulmonary and arterial catheters, Crit Care Med 10:736-739, 1982.

Singh S et al: Catheter colonization and bacteremia with pulmonary and arterial catheters, Crit Care Med 11:736-739, 1983.

Sise MJ, Hollingsworth P, and Brimm JE: Complications of the flow-directed pulmonary artery catheter: a prospective analysis in 219 patients, Crit Care Med 9:315-317, 1981.

Skarvan K, Hasse J, and Wolff G: Myocardial transmural pressure in ventilated patients, Intensive Care Med 7:277-283, 1981.

Sketch MH et al: Use of percutaneously inserted venous catheters in coronary care units, Chest 62:684-689, 1972.

Smith P et al: Cardiovascular effects of ventilation with positive airway pressure, Ann Surg 195:121-130, 1982.

Sommers MS, Baas LS, and Beiting AM: Nosocomial infections related to four methods of hemodynamic monitoring, Heart & Lung 16:13-19, 1987.

Sprung CK et al: Prophylactic use of lidocaine to prevent advanced ventricular arrhythmias during pulmonary artery catheterization, Am J Med 75:906-910, 1983.

Stone, JG, Khambatta HJ, and McDaniel DD: Catheter induced pulmonary artery trauma: can it always be averted? J Thorac Cardiovasc Surg 86:146-155, 1983.

Swan HJC: Guidelines for use of balloon-tipped catheter, Am J Cardiol 34:119-120, 1974.

Swan HJC: Balloon flotation catheters: their use in hemodynamic monitoring in clinical practice, JAMA 233:865-867, 1975.

Swan HJC and Shah PK: The rationale for bedside hemodynamic monitoring, J Crit Illness 1:24-28, 1986.

Thomson IR et al: Right bundle-branch block and complete heart block caused by the Swan-Ganz catheter, Anesthesiology 51:359-362, 1979.

Tooker J, Huseby J, and Butler J: The effects of Swan-Ganz catheter height on the wedge pressure—left atrial pressure relationship in edema during positive-pressure ventilation, Am Rev Respir Dis 117:721-726, 1978.

Tuchschmidt J, Mecher C, Wagers P, and Jung R: Elevated pulmonary capillary wedge pressure in a patient with hypovolemia, J Clin Mtrg 3:67-69, 1988.

Tuchschmidt J, and Sharma OP: Impact of hemodynamic monitoring in a medical intensive care unit, Crit Care Med 15:840-843, 1987.

Vaitkus L: Discontinuing PEEP to measure pulmonary capillary wedge pressures (correspondence), N Engl J Med 308:776, 1983.

Weinstein RA: Pressure monitoring devices: overlooked source of nosocomial infection, JAMA 236:936-938, 1976.

West JB, Dollery CT, and Naimark A: Distribution of blood flow in isolated lung: relation to vascular and alveolar pressures, J Appl Physiol 19:713-724, 1964.

West JB: Regional differences in lung, New York, 1977, Academic Press, Inc.

Whalley DG: Hemodynamic monitoring: pulmonary artery catheterization, Can Anesth Soc J 32:299-305, 1985.

Wiedmann HP, Matthay MA, and Matthay RA: Cardiovascular-pulmonary monitoring in the intensive care units, Chest 85:537-549 and 656-668, 1984.

Williams WH et al: Use of blood gas values to estimate the source of blood withdrawn from a wedged flow-directed catheter in critically ill patients, Crit Care Med 10:636-640, 1982.

Yang SS, Bentivoglio L, Maranhao V, and Goldberg H: From cardiac catheterization data to hemodynamic parameters, Philadelphia, 1972, FA Davis Co.

Chapter 6

Intra-arterial Pressure Monitoring

In 1733 the Reverend Stephen Hales cannulated the femoral artery of a horse and recorded the first direct intra-arterial pressure measurement. With the use of a 12-foot brass pipe, he measured the height to which the blood rose (8 feet 3 inches, which is equivalent to 190 mm Hg). This manometrically measured pressure represented the mean femoral arterial pressure. Although numerous other techniques for measurement of arterial blood pressure were developed after that time, they all measured only the mean arterial pressure. It was not until the beginning of the twentieth century that Otto Frank, a German scientist, developed an optical-recording system that was able to measure the high-fidelity components of the pulsatile arterial pressure (systole, diastole, dicrotic notch). Today, intra-arterial measurement of blood pressure has become a cornerstone in the care and management of critically ill patients. Directly measured arterial pressure is not only more accurate, but the ability to visually assess the arterial pulse waveform can often provide important diagnostic information. Additionally, quick access to arterial blood significantly facilitates assessment of blood gases.

PHYSIOLOGIC REVIEW

The arterial blood pressure is generated by the ejection of blood into the arterial vasculature from the LV. The amount of pressure generated is determined by the volume of blood ejected as well as the resistance to ejection within the systemic vascular network. This is best expressed as:

$$\text{Pressure} = \text{Flow} \times \text{Resistance}$$

As blood is ejected into the proximal portion of the aorta, the vessel wall stretches and distends to accommodate the increase in volume. This stretching of an aortic segment is transmitted peripherally along adjacent segments of the aorta, producing a pulse wave that is transmitted through the arterial circulation and felt peripherally as a pulse. The rate at which the pulse wave travels down the aorta is determined by the compliance or distensibility of the arterial system. Decreases in compliance (as seen in elderly patients with arteriosclerosis) result in a rapid transmission of pulse wave. (In a completely rigid tube, the velocity or speed of pulse wave transmission would be extremely fast—approximately the speed of sound in blood!)

As the pulse wave travels peripherally from the central aorta, it changes in shape as well as value. This occurs as a result of reflected waves which summate on the primary systolic wave. (This is somewhat analogous to the phenomenon of dropping a stone in a shallow pond producing ripples or waves that travel peripherally to the shore. Waves that have already reached the shore are reflected backward and on encountering a forward wave, summate it, resulting in a somewhat amplified wave.)

Arterial Pulse Waveform

The arterial pressure waveform resembles the PA pressure waveform in contour, since the same physiologic events occur on the left side of the heart as on the right side of the heart. The value, however, is normally six times greater on the left side of the heart. The arterial pressure is divided into two phases: systole and diastole (Fig. 6-1). Arterial systole begins with the opening of the aortic valve and

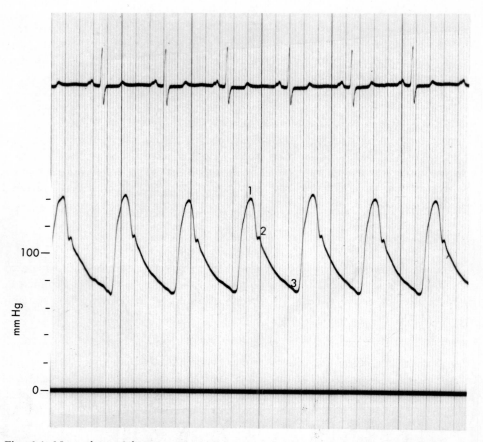

Fig. 6-1. Normal arterial pressure tracing. *1*, Systole; *2*, dicrotic notch; *3*, diastole. (From Daily EK, and Schroeder JS: Hemodynamic waveforms: exercise in identification and analysis, St Louis, 1983, The CV Mosby Co.)

rapid ejection of blood into the aorta. This is followed by runoff of blood from the proximal aorta to the peripheral arteries. On the arterial pressure waveform this is seen as a sharp rise in pressure followed by a decline in pressure. As the pressure falls, the aortic valve snaps shut, causing a small rise in arterial pressure that appears as a dip on the downslope and is termed the *dicrotic notch*. The *peak systolic pressure* (which reflects LV systolic pressure) is normally 100 to 140 mm Hg. Children 10 years old and under have lower systolic blood pressures of less than 100 mm Hg.

Diastole follows closure of the aortic valve and continues until the next systole. During this time, run-off to the peripheral arteries occurs without further flow from the LV. On the arterial pressure waveform this is seen as a gradual decrease in pressure. The lowest point of diastole (actually, end-diastole) is referred to as the *arterial diastolic pressure* and is normally 60 to 80 mm Hg.

The mean arterial pressure represents the average arterial pressure during

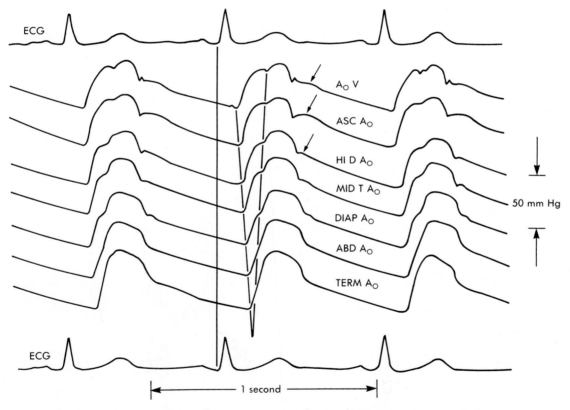

Fig. 6-2. Arterial pressure waveforms as a function of location from the ascending aorta to the iliac bifurcation in one patient. Figure constructed from single or pairs of pulses selected from cardiac cycles with equal R-R intervals and from similar phases of respiration. AoV = sensor just above aortic valve; Asc Ao = ascending aorta; Hi D. Ao = high descending aorta; Mid T. Ao = midthoracic aorta; Term Ao = terminal abdominal aorta just before iliac bifurcation. (From Murgo JP, Westerfol N, Giolma JP, and Altobelli SA: Aortic impedance in normal man: relationship to pressure waveforms, Circ 62:105-116, 1980.)

systole and diastole. Normal mean arterial pressure is 70 to 90 mm Hg. The mean arterial pressure (MAP) is dependent on two factors: (1) the volume of bloodflow through the vessel (cardiac output) and (2) the elasticity or resistance of the vessels (systemic vascular resistance). This interrelation can be expressed as:

$$MAP = Cardiac\ output\ (CO) \times Systemic\ vascular\ resistance\ (SVR)$$

The pulse pressure is the difference between the systolic and diastolic pressure and is largely reflective of the stroke volume and arterial compliance. Wide pulse pres-

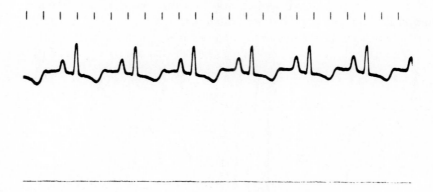

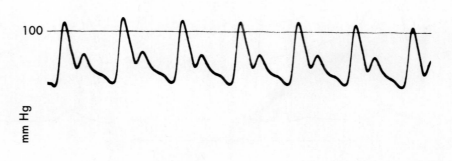

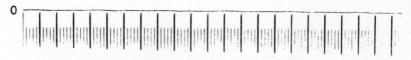

Fig. 6-3. Normal radial arterial waveform.

sures are associated with large stroke volumes, while a narrow pulse pressure is seen in patients with low stroke volume.

The arterial pressure differs in both contour and value in various arterial locations (Fig. 6-2). As mentioned previously, the systolic pressure is higher in the femoral artery than in the radial or brachial artery, by as much as 25 to 50 mm Hg. Generally, the diastolic and mean values remain nearly the same. Additionally, the more distal the location of the arterial catheter, the sharper and later the upstroke and the less defined the dicrotic notch (Fig. 6-3).

ECG correlation

The systolic arterial pressure rise occurs immediately following ventricular depolarization, that is, after the QRS complex on the ECG. Again, there may be some delay, depending on the catheter location and length of tubing used. The dicrotic notch occurs after the T wave of the ECG.

In atrial fibrillation the arterial pressure value varies considerably (Fig. 6-4), depending on the RR intervals and length of time for ventricular filling. However, the normal characteristics of the waveform are still present.

When a PVC occurs, ventricular systole is initiated early, before the LV has had time to fill with blood. This results in a diminished stroke volume and lowered arterial pulse pressure (Fig. 6-5). Isolated PVCs are usually well compensated for by a pause and an increase in stroke volume and arterial pressure with the succeeding contraction. Runs of PVCs, however, can be devastating, since there is virtually no opportunity for LV filling and, therefore stroke volume and arterial pressure fall precipitously (Fig. 6-6).

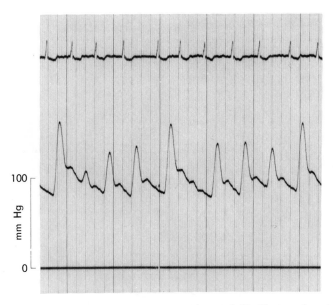

Fig. 6-4. Arterial pressure tracing of a patient with atrial fibrillation showing the marked beat-to-beat variation in peak systolic pressure, dependent on the length of the previous R-R interval.

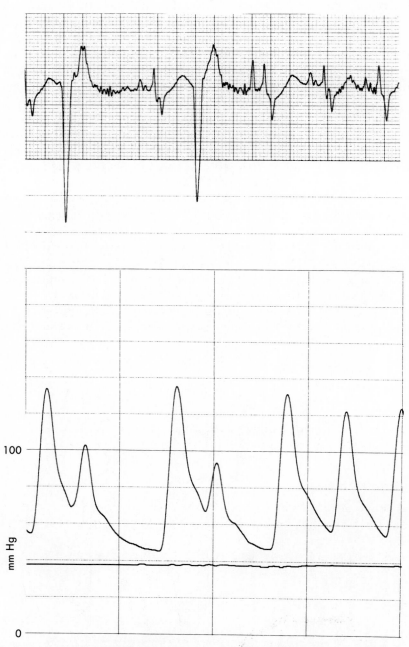

Fig. 6-5. Arterial pressure waveform demonstrating decreased pulse pressure associated with a PVC. Arterial hypertension and waveform contour reflect aortic regurgitation.

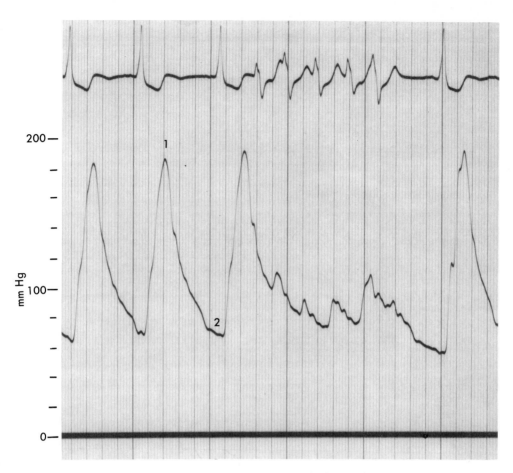

Fig. 6-6. Arterial pressure waveform demonstrating marked reduction in stroke volume and pulse pressure associated with a run of PVC's. (1 = systole; 2 = end-diastole.)

Abnormal findings

In addition to undergoing changes as it travels distally, or in association with certain dysrhythmias, the arterial pulse wave can exhibit changes that are related to specific underlying pathology.

The arterial pressure is elevated in the following conditions:
1. Systemic hypertension
2. Arteriosclerosis
3. Aortic insufficiency

The arterial pressure waveform with aortic insufficiency classically reveals a wide pulse pressure with an elevated systolic pressure and a lowered diastolic pressure (Fig. 6-7). This is a result of rapid ejection of a large stroke volume (the normal stroke volume plus the regurgitant volume), with regurgitation of blood across the incompetent aortic valve during diastole. Also, the dicrotic notch on the downslope of the arterial pressure is usually absent.

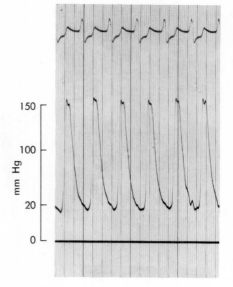

Fig. 6-7. Arterial pressure tracing in patient with aortic insufficiency. Note the wide pulse pressure with elevated systolic pressure of 150 mm Hg and low diastolic pressure of 20 mm Hg.

Additionally, certain drugs, including vasopressors and certain positive inotropic agents, can markedly increase arterial pressure by increasing systemic vascular resistance and/or increasing cardiac output.

The arterial pressure may be abnormally low in the following conditions:

1. Low cardiac output
2. Aortic stenosis
3. Arrhythmias

The contour of the arterial pressure waveform with low cardiac output or even the state of shock is normal, but the systolic value is abnormally low. However, the pulse pressure is narrow because of the small stroke volume ejected each beat. This is called pulsus parvus (Fig. 6-8).

Both the contour and the value of the arterial pressure are altered with aortic stenosis. Because of the increased resistance to ejection of blood through the narrowed aortic valve orifice, the upstroke of the arterial pressure waveform is slow and appears to rise at an angle rather than straight up (Fig. 6-9). Often the dicrotic notch is not well defined and may appear as a "bend" on the downslope of the arterial pressure waveform. This is caused by the stiff closing movement of diseased aortic valve leaflets, which does not produce a rise in pressure. The value of the arterial pressure is low with a narrow pulse pressure, indicating a low stroke volume. It should be mentioned here that the contour of a damped arterial waveform closely resembles the arterial waveform of aortic stenosis (Fig. 6-10).

Other distinct pathological changes in the configuration of the arterial pressure waveform include:

1. Pulsus bisferiens
2. Pulsus alternans
3. Pulsus paradoxus

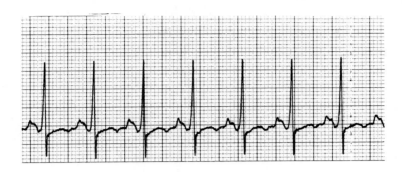

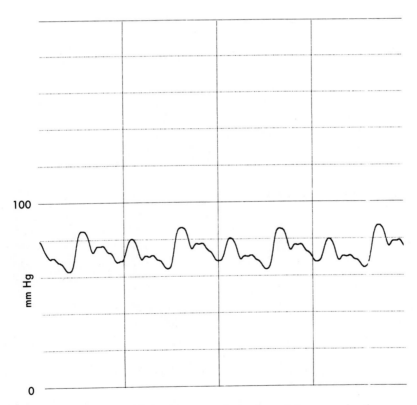

Fig. 6-8. Arterial pressure waveform demonstrating pulsus alternans and pulsus parvus as a result of a low stroke volume in a patient suffering an acute MI.

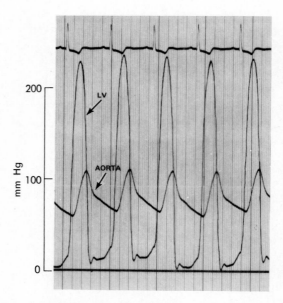

Fig. 6-9. Simultaneous LV and aortic pressure tracings showing marked pressure difference during systole because of severe aortic stenosis. Note the slow upstroke of the aortic pressure tracing.

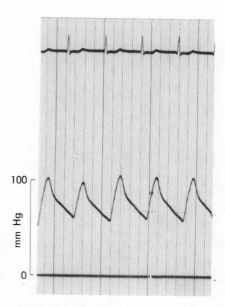

Fig. 6-10. Overdamped arterial pressure waveform with poor upstroke and loss of dicrotic notch. Note similarity to pressure waveform of aortic stenosis.

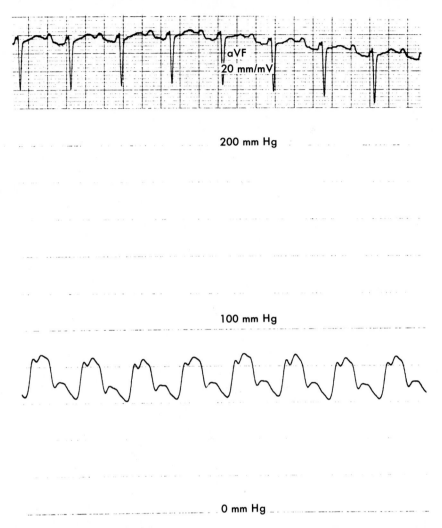

aVF
20 mm/mV

200 mm Hg

100 mm Hg

0 mm Hg

Fig. 6-11. Arterial pressure waveform demonstrating bisferiens or "double-peaked" systolic waveform in a patient with hypertrophic cardiomyopathy.

Pulsus bisferiens describes an arterial pulse with two distinct systolic peaks (Fig. 6-11). This characteristic feature may be found in patients with aortic regurgitation or, more commonly, hypertrophic cardiomyopathy. The first peak is produced by rapid, forceful ejection of blood into the aorta. The pressure then declines slightly (in hypertrophic cardiomyopathy this is because of a severe obstruction during midsystole) and is followed by a smaller pressure rise produced by continued ventricular contraction.

Pulsus alternans refers to a regular, alternating pattern of changes in pressure pulse amplitude, with every other pulse being slightly greater than the previous one (Fig. 6-12). Generally, it is a result of alternating ventricular contractility and subsequent stroke volume, and it commonly occurs in patients with severe LV failure.

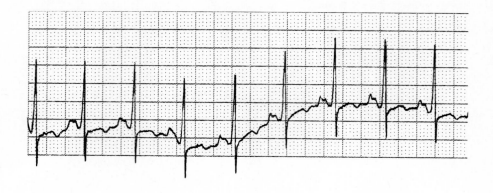

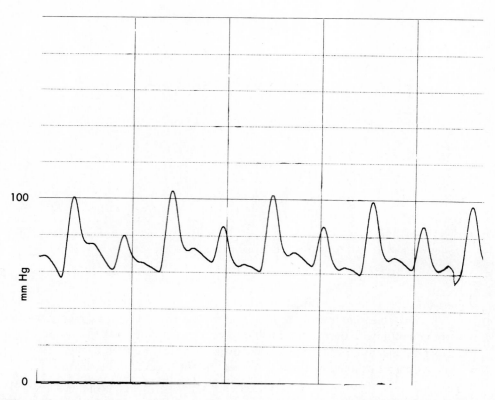

Fig. 6-12. Arterial pressure waveform demonstrating pulsus alternans as a result of alternating stroke volume.

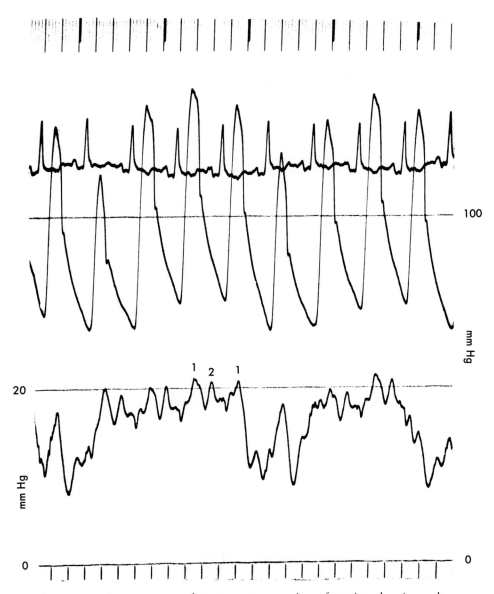

Fig. 6-13. Arterial pressure waveform on upper portion of tracing showing pulsus para-doxus of approximately 18 mm Hg in a patient with cardiac tamponade. On the lower por-tion of the tracing is a simultaneous RA waveform demonstrating an elevated pressure and an Xy pattern (*1* = *a* wave; *2* = *v* wave.)

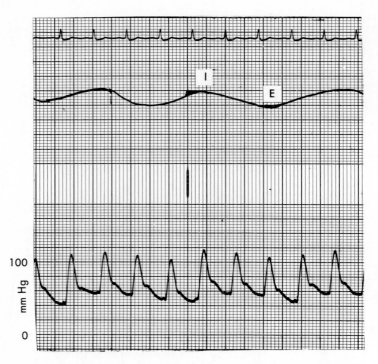

Fig. 6-14. Arterial pressure waveform demonstrating mild reversed pulsus paradoxus with an increase of approximately 14 mm Hg during mechanical inhalation. (Note pneumotachograph on upper portion of tracing indicating inhalation *(I)* and exhalation *(E)*.)

Pulsus alternans can also occur transiently following temporary arrhythmic episodes.

Pulsus paradoxus was first described by Kussmaul as a paradoxical disappearance of peripheral arterial pulsations during inspiration despite continued regular heart beats. When the systolic arterial pressure declines more than 10 mm Hg during normal spontaneous inspiration, pulsus paradoxus is said to exist (Fig. 6-13). (This phenomenon is observed most easily from the displayed intra-arterial pressure; however, it can also be obtained, although less easily, from the noninvasive indirect blood pressure measurement.) Pulsus paradoxus is classically seen in cases of cardiac tamponade (about 70% to 80%), but can also be seen in patients with obstructed airway disease and, less commonly, in hypovolemic shock and pulmonary embolism.

Reversed or positive pulsus paradoxus is a phenomenon describing an exaggerated *rise* in systolic arterial pressure (>10 mm Hg) during inspiration in patients receiving positive pressure ventilation (Fig. 6-14). This variation in systolic pressure is thought to accurately reflect hypovolemia in patients on positive pressure ventilation and usually disappears with appropriate volume therapy.

The effects of arrhythmias on the arterial pressure waveform are discussed under the ECG correlation section.

Certain drugs, including vasodilators and certain calcium antagonists, can also decrease arterial blood pressure by decreasing systemic vascular resistance.

Abnormalities of the arterial pressure waveform may result from mechanical causes of damping, fling, or whip or inaccurate zeroing or calibrating. Damping produces an arterial pressure waveform similar to that of aortic stenosis, that is, a slow upstroke, rounded appearance, poorly defined dicrotic notch, and narrow pulse pressure (see Fig. 6-10). A clot at the tip of the catheter or lodging of the catheter tip against the vessel wall is usually the cause, and gentle flushing or repositioning of the catheter tip eliminates this problem. Fling or whip in the arterial pressure waveform may be a result of excessive movement of the catheter tip or an underdamped monitoring system.

Because of the high frequency components within the arterial pulse wave, distortion caused by inadequate dynamic response characteristics of the monitoring system is the major reason for inaccuracies in direct arterial pressure monitoring. This becomes emphasized in the presence of tachycardia, which further increases the frequency response requirements of the monitoring system. Since the resonant or natural frequency and the damping coefficient of the monitoring system can be assessed in such a practical and simple way at the bedside, (see the discussion in Chapter 3) it is highly recommended that frequent checks of the system be performed.

Fling occurs in the pressure waveform when there is excessive catheter movement in the artery or, more commonly, when the catheter tip faces "upstream" into the flow. It can also occur when excess tubing is used, when the heart rate is very rapid, or when the rate of pressure rise (dP/dT) is rapid. Fling is characterized by rapid, sharp negative or positive waves, particularly during systole (Fig. 6-15).

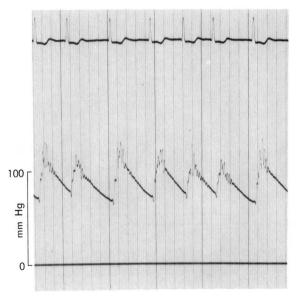

Fig. 6-15. Aortic pressure tracing showing fling caused by turbulent blood flow resulting in vibration during each systole.

Fling can usually be reduced or eliminated by moving the catheter tip, reducing the tubing length, or using a damping device.

Table 6-1 describes some causes of inaccurate arterial pressure measurement.

Vasodilators (including certain calcium antagonists) affect both the contour and the value of the arterial pressure waveform. The decreased systemic vascular resistance and impedance to flow during afterload reduction cause a rapid upstroke of the arterial systolic pressure, a rapid decline in systolic pressure during the reduced ejection phase, and less change in pressure during diastole (the period of resistance-reduced runoff) (Fig. 6-16). The value of both the systolic and diastolic

Table 6-1. Inaccurate arterial pressure measurements

Problem	Cause	Prevention	Treatment
Damped pressure tracing	Catheter tip against vessel wall	Usually cannot be avoided.	Pull back, rotate, or reposition catheter while observing pressure waveform.
	Partial occlusion of catheter tip by clot	Use continuous drip under pressure. Briefly "fast flush" after blood withdrawal (<2 to 4 ml) Adding 1 unit heparin/1 ml IV fluid may help.	Aspirate clot with syringe and flush with heparinized saline (<2 to 4 ml).
	Clot in stopcock or transducer	Carefully flush catheter after blood withdrawal and reestablish IV drip. Use continuous flush device.	Flush stopcock and transducer; if no improvement, change stopcock and transducer.
Abnormally high or low readings	Change in transducer reference level	Maintain air-reference port of transducer at midchest and/or catheter tip level for serial pressure measurements.	Recheck patient and transducer positions.
Damped pressure without improvement after flushing	Air bubbles in transducer or connector tubing	Carefully flush transducer and tubing when setting up system and attaching to catheter.	Check system; flush rapidly; disconnect transducer and flush out air bubbles.
	Compliant tubing	Use stiff, short tubing.	Shorten tubing or replace softer tubing with stiffer tubing.
No pressure available	Transducer not open to catheter Settings on monitor amplifiers incorrect—still on *zero, cal,* or *off*	Follow routine, systematic steps for setting up system and turning stopcocks.	Check system— stopcocks, monitor, and amplifier setup.
	Incorrect scale selection	Select scale appropriate to expected range of physiologic signal.	Select appropriate scale.

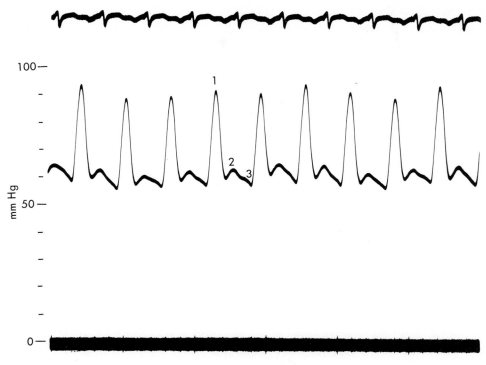

Fig. 6-16. Arterial pressure waveform in a patient receiving nitroprusside infusion. Note the rapid upstroke and decline of the arterial waveform as a result of afterload reduction. (1 = systole; 2 = dicrotic notch; 3 = end-diastole.)

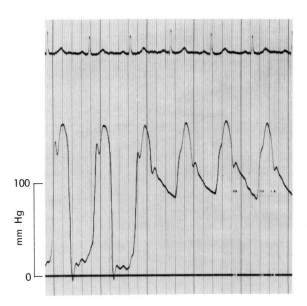

Fig. 6-17. Pullback tracing of a catheter from the left ventricle across the aortic valve into the aorta. Note that the systolic pressures are the same and that there is no LV-aortic pressure gradient.

pressures are often reduced, although it is possible to greatly enhance the cardiac output and thereby cause little change in the arterial pressures.

CLINICAL APPLICATIONS

Data obtained from direct arterial pressure provide important information regarding cardiac performance as well as vascular conditions.

In the absence of aortic stenosis, the peak systolic arterial pressure reflects the maximum pressure generated by the LV (Fig. 6-17). In addition, systolic pressure is frequently used to monitor *afterload*. Afterload is defined as LV wall tension during systole. The two principal determinants are systolic pressure and the radius of the left ventricle. During hemodynamic monitoring, the radius or size of the left ventricle (related to LV volume) is assumed to remain relatively constant, and therefore the systolic arterial pressure is the single parameter used to clinically monitor afterload.

The *diastolic arterial pressure* reflects both the velocity of runoff and the elasticity of the arterial system. The elastic properties of the vessels affect the arterial system's ability to change luminal dimensions as the blood volume changes. Heart rate also affects the diastolic pressure, since it determines the duration of diastole in the cardiac cycle. The longer the period of diastole (bradycardia), the further the fall of the diastolic pressure. Conversely, the shorter the diastolic period (with tachycardia), the higher the diastolic pressure.

The diastolic arterial pressure is also important in determining coronary artery perfusion, particularly to the left ventricle, where most flow occurs during diastole. Coronary artery perfusion pressure (CPP) is calculated as:

$$CPP = \text{Diastolic Arterial Pressure} - \text{LVEDP (or PAWp)}$$

Normal coronary artery perfusion pressure is 60 to 80 mm Hg. Perfusion pressures below 50 mm Hg threaten myocardial perfusion. Efforts to maintain adequate CPP include increasing the diastolic arterial pressure, and/or decreasing the PAW pressure.

The mean arterial pressure (MAP) represents the average pressure within the arterial system. Since diastole typically lasts approximately two thirds of the entire cardiac cycle, the mean pressure value is closer to the diastolic value than the systolic value. The mean pressure can be mathematically estimated by the following equation:

$$\text{Mean arterial pressure (MAP)} = \frac{\text{Systolic pressure} + (\text{Diastolic pressure} \times 2)}{3}$$

Mean arterial pressure is determined by flow and resistance in the following way:

$$\text{MAP} = \text{Cardiac output (CO)} \times \text{Systemic vascular resistance (SVR)}$$

Looking at the above formula, it is clear that a change in flow or CO without a change in SVR will cause a corresponding change in mean arterial pressure. This is true whether the increase in CO is accomplished by an increase in stroke volume, an increase in heart rate, or both.

EXAMPLE: If the patient's cardiac output is 5 L/min and SVR is 20 units, the MAP is 100 mm Hg.

$$MAP = CO \times SVR$$

$$100 = 5 \times 20$$

A sudden increase in the CO to 8 L/min without a change in the SVR would increase the MAP to 160 mm Hg.

$$160 = 8 \times 20$$

According to Poiseuille's law, resistance (SVR) is determined by length, viscosity, and the reciprocal of the radius raised to the fourth power (R^4) as follows:

$$SVR = \frac{8 \text{ Length} \times \text{Viscosity}}{\pi R^4}$$

Since length does not alter after completion of growth and viscosity remains relatively constant (except in hemorrhage, polycythemia, or marked temperature changes), the radius of the arterial vessels remains the primary determinant of changes in resistance. The formula for mean arterial pressure can therefore be rewritten as

$$MAP = CO \times \text{Viscosity} \times (L/R^4)$$

Clearly, even very small changes in the diameter of the major resistance vessels (the arterioles) result in large changes in pressure. For example, doubling the radius of the arterial vessels (with an arterial vasodilator) would decrease the mean arterial pressure by a factor of 16 if the CO remained constant.

Rapid adjustment of the SVR in response to changes in position, activity, and stress normally maintains a narrow range of blood pressure. In the patient with cardiac disease, however, as the left ventricle fails and cardiac output falls, stimulation of the baroreceptors causes vasoconstriction and the SVR rises in an attempt to maintain adequate blood pressure. This increase in afterload or impedance to LV ejection can aggravate the failing heart and further decrease the stroke volume. With pharmacologic afterload reduction, a decrease in resistance may allow an increase in stroke volume without a significant fall in blood pressure, as shown in the following example:

EXAMPLE: Afterload reduction decreased SVR to 15 units and increased CO to 7 L/min, resulting in a MAP of 105 mm Hg, essentially unchanged from the original MAP of 100 mm Hg.

$$105 \text{ mm Hg} = 7 \text{ L/min} \times 15 \text{ units}$$

Direct measurement of the SVR is not possible but can be simply calculated using the previous formula rewritten as:

$$SVR = \frac{MAP}{CO}$$

EXAMPLE: If the patient's CO is 5 L/min and MAP is 100 mm Hg, the SVR is 20 units.

$$SVR \text{ (units)} = MAP \text{ (mm Hg)} \div CO \text{ (L/min)}$$

$$20 \text{ units} = 100 \text{ mm Hg} \div 5 \text{ L/min}$$

Resistance is also expressed in absolute resistance units (dynes/sec/cm^{-5}). This is achieved simply by multiplying the number of units by 80.

EXAMPLE: 20 units $\times$ 80 = 1600 dynes/sec/cm^{-5}

More accurate calculation of SVR is obtained when the pressure difference between the proximal and distal ends of the cardiovascular system (arterial and venous) is divided by the CO. The formula is:

$$SVR = \frac{MAP - RAm}{CO}$$

Since the RA pressure is generally quite low, the venous pressure may not be included in calculating SVR. If, however, the RA pressure is significantly elevated, it should be subtracted from the MAP to obtain a true driving pressure.

NORMAL VALUES FOR SVR: 15 to 20 units
900 to 1400 dynes/sec/cm^{-5}

The systemic arterial pressure determines the perfusion of the body tissues, including not only muscle, skin, and extremities but more critical organs such as the brain, heart, and kidneys. By varying the degree of vasoconstriction or vasodilation, some organs can partially regulate the amount of blood flow through them. Over 70% of the coronary blood flow occurs during diastole. Because of this and because the heart tissues have a very high extraction ratio of oxygen from hemoglobin, the heart is quite sensitive to hypotension. There are no clinically applicable bedside techniques presently available for monitoring the amount or sufficiency of coronary blood flow. Renal blood flow and perfusion may be partially monitored by urinary flow, but renal autoregulation of this flow does not allow a direct correlation between the two. Thus the health of the body tissues depends on an adequately functioning heart and vascular system to supply an appropriate flow *and* perfusion pressures that are adequate to deliver blood throughout the body.

INTRA-ARTERIAL PRESSURE MEASUREMENT

Arterial pressure can be measured indirectly (with an occluding cuff or with Doppler flow techniques) or directly via a catheter placed into an artery. Automated blood pressure equipment is also now in use in many areas of the hospital for patients who require frequent blood pressure checks. This method is very useful and reliable in patients who are normotensive and clinically stable but is not useful in critically ill patients. In these patients direct arterial pressure monitoring is necessary to accurately measure systolic and diastolic pressure, particularly in the presence of vasoconstriction, which makes indirect measurements difficult to obtain.

Direct arterial pressure can be measured via a transducer or an anaeroid manometer connected to a small Teflon catheter inserted into a peripheral artery. Transduced pressures provide systolic, diastolic, and mean values as well as a displayed arterial waveform. Use of an anaeroid manometer is a simple, practical way of measuring the MAP.

Use of a Transducer

A pressure transducer, monitoring equipment, and an oscilloscope permit direct monitoring of systolic, diastolic, and mean arterial pressure on a continuous basis (Fig. 6-18). Equipment preparation and setup is the same as for PA monitoring (see p. 132). Ideally, the transducer should be placed as close to the catheter as is practically possible. Special attention should also be made to carefully remove even the smallest of air bubbles from the system. This is not only to prevent the inadvertent injection of air into the arterial system, but also to improve the dynamic response of the monitoring system. Even a very tiny air bubble can reduce the resonant frequency to approximately 10 Hz (which is well within the frequency range of the arterial pressure wave) producing an inaccurate pressure reading (see the discussion in Chapter 3).

Discrepancies frequently exist between cuff and directly measured arterial pressures. An "occluded blood pressure" measurement is sometimes used to determine the actual systolic blood pressure. In this technique, a blood pressure cuff is placed over the brachial artery on the ipsilateral arm of the cannulated artery. While observing the arterial waveform on the oscilloscope, the cuff is inflated until the char-

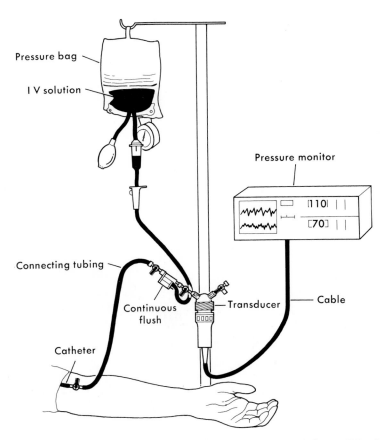

Fig. 6-18. Connections between the arterial catheter, pressure transducer, IV solution, and pressure monitor.

acteristic waveform is no longer present. The cuff is then slowly released until the arterial waveform reappears. The mercury and gauge reading noted when the waveform reappears represents the systolic arterial pressure. While this technique may provide some idea regarding the discrepancy between the direct and indirect blood pressure measurements, assessment of the dynamic response of the monitoring system should also be checked and the system optimized following the directions in Chapter 3.

Another described method to determine the actual arterial systolic pressure when a discrepancy exists between cuff and directly measured arterial pressures involves the use of the pulse oximeter. Using this technique, the blood pressure cuff, placed on the same arm as the pulse sensor, is inflated until the pulse oximeter ceases to sense pulsations. The mercury or gauge reading noted at this precise point is thought to reflect the actual systolic arterial pressure. However, this technique needs to be tried in a variety of critical care settings and on a larger number of patients before it can be recommended as a reliable method.

Significant differences may also exist between the digitally displayed arterial systolic pressure and that recorded on a paper writeout or strip recorder. Some of

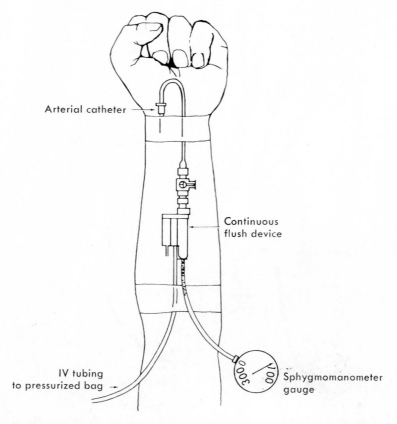

Fig. 6-19. Mean arterial pressure monitoring device with a sphygmomanometer gauge and a continuous flush device.

this may be the result of large changes during portions of the respiratory cycle, but greater differences have been noted in the presence of hypertension, hypotension, or dysrhythmias. As with the PA and PAW pressures, measurement of arterial pressures should be obtained at end-expiration from a strip chart recording.

Monitoring with a standard anaeroid sphygmomanometer gauge. A simple, inexpensive method of continuously monitoring mean intra-arterial pressure is to connect a standard anaeroid sphygmomanometer gauge to an intra-arterial catheter (Fig. 6-19). The manometer is protected from the fluid by an air column in the proximal part of a connecting tubing. This arrangement results in a damped or mean pressure that can be read directly from the manometer. Problems with catheter patency are the same as those with other intra-arterial pressure systems. A continuous flush device can be attached for improved patency. Thus, in addition to continuous mean pressure measurement, this arterial catheter system permits blood sampling and flushing through a stopcock and continuous IV flow and flushing.

The advantages of this system are its simplicity, low cost, avoidance of expensive and complex electronic equipment, continuous availability of the measurement, and avoidance of connectors away from the patient.

Table 6-2. Problems encountered with arterial catheters

Problem	Cause	Prevention	Treatment
Hematoma after withdrawal of needle	Bleeding or oozing at puncture site	Maintain firm pressure on site during withdrawal of catheter and for 5 to 15 min (as necessary) after withdrawal. Apply elastic tape (Elastoplast) firmly over puncture site.	Continue to hold pressure to puncture site until oozing stops.
		For femoral arterial puncture sites, leave a sandbag on site for 1 to 2 hr to prevent oozing. If patient is receiving heparin, discontinue 2 hr before catheter removal.	Apply sandbag to femoral puncture site for 1 to 2 hr after removal of catheter.
Decreased or absent pulse distal to puncture site	Spasm of artery	Introduce arterial needle cleanly, nontraumatically.	Inject lidocaine locally at insertion site and 10 mg into arterial catheter.
	Thrombosis of artery		Arteriotomy and Fogarty catheterization both distally and proximally from the puncture site result in return of pulse in more than 90% of cases if brachial or femoral artery is used.

(Continued)

Table 6-2. Problems encountered with arterial catheters—cont'd

Problem	Cause	Prevention	Treatment
Bleedback into tubing, dome, or transducer	Insufficient pressure on IV bag Loose connections	Maintain 300 mm Hg pressure on IV bag. Use Luer-Lok stopcocks.	Replace transducer. "Fast flush" through system. Tighten all connections.
Hemorrhage	Loose connections	Keep all connecting sites visible. Observe connecting sites frequently. Use built-in alarm system. Use Luer-Lok stopcocks.	Tighten all connections.
Emboli	Clot from catheter tip into bloodstream	Always aspirate and discard before flushing. Use continuous flush device. Use 1 unit heparin/1 ml IV fluid. Gently flush <2 to 4 ml.	Remove catheter.
Local infection	Forward movement of contaminated catheter Break in sterile technique Prolonged catheter use	Carefully suture catheter at insertion site. Always use aseptic technique. Remove catheter after 72 to 96 hr. Inspect and care for insertion site daily, including dressing change and antibiotic or iodophor ointment.	Remove catheter. Prescribe antibiotic.
Sepsis	Break in sterile technique Prolonged catheter use Bacterial growth in IV-fluid	Use percutaneous insertion. Always use aseptic technique. Remove catheter after 72 to 96 hr. Change IV fluid bag, stopcocks, dome, and tubing every 24 to 48 hr. Do not use IV fluid containing glucose. Sterilize transducers before use (if nondisposable transducers used). Use sterile dead-ender caps on all ports of stopcocks. Carefully flush remaining blood from stopcocks after blood sampling.	Remove catheter. Prescribe antibiotic.

The disadvantages include difficulties maintaining sterility, ease of retrograde flow of blood or IV fluid into the manometer, and damping of the pressure yielding a "mean" pressure only. Several commercial units are available that provide more complex methods of preventing retrograde flow of fluid.

Sterilization of the pressure gauge before its connection to the arterial catheter is recommended. The pressure gauge may be gas sterilized with ethylene oxide but should not be autoclaved or submerged in cold disinfectant.

Tables 6-2 and 6-3 describe the causes, prevention, and treatment of problems frequently encountered with intra-arterial catheters and suggestions for optimizing arterial monitoring.

Maintenance of catheter patency. Maintaining catheter patency can be a greater problem with an arterial catheter than with a venous catheter, since the arterial catheter is a high-pressure system.

An effective method of maintaining catheter patency is to use a pressure bag setup and continuous flush device, as shown in Fig. 6-18. The setup is the same as for the PA catheter outlined on p. 132. The continuous flush device allows a flow of approximately 2 to 5 ml/hr of IV fluid into the arterial catheter; this amount of fluid is usually sufficient to maintain catheter patency while not altering the measured pressure. Additionally, most continuous flush devices allow the rapid delivery of fluid (between 0.75 and 1.5 ml/sec) when the flush valve is completely open.

Thrombus formation almost invariably occurs, to at least a small degree, on the catheter tip and on the entire catheter surface. Flushing of this material creates an embolus that is carried distally and may occlude a small critical artery (for example, to a finger). To prevent this serious complication, the catheter should be aspirated before flushing, and the blood, which may contain a clot from the catheter tip in it, should be discarded. This should be followed by gentle flushing of small volumes (2 to 4 ml) of solution to prevent embolization. If flushing is performed

Table 6-3. Guide for optimal arterial monitoring

Procedure	Reason
Label IV tubing of arterial line as "artery" or "arterial line."	Visual aid may help to avoid confusion with venous lines.
Keep pressure bag inflated to pressure greater than patient's arterial pressure.	Slow deflation of bag will result in blood flow back into tubing.
Maintain constant fluid flow with continuous flush device (2 to 4 ml/hr).	Constant fluid flow maintains patency and prevents clotting.
Check all connections.	Loose connections can introduce air or allow blood loss.
Immobilize extremity.	Extremity movement can result in needle or catheter displacement.
Keep all connectors and puncture sites visible.	Possible bleeding may be observed.
Frequently check pulse distal to puncture site.	Weakening or loss of pulse may indicate thrombosis.
Check circulation, movement, and sensation of extremity distal to puncture site.	Any changes in circulation, movement, or sensation may indicate hematoma formation.
Label date of catheter insertion on dressing.	Removal of catheter after 72 to 96 hr may reduce risk of infection.

with the continuous flush device, the flush valve should be opened only for a few seconds. This precaution is based on Lowenstein, Little, and Low's study showing that a vigorous flush of as little as 7 ml of fluid into a radial artery catheter could reach the aortic arch and possibly result in cerebral embolization.

It is very important that the extremity with the arterial line be left uncovered, so that it may be easily observed for bleeding caused by loose connections in the line. An alarm should also be built into the monitoring system to alert the nurse if the arterial line should become disconnected. An arterial line requires close and frequent observation, since a loose connection could allow potentially fatal bleeding from the catheterized artery. The pulse distal to the arterial catheters should be checked every 2 hours for early signs of compromise or absence that may indicate thrombosis. Circulation and movement of the extremity distal to the arterial catheter should also be checked every 2 hours.

The transducer should be kept filled with IV fluid during use and free of air bubbles and blood. If blood does back up into the transducer for any reason, the transducer should be disconnected from the patient and carefully flushed or replaced. (Disposable domes must be replaced after defibrillation that damages the dome membrane and renders it unsterile.)

Prevention of Infection of Arterial Lines

Studies of the bacterial contamination of stopcocks connected to arterial lines have reported positive cultures in 15% to as high as 50% of patients with arterial lines. In many instances this high contamination rate most likely reflects nosocomial contamination during blood sampling. Cultures from arterial site catheters have also shown contamination at the tip of the catheter, although these studies have been of limited value because of the difficulty in determining whether contamination was present while the catheter was indwelling or at the time of withdrawal for study or replacement. The recommendations made for arterial sampling procedures outlined in the next section therefore should be followed.

Arterial Blood Sampling

Arterial blood gas measurements are frequently obtained in the critically ill patient to monitor and identify any dysfunctions of the metabolic, respiratory, or cardiovascular systems. An indwelling arterial catheter facilitates frequent evaluation of these parameters. The steps for obtaining arterial blood from an arterial catheter for blood gas analysis are the following:

1. Turn the arterial stopcock off to the IV solution, remove the dead-ender cap from the sideport, and withdraw and *discard* 5 ml of blood. This will rid the catheter of IV solution. A study by Molter indicates that withdrawal of a lesser amount of volume (as little as 1 ml) is sufficient to adequately clear the line of IV solution. The requisite amount of blood to be withdrawn and discarded depends, of course, on the amount of dead space volume between the catheter tip and the sampling site. This study indicates that withdrawal of 2.5 times the dead space volume before blood sampling is sufficient for accurate blood gas analysis.

2. Through the same port, withdraw 5 ml of arterial blood using a sterile, heparin-coated syringe.

3. Remove the syringe, turn the arterial catheter stopcock to resume IV flow, and

briefly "fast flush" the line with the use of the continuous flush device.

4. Immediately remove any air bubbles from the arterial blood sample. (Presence of air bubbles in the sample would alter the values.)

5. Place a cap on the syringe of the arterial blood sample and gently rotate the syringe to mix the blood with the heparin.

6. Place an identification label on the syringe.

7. Immerse the arterial blood sample syringe in an ice bed. (This will reduce oxygen metabolism.)

8. Turn the arterial catheter stopcock off to the catheter and activate the fast flush device to flush blood out of the withdrawal port of the stopcock.

9. Replace a sterile dead-ender cap on the sideport of the stopcock.

10. Turn the arterial catheter stopcock to resume IV flow through the catheter.

REFERENCES

Amato JJ, Solod E, and Cleveland RJ: "Second" radial artery for monitoring perioperative pediatric cardiac patient, J Pediatr Surg 12:715-717, 1977.

Band JD, and Maki DG: Infections caused by arterial catheters used for hemodynamic monitoring, Am J Med 67:735-741, 1979.

Barr PO: Percutaneous puncture of the radial artery with a multipurpose Teflon catheter for indwelling use, Acta Physiol Scand 51:343-347, 1961.

Bartlett RH, and Munster AM: An improved technique for prolonged arterial cannulation, N Engl J Med 279:92-93, 1968.

Bedford RF: Radial arterial function following percutaneous cannulation with 18- and 20-gauge catheters, Anesthesiology 47:37-39, 1977.

Brown AE, Sweeney DB, and Lumley J: Percutaneous radial artery cannulation, Anesthesia 24:532-536, 1969.

Bruner JMR, Krenis LJ, Kunsman JM, and Sherman AP: Comparison of direct and indirect methods of measuring arterial blood pressure, Med Instrum 15:11-21, 1981.

Centers for Disease Control: Nosocomial bacteremia for intravascular pressure monitoring systems. In National nosocomial infections study report, 1977 (6-month summaries), Atlanta, 1979, U.S. Department of Health, Education, and Welfare.

Coyle JP, Teplick RS, Long MS, and Davison JK: Respiratory variations in systemic arterial pressure as an indicator of volume status, Anesthesiology 58:A53, 1983.

Crossland SG, and Neviaser RJ: Complications of radial artery catheterization, Hand 9:287-290, 1977.

Curtiss EI, Reddy PS, Uretsky BF, and Cecchetti AA: Pulsus paradoxus: definition and relation to the severity of cardiac tamponade, Am Heart J 115:391-398, 1988.

Davis FM: Radial artery cannulation: influence of catheter size and material on arterial occlusion, Anaesth Intensive Care 6:49-53, 1978.

Donowitz LG et al: Serratia marcescens bacteremia from contaminated pressure transducers, JAMA 242:1749-1751, 1979.

Downs JB, Chapman RL, Jr, and Hawkins IF, Jr: Prolonged radial-artery catheterization: an evaluation of heparinized catheters and continuous irrigation, Arch Surg 108:671-673, 1974.

Friedman HS, Sakura H, and Lajam F: Pulsus paradoxus: a manifestation of a marked reduction of left ventricular end-diastolic volume in cardiac tamponade, J Thoracic Cardiovasc Surg 79:74-82, 1980.

Furman EB, Hairabet JK, and Roman DG: The use of indwelling radial artery needles in paediatric anesthesia, Br J Anaesth 44:531-532, 1972.

Gardner RM: Direct blood pressure dynamic response requirements, Anesthesiology 54:227-236, 1981.

Gardner RM, Schwartz R, Wong HC, and Burke JP: Percutaneous indwelling radial artery catheters for monitoring cardiovascular function: prospective study of the risk of thrombosis and infection, N Engl J Med 290:1227-1231, 1974.

Gardner RM, Warner HR, Toronto AF, and Gaisford WD: Catheter-flush system for continuous monitoring of central arterial pulse waveform, J Appl Physiol 29:911-913, 1970.

Gelberman RH, and Blasingame JP: The timed Allen's test, J Trauma 21:477-479, 1981.

Gloyna DF et al: A comparison of blood pressure measurement techniques in the hypotensive patient, Anesth Analg 63:222, 1984.

Gravlee GP et al: Comparison of brachial, radial, and aortic arterial pressure monitoring during cardiac surgery, Circ VII 61:A69, 1984.

Jones RM et al: The effect of method of radial artery cannulation on post cannulation blood flow and thrombus formation, Anesthesiology 55:76-78, 1981.

Kaye W: Catheter- and infusion-related sepsis: the nature of the problem and its prevention, Heart Lung 11:221-227, 1982.

Kaye W: Invasive monitoring techniques: arterial cannulation, bedside pulmonary artery catheterization, and arterial puncture, Heart Lung 12:395-428, 1983.

Kim JM, Arakawa K, and Bliss J: Arterial cannulation: factors in the development of occlusion, Anesth Analg 54:836-841, 1975.

Lantiegne KC, and Civetta JM: A system for maintaining invasive pressure monitoring, Heart Lung 7:610-621, 1978.

Little JM, Clarke B, and Shanks C: Effects of radial artery cannulation, Med J Aust 2:791-793, 1975.

Llamas R, Gupta S, and Baum G: A simple technique for prolonged arterial cannulation, Schweiz Med Wochenschr 101:1057-1061, 1971.

Loubser PG: Comparison of intra-arterial and automated oscillometric blood pressure measurement in postoperative hypertensive patients, Med Instrum 20:255-259, 1986.

Lowenstein E, Little JW, and Lo HH: Prevention of cerebral embolization from flushing radial-artery cannulas, N Engl J Med 285:1414-1415, 1971.

Maki DG and Hassemer CA: Endemic rate of fluid contamination and related septicemia in arterial pressure monitoring, Am J Med 70:733-738, 1981.

Maloy L, and Gardner RM: Monitoring systemic arterial blood pressure: strip chart recording versus digital display, Heart & Lung 15:627-635, 1986.

Mandel MA, and Dauchot PJ: Radial artery cannulation in 1,000 patients: precautions and complications, J Hand Surg 2:482-485, 1977.

Molter N: Arterial blood gas analysis: a study of sampling techniques from indwelling arterial catheter systems (abstract), Heart Lung 12:428, 1983.

Nystrom E et al: A comparison of automated indirect arterial blood pressure meters: with recordings from a radial arterial catheter in anesthetized surgical patients, Anesthesiology 62:526, 1985.

O'Rourke MF: Pressure and flow waves in systemic arteries and the anatomical design of the arterial system, Jour Appl Physiol 23:139-149, 1967.

Perel A, Pizov R, and Cotev S: The systolic blood pressure variation is a sensitive indicator of hypovelemia in ventilated dogs subjected to graded hemorrhage, Anesthesiology 67:498-502, 1987.

Rothe CF, and Kim KC: Measuring systolic arterial blood pressure. Possible errors from extension tubes or disposable transducer domes, Crit Care Med 8:683-689, 1980.

Rushmer RF: Structure and function of the cardiovascular system, Philadelphia, 1972, WB Saunders Co.

Sabin S, Taylor JR, and Kaplan AI: Clinical experience using a small-gauge needle for arterial puncture, Chest 69:437-439, 1976.

Samaan HA: The hazards of radial artery pressure monitoring, J Cardiovasc Surg 12:342-347, 1971.

Seldinger SI: Catheter replacement of the needle in percutaneous arteriography, Acta Radiol 39:368-376, 1953.

Shinozaki R et al: Bacterial contamination of arterial lines, JAMA 249:223-225, 1983.

Singh S et al: Catheter colonization and bacteremia with pulmonary and arterial catheters, Crit Care Med 10:736-739, 1983.

Slogoff S, Keats AS, and Arlund C: On the safety of radial artery cannulation, Anesthesiology 59:42-47, 1983.

Stamm WE, Colella JJ, Anderson RL, and Dixon RE: Indwelling arterial catheters as a source of nosocomial bacteremia, N Engl J Med 292:1099-1102, 1975.

Yang SS, Bentivoglio L, Maranhao V, and Goldberg H: From cardiac catheterization data to hemodynamic parameters, Philadelphia, 1972, FA Davis Co.

Chapter 7

Cardiac Output Measurements

Cardiac output is the amount of blood ejected by the heart per unit of time and is reported as liters per minute. Although there may be slight discrepancies, the cardiac output of both right and left ventricles is the same unless there is an intracardiac shunt. The importance of considering cardiac output in the evaluation of overall cardiac status and LV performance, as well as its value in the determination of valve areas and resistances, has long been recognized. Even more important is the use of repeated cardiac output measurements to assess a patient's response to therapy.

Three methods of determining cardiac output are (1) the Fick method, (2) the indicator-dilution method, and (3) the thermodilution method. Although each method is sound and has particular advantages and disadvantages (Table 7-1), the thermodilution method is used most commonly at bedside.

PHYSIOLOGIC REVIEW

The function and viability of all body tissues are dependent on an adequate supply of oxygen and nutrients from the circulating blood. This supply is dependent on the flow rate of blood and local tissue diffusion. The heart itself extracts the greatest amount of oxygen from the blood (approximately 70% of the oxygen present in every milliliter of blood). The brain is the next highest extractor of oxygen per milliliter of blood. Deprivation of oxygen supply to brain tissue for more than 2 to 4 minutes can result in severe, irreversible brain damage.

A demand for increased tissue oxygen can be met in two ways: (1) by an increase in flow rate (cardiac output) or (2) by an increase in oxygen extraction from the blood.

Cardiac output is the product of heart rate and stroke volume (CO = HR × SV). Stroke volume is the volume of blood ejected with each heartbeat and is the difference between the volume of the left ventricle at end-diastole (the end of the filling period) and the volume remaining in the ventricle at end-systole (the end of ejection) (Fig. 7-1). Most ventricular filling occurs rapidly early in diastole and is affected by the filling pressure of the left atrium and the distensibility of the ventricular wall. Systolic ejection occurs during contraction of the ventricle and is

Table 7-1. Advantages and disadvantages of the three major methods for determining cardiac output

Method	Advantages	Disadvantages
Fick	Gives accurate results even in presence of low cardiac output states, valvular insufficiencies, and shunts. Gives an indication of patient's pulmonary status. Is considered "gold standard" because of accuracy.	Requires patient to be in constant or steady state. Requires withdrawal of both arterial and venous blood samples (10 to 20 ml). Requires cooperation in collecting expired air (this cooperation may be diffiuclt to get from acutely ill patient). Requires at least two people for simultaneous collection of expired air and blood samples. Requires more time in analyzing samples. Oxygen administraton affects results.
Indicator-dilution	Is more rapidly performed than Fick method. Serial outputs are more easily performed than Fick method. Use of small computer can give results immediately. Is not affected by oxygen administration.	Requires venous and arterial catheters. Is less accurate in patients with low cardiac output, valvular insufficiency, or shunts. Rapid recirculation may affect calculation. Requires proper recording device. Requires withdrawal of arterial blood for each determination. If computer analysis is not available, requires hand measurement and calculation of time-concentration curves.
Thermodilution	Requires only one catheter. Catheter can be inserted at bedside. Does not require blood withdrawal. Is rapidly performed. Gives good reproducibility. Is minimally affected by recirculation. Requires only one person. Is not affected by oxygen administration.	Presents possible electrical hazard if there are damaged thermistor wires in catheter. Indwelling pulmonary artery catheter can be a hazard. Requires proper recording device and computer for calculations. May be inaccurate in low cardiac output state. Is not accurate in presence of shunts or pulmonary or tricuspid insufficiency. Specific heat and gravity of blood changes with hematocrit changes.

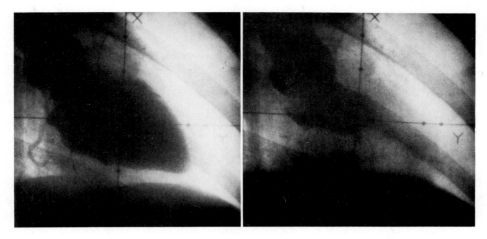

Fig. 7-1. LV angiogram showing the volume of the left ventricle at end-diastole *(left)* and end-systole *(right)*. The upper left corners show the aorta filled with radiopaque dye.

partly dependent on the degree of muscle fiber shortening attained by the ventricle. Starling and his associates found a direct correlation between the diastolic volume (increasing volume causing lengthening of muscle fibers) and the energy released in the following systole (the shortening of muscle fibers). Therefore one way the heart can increase stroke volume is by increasing the diastolic volume and length of muscle fibers, which will result in a greater ejection fraction and stroke volume. This is one of the primary compensatory mechanisms the heart inherently uses to increase cardiac output.

Actual measurements of LV volume are difficult because of the nonsymmetrical shape of the left ventricle and its constantly changing volume during the cardiac cycle. However, a mean stroke volume can be calculated by dividing the cardiac output by the ventricular rate during that period. The normal range of stroke volume is 60 to 130 ml.

Unlike a mechanical pump, whereby a specific amount of fluid is ejected regardless of any change in rate, the heart adapts itself to changes in heart rate. For example, the increased time of diastole that occurs with a slow heart rate allows greater ventricular filling with resultant greater lengthening of the muscle fibers. According to the Frank-Starling law, the result is increased muscle shortening, an increased ejection fraction, and increased stroke volume. Therefore the decrease in heart rate is compensated for by an increase in stroke volume, maintaining a constant average blood flow, or normal cardiac output. Tachycardia, on the other hand, decreases the duration of diastole with minimal effect on the systolic time period. If the tachycardia is excessive, it prevents sufficient time for adequate filling of the LV to occur. This decrease in LV filling results in a reduced stroke volume and a reduced cardiac output in spite of the rapid heart rate. A failing heart will also increase in size (dilate) to try to compensate for a lower efficiency by increasing diastolic volume to effect increased muscle shortening and to improve stroke volume. Tachycardia and cardiac arrhythmias can significantly reduce stroke volume and cardiac output by preventing adequate time for LV filling.

Cardiac output is affected not only by the factors within the heart but by resistance to ejection of the blood from the ventricle (afterload). The higher the systolic blood pressure, the higher is the resistance to ejection of an adequate stroke volume. This factor is particularly serious in a patient with a failing heart and low stroke volume. Reducing peripheral resistance (afterload reduction) increases stroke volume sufficiently so that little or no reduction in blood pressure occurs. This is particularly clear when the formula BP = CO × SVR is reviewed. If the resistance is decreased and the cardiac output is increased, the blood pressure remains nearly the same.

Normal resting cardiac output is 4 to 8 L/min. These values, however, do not take into account the needs of the individual's tissues according to actual body size. Whereas a cardiac output of 4 L/min might be adequate for a person of small stature, it would not be adequate for a larger person. A more specific measurement is the cardiac index, which is the cardiac output per square meter of body surface area (BSA). The body surface area can be obtained from Dubois's height-weight formula (Appendix D). A normal resting cardiac index is 2.5 to 4 L/min/m².

EXAMPLE: A 77 kg man has a cardiac output of 6.7 L/min. He is 180 cm tall and according to the Dubois body surface chart has a BSA of 1.96 m². His cardiac index (CI) is therefore 3.4 L/min/m².

$$CI = \frac{6.7}{1.96} = 3.4 \text{ L/min/m}^2$$

A low cardiac output may be the result of poor filling of the ventricle or poor forward emptying of the ventricle (Table 7-2). A common cause of low resting cardiac output is diminished myocardial function resulting from myocardial infarction.

FICK METHOD
Principle

The Fick method of cardiac output determination (Fig. 7-2) is based on Adolph Fick's principle that the difference between the arterial and mixed venous oxygen concentration reflects oxygen uptake per unit of blood as it flows through the lungs.

Table 7-2. Factors causing low cardiac output

Inadequate LV filling	Inadequate LV ejection
Tachycardia	Coronary artery diseases causing LV ischemia or infarction
Rhythm disturbance	Primary myocardial disorders such as myocarditis, cardiomyopathy
Hypovolemia	
Mitral or tricuspid stenosis	
	Increased afterload
Pulmonic stenosis	Aortic stenosis
Constrictive pericarditis or tamponade	Hypertension
Restrictive cardiomyopathy	Mitral regurgitation
	Drugs with negative inotropic effect
	Metabolic disorders

The amount of oxygen removed from inspired air over a given time period reflects the oxygen consumption of the tissues. If the oxygen saturations of mixed venous blood (flowing into the lungs) and arterial blood (leaving the lungs) are measured, the amount of blood flowing through the lungs can be calculated. The following formula is used to calculate cardiac output:

$$CO \text{ (ml/min)} = \frac{O_2 \text{ consumption (ml/min)}}{\text{Arterial } O_2 \text{ content (vol\%)} - \text{Venous } O_2 \text{ content (vol\%)}}$$

(Vol% = ml O_2/100 ml blood)

EXAMPLE: O_2 consumption = 250 ml/min
Arterial O_2 content = 20 vol%
Mixed venous O_2 content = 15 vol%
Arteriovenous O_2 difference = 5 vol% (20 vol% − 15 vol%)

Using the above formula, the calculation for cardiac output would be:

$$CO = \frac{250 \text{ ml/min}}{20 \text{ vol\%} - 15 \text{ vol\%}} = \frac{250 \text{ ml/min}}{5 \text{ vol\%}} = \frac{250}{0.05} = 5000 \text{ ml/min} = 5 \text{ L/min}$$

Since accurate calculation of the cardiac output with the Fick method requires collection of expired air and P_{O_2} and P_{CO_2} measurements, this method is rarely used for bedside monitioring. Rather, it is the standard against which other methods are validated.

Various instruments, including pulse oximeters and fiberoptic catheters, are available for measuring the oxygen saturation of blood. Since most of these instruments provide a reading in direct percentage of saturation, it is necessary to convert the data to volume percent saturation (oxygen saturation per 100 ml blood) or oxygen content for use in the Fick formula of cardiac output determination. Some instruments that measure oxygen saturation also measure hemoglobin in grams per 100 ml blood. Each gram of hemoglobin is able to carry 1.34 ml of oxygen. This represents the total amount of oxygen that can combine with each gram of hemoglobin. If the oxygen saturation and hemoglobin concentration of the patient's

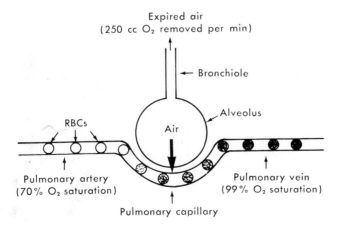

Fig. 7-2. Uptake of oxygen from the alveolus by red blood cells *(RBCs)* in the pulmonary capillary in a person with an oxygen consumption of 250 ml/min. The oxygen taken up is measured in the expired air and represents the body's oxygen consumption.

blood are known, the following formula can be used to calculate volume percent oxygen content:

$$\text{Hemoglobin (g/100 ml)} \times 1.34 \times O_2 \text{ saturation} = \text{vol\% } O_2 \text{ content}$$

> **EXAMPLE:** A patient's venous oxygen saturation is 75%, and the hemoglobin concentration is 15 g/100 ml.
> $$15 \text{ g/100 ml} \times 1.34 \times 0.75 = 15.06 \text{ vol\% } O_2 \text{ content}$$

Some oxygen also combines with the plasma portion of blood and is referred to as dissolved oxygen. (See the discussion on p. 202.) However, the contribution of dissolved oxygen to the cardiac output calculation is minimal and for the purpose of bedside hemodynamic monitoring is usually not included.

The arteriovenous oxygen difference (a-vDo$_2$) is obtained by subtracting the volume percent saturation of mixed venous blood from the volume percent saturation of arterial blood. The normal range of the a-vDo$_2$ is 3 to 5.5 vol%. An arteriovenous oxygen difference greater than 5.5 vol% is seen in patients with a low cardiac output, where an increase in extraction of oxygen by the tissues reduces the venous blood oxygen saturation and thereby widens the a-vDo$_2$.

> **EXAMPLE:** A patient's arterial blood oxygen saturation is 95%, the mixed venous oxygen saturation is 75%, and the hemoglobin concentration is 15 g/100 ml.
> $$15 \text{ g/100 ml} \times 1.34 \times 0.95 = 19.10 \text{ vol\% } \textit{arterial} \text{ } O_2 \text{ content}$$
> $$15 \text{ g/100 ml} \times 1.34 \times 0.75 = 15.06 \text{ vol\% } \textit{venous} \text{ } O_2 \text{ content}$$
>
> $$\text{Arterial } O_2 \text{ content} - \text{Venous } O_2 \text{ content} = \text{a-vDo}_2$$
> $$19.10 \text{ vol\%} - 15.06 \text{ vol\%} = 4.04 \text{ vol\% a-vDo}_2$$

Estimated Calculation of Fick Cardiac Output

At times, an estimation of the cardiac output according to the Fick method is obtained using an expected or normal value for oxygen consumption and a measured arteriovenous oxygen difference (a−vDo$_2$).

The a-vDo$_2$ varies inversely with the cardiac output; that is, the greater the blood flow, the less oxygen is removed per unit of blood and the smaller the arteriovenous oxygen difference. As blood flow decreases, oxygen extraction by tissues will increase and venous blood returning to the heart will be less saturated with oxygen; thus a wide arteriovenous oxygen difference (>5.5 vol%) usually reflects a low cardiac output.

Oxygen consumption, the other factor in this estimated calculation of cardiac output, is presumed to be relatively constant and within the normal range of 110 − 150 ml/min/m^2 (average 125 ml/min/m^2). However, oxygen consumption can vary with changes in body temperature, external work, and restlessness. (See Table 8-5.)

The following steps are taken to *estimate* the cardiac output by the Fick method. The example used is a 180 cm man weighing 80 kg.

1. Using the patient's height and weight, calculate his BSA from Dubois's chart (Appendix D). A man weighing 80 kg who is 180 cm tall has a BSA of 2.00 m^2.
2. Multiply BSA times 125 ml oxygen/min/m^2.

$$2.00 \times 125 = 250 \text{ ml } O_2/\text{min} = \text{Estimated } O_2 \text{ consumption}$$

3. Calculate arterial and venous oxygen contents and hemoglobin (see example above for steps in calculation).

4. Divide the estimated oxygen consumption by the arteriovenous oxygen difference.

$$\frac{250}{4.04} = 61.88 \times 100 = 6188 \text{ ml/min} = 6.19 \text{ L/min CO}$$

THERMODILUTION METHOD
Principle

Fegler described the measurement of cardiac output by thermodilution as early
as 1954. This method applies the indicator-dilution principle, whereby a solution
having a known temperature is injected into the bloodstream and the resulting
temperature change is recorded downstream. Both indicator-dilution and thermodilution involve marking or "tagging" blood elements with either dye or a different temperature and observing the speed with which these particles move over
time. The resultant answer is averaged for an entire minute, giving the average rate
of flow in L/min. The thermodilution method did not gain popular acceptance until
Swan and Ganz introduced a flow-directed, thermal-sensitive catheter, which resulted in a simple, safe, and accurate measurement of cardiac output that could be
easily used in the clinical setting. Its results compare favorably with the Fick and
indicator-dilution methods of measuring blood flow. Because of its rapidity and
minimal recirculation, measurements can be made as frequently as every 60 seconds, and reproducibility is good. An injection of solution, either cold or at room
temperature, can be used as the indicator. The use of room temperature solution
results in less temperature change and requires greater amplification of the temperature-time curve. The principal for both methods is the same.

Technique

A bolus of cold or room temperature fluid is injected into the right atrium
through the proximal lumen of a thermodilution catheter; the resulting temperature change is detected by the thermistor in the catheter tip in the pulmonary artery
and is recorded as a temperature-time curve by the cardiac output computer (Fig.
7-3).

The formula used in calculating the blood flow or cardiac output is based on
the premise that the heat gain recorded when the injectate is mixed with the blood
equals the heat lost by the blood. A certain amount of heat is naturally lost
through handling of the syringe and through the catheter itself before entry into
the right atrium. Although the cardiac output computer adds a constant factor to
the calculations to offset this heat loss, the actual amount of heat lost is not constant and may be responsible for some of the error encountered with the thermodilution method of cardiac output determination. Details of the formula and calculations are not discussed here. They can, however, be found in the article by Forrester and co-workers listed at the end of this chapter.

Equipment

1. Quadruple-lumen, flow-directed thermodilution catheter
2. Closed injectate system (optional if room temperature injectate used)
3. Sterile plastic 10 ml syringe for injection of solution
4. Thermodilution cardiac output computer (COC) with connecting cable

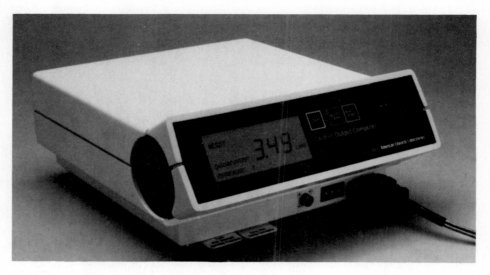

Fig. 7-3. Cardiac output computer for immediate analysis of the thermodilution curve and calculation of the cardiac output. (Courtesy American Edwards Laboratories, Santa Ana, Calif.)

5. Sterile IV solution at room temperature or at 0° to 4° C.
6. Injectate temperature probe
7. IV tubing
8. Ice (if iced injectate used)

   Thermodilution catheters are precalibrated. Immediately before the catheter is inserted, however, its electrical continuity should be tested by connecting the thermistor connector cable to the appropriate catheter hub and depressing the *self-test* button of the COC. If there is some fault with the catheter or the connection, the computer will signal "Faulty catheter." A new catheter should then be used. The balloon of the catheter should also be tested by being filled with the designated amount of air and immersed in sterile water. The appearance of any air bubbles in the water indicates a leak in the balloon, and it should not be used.

Procedure

1. Insert the spiked end of the IV tubing into the solution bag and hang it from an IV pole.
2. If iced injectate solution is used, run the tubing through the prepared closed injectate system (Fig. 7-4).
3. Attach the in-line temperature probe to the distal end of the tubing.
4. Attach a 10 ml syringe to the stopcock port opposite the temperature probe.
5. Attach the distal end of the temperature probe cable to the COC.
6. Completely fill the tubing and ports with IV fluid.
7. Attach the injectate system to the proximal port of the PA catheter via a three-way Luer-Lok stopcock.
8. Attach the thermistor connector cable from the COC to the thermistor hub of the catheter.

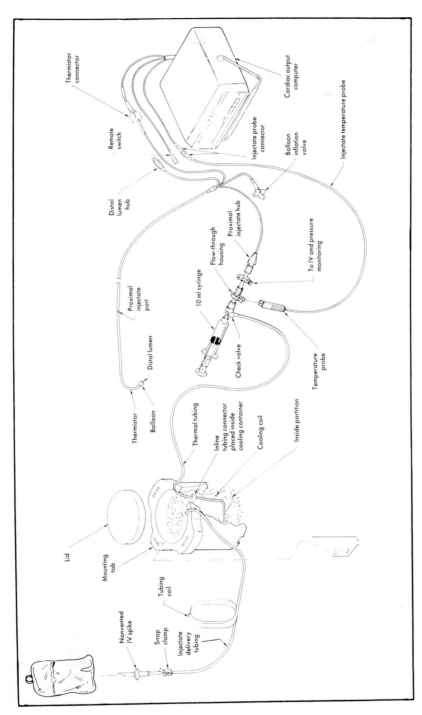

Fig. 7-4. Schematic illustration of a closed injectate delivery system (CO-Set) for use with cold injectate. (Courtesy American Edwards Laboratories, Santa Ana, Calif.)

Table 7-3. Problems with thermodilution cardiac output measurements

Problem	Cause	Action
Cardiac output values lower than expected	Injectate volume greater than designated amount	Inject exact volume to correspond to computation constant used.
	Catheter tip in RV or RA	Verify PA waveform from distal lumen. Reposition catheter.
	Incorrect computation constant (CC)	Reset computation constant. Correct prior CO values: Incorrect CO value $\times$ $\dfrac{\text{Correct CC}}{\text{Wrong CC}} = \text{Correct CO}$
	Left-to-right shunt (VSD)	Check RA & PA oxygen saturations. Use alternative CO measurement technique.
	Catheter kinked or partially obstructed with clot	Check for kinks at insertion site; straighten catheter; aspirate and flush catheter.
	Faulty catheter (communication between proximal and distal lumens)	Replace catheter.
Cardiac output values higher than expected	Injectate volume less than designated amount	Inject exact volume to correspond to computation constant. Carefully remove all air bubbles from syringe.
	Catheter too distal (PAW)	Verify PA waveform from distal lumen. Pull catheter back.
	RA port lies within sheath	Advance catheter.
	Thermistor against wall of PA	Reposition patient. Rotate catheter to turn thermistor away from wall. Reposition catheter.
	Fibrin covering thermistor	Check a-v_{O_2} difference; change catheter.
	Incorrect computation constant (CC)	Correct prior CO values (see formula above). Reset computation constant.
	Right-to-left shunt (VSD)	Use alternative CO measurement technique.
	Incorrect injectate temperature	Use closed injectate system with in-line temperature proble. If syringes used, handle minimally. Do not turn stopcock to reestablish IV infusion through proximal port between injections: reduce or discontinue IV flow through VIP port.

Continued.

Table 7-3. Problems with thermodilution cardiac output measurements—cont'd

Problem	Cause	Action
	Magnetic interference producing numberous spikes in CO curve	Try to determine cause of interference. Wipe CO computer with damp cloth.
	Long lag time between injection and upstroke of curve	Press "START" button *after* injection completed to delay computer sampling time.
Irregular upslope of CO curve	Uneven injection technique	Inject smoothly and quickly (10 ml in ≤4 sec).
	RA port partially occluded with clot	Always withdraw, then flush proximal port before CO determinations.
	Catheter partially kinked	Check for kinks, particularly at insertion site; straighten catheter; reposition patient.
Irregular downslope of CO curve	Cardiac arrhythmias (PVCs, AF, etc.)	Note ECG during CO determinations. Try to inject during a stable period. Increase the number of CO determinations.
	Marked movement of catheter tip	Obtain x-ray film to determine position of tip. Advance catheter tip away from pulmonic valve.
	Marked variation in PA baseline temperature	Use iced temperature injectate to increase signal/noise ratio. Increase the number of CO determinations. Inject at various times during respiratory cycle.
	Curve prematurely terminated	Press START button *after* injection completed to delay computer sampling time.
	Right-to-left shunt	Use alternative CO measurement technique.

9. Turn on the power of the COC. (An RDY signal should be displayed after approximately 2 seconds indicating that the computer is ready.)
10. Depress the SELF-TEST button to check the patency of the system (once each day).
11. Check the blood temperature and the injectate temperature by depressing the appropriate button on the COC. Cardiac output determinations should not be performed if the injectate temperature is unstable. It is necessary to wait for the temperature to stabilize to obtain accurate readings. This may take up to 45 to 60 minutes if the injectate solution has not been prechilled.
12. Enter the correct computation constant by turning the thumbwheel on the side panel of the computer. The correct computation constant (CC) is included in

the package insert of each catheter. Most institutions tape one of these inserts to the top of each cardiac output computer. If the wrong computation constant has been entered, the data may still be used according to the formula listed in Table 7-3.

13. Depress the CARDIAC OUTPUT button on the COC and wait for a RDY signal to appear.
14. Check the pressure waveform from the distal lumen of the PA catheter to verify a good PA waveform.
15. Start the strip chart recorder.
16. Slowly withdraw the plunger of the syringe and fill it with exactly 10 ml of injectate.
17. Turn the stopcock closed to the IV solution and open from the injectate syringe to the proximal lumen of the catheter.
18. Press the START button and rapidly and evenly inject the solution in the syringe through the proximal lumen of the catheter. This should be done smoothly in less than 4 seconds either manually or automatically with a CO_2 injector. The advantage of the CO_2 automatic injector is that it minimizes handling of the syringe, which can warm the injectate, and allows for a rapid, even injection.
19. Check the CO curve on the paper writeout observing for the presence of a smooth, rapid upstroke indicating a rapid, even injection (Fig. 7-5).
20. Repeat steps 13 through 18 for repeated CO measurements. Usually the first cardiac output reading is discarded and at least three cardiac output determinations are performed to obtain an average reading. If these readings vary significantly, up to five or six determinations may be necessary to obtain a more accurate mean value.

The obvious advantage of the closed system is that it is completely closed, eliminating the need to frequently open the system with the inherent risks of contamination that accompany each entry. The primary disadvantage is the increased bulk on or near the patient, since the entire system must remain attached to the catheter.

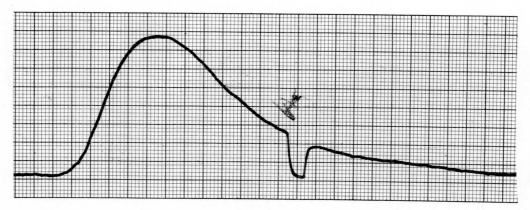

Fig. 7-5. Normal thermodilution cardiac output curve demonstrating a smooth, rapid upstroke and even downslope. (Dip on the downslope indicates end of the computer sampling period)

This can potentially interfere with patient movement and be inadvertently loosened or dislodged, resulting in bleedback, introduction of air, and/or contamination. Special care is required to prevent these complications.

Sources of Error

The thermodilution measurement of cardiac output provides information over a very brief "window" of time, that is, only several seconds of actual measurement. This number, then, is used as a reflection of the patient's flow rate per minute of time, and depending on how frequently measurements are performed, they are assumed to reflect the patient's cardiac output over the ensuing hours. Obviously, these assumptions can frequently be erroneous. In addition to the patient's changing condition, the technique itself can introduce errors that further compound the problem.

Technical Considerations

Since thermodilution cardiac output measurement is calculated from a resultant change in blood temperature, it is paramount that the temperature of both the blood and the injectate solution be accurate and stable. Improvements in cardiac output equipment, specifically a closed injectate system with an in-line thermistor that measures the injectate's temperature as it leaves the syringe (see Fig. 7-4), have reduced, but certainly not eliminated, this source of error. Heat from the injectate, whether iced or room temperature, is lost through handling of the injectate syringe and throughout the catheter itself as it travels to the RA. (This loss is relatively greater with the use of iced temperature injectate than with room temperature injectate.) A warm environment or the use of heat lamps can appreciably alter the injectate temperature. Some ways to minimize injectate heat transfer or loss include the following:

1. Use a closed-injectate system with an in-line temperature probe. This reduces exposure to environmental influences and minimizes the amount of hand contact with the injectate. Additionally, the in-line temperature probe measures the temperature of the injectate *after* it leaves the syringe.
2. Inject an initial volume of injectate to "cool the catheter" and reduce the heat loss of subsequent injections. It is not necessary to perform a cardiac output measurement on this initial injection.
3. Use room temperature rather than iced temperature injectate. Numerous studies have demonstrated similar results between room temperature and ice temperature cardiac output determinations in a number of patient populations. In addition, room temperature injectate is less likely to cause a slowing of the heart rate, as can occur with cold injectate. However, to ensure a minimum temperature difference of 12° between blood temperature and injectate temperature, it may be necessary to use iced injectate in patients who are very hypothermic.
4. Keep injectate solution and tubing, as well as the catheter, away from direct sunlight or heat lamps.

Since the thermodilution measurement of cardiac output integrates a change in blood temperature produced by a bolus of fluid of different temperature, it is essential that the injectate be administered rapidly (10 ml in 4 seconds or less) and evenly. Slow or uneven injection techniques will produce inaccurate data and fre-

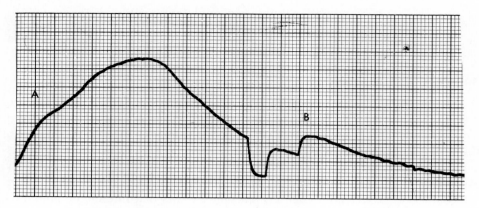

Fig. 7-6. Irregular thermodilution cardiac output curve demonstrating an uneven upslope *(A)* as a result of poor injection technique. The reappearance of thermal indicator *(B)* following cessation of computer sampling could be because of a left-to-right intracardiac shunt (VSD).

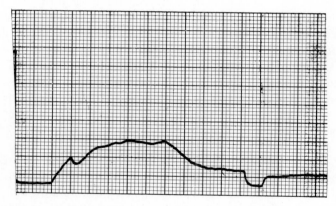

Fig. 7-7. Irregular thermodilution cardiac output curve demonstrating very uneven, slow injection technique as indicated by the irregular upstroke. Data from such a CO curve would be inaccurate.

quently are responsible for discrepancies between serial cardiac output readings. Faulty injection techniques are visually apparent on the corresponding cardiac output curve, showing a slow or uneven upstroke similar to that seen in Fig. 7-6. When such a cardiac output curve is produced, the data should be discarded from calculations of cardiac output. Accurate thermodilution cardiac output determinations require careful inspection of each cardiac output curve to assess technical adequacy. This requires a paper printout of each curve. Figs. 7-7 to 7-9 depict other errors apparent in the cardiac output curves resulting in erroneous measurements. If reliance is placed solely on the digitally displayed value, no assessment of technical accuracy can be made. This would be like monitoring the numerical value of the PA or PAW pressure without assessing the corresponding waveform!

While the upslope of the cardiac output curve indicates injection technique, the

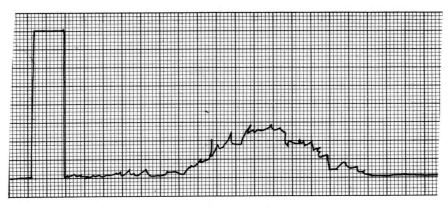

Fig. 7-8. Irregular thermodilution cardiac output curve demonstrating marked electromagnetic interference as demonstrated by the numerous spikes on the curve. Data from such a CO curve is inaccurate.

downslope, as well as the area under the curve, relates to the rate of blood flow through the right side of the heart. A slow, prolonged downslope producing a large area beneath the curve is associated with a low flow rate, or low cardiac output (Fig. 7-10). This is in contrast to the rapid downslope and smaller area seen in patients with high cardiac outputs (Fig. 7-11). If the digital display on the cardiac output computer does not correlate with this curve depiction, troubleshooting steps should be initiated to determine the cause of error (see Table 7-3). In this way analysis of the cardiac output curve, including the upslope, downslope, and area beneath the curve, are used to assess the accuracy of cardiac output determinations.

All cardiac output computers measure temperature changes over a limited amount or window of time. This measurement begins when the *start* button is initiated and continues until the slope returns to 30% of baseline, or until some specific time period has elapsed. Usually the *start* button is depressed at the beginning of each injection, signaling the computer to begin analysis. However, in patients with very low stroke volumes in whom blood moves very slowly from RA to PA, the cardiac output computer can have completed its period of analysis before maximum temperature difference has been sensed in the PA. The result would be a cardiac output curve with a small area and an erroneously high cardiac output reading. This problem can be eliminated by delaying the cardiac output computer's period of analysis until after injection is completed. The START button is not depressed until after the injectate is fully administered. Once again, careful analysis of the cardiac output curve is necessary to ensure that accurate measurements are obtained.

The formula used by the COC to measure cardiac output is based on the specific properties of 5% dextrose in water. To avoid the possible bacterial growth that can occur with dextrose solutions, it is not uncommon to substitute a saline solution for the injectate. However, the specific properties, including the density, of saline differ from dextrose and can introduce a small error (probably less than 1%) in the cardiac output determinations.

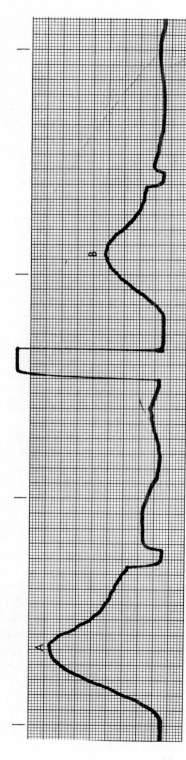

Fig. 7-9. Two varying thermodilution cardiac output curves obtained in sequence in the same patient. The second curve (B), although technically acceptable, was performed less than 30 seconds after the first determination (A), while the PA temperature had not yet returned to a stable baseline.

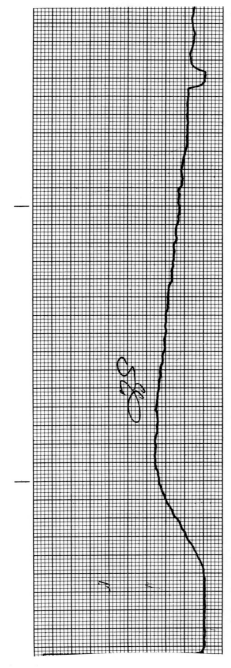

Fig. 7-10. Very low cardiac output (2.5 L/min) as indicated by a slow upstroke and downslope producing a large area beneath the curve. PA temperature changes were sensed for more than 25 seconds as a result of a very low flow rate (stroke volume).

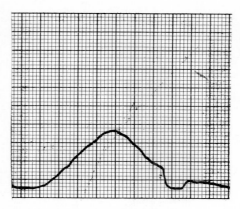

Fig. 7-11. High cardiac output (7.3 L/min) as indicated by a normal, smooth upstroke and rapid downslope producing a small area beneath the curve.

Errors in measurement of cardiac output via a thermodilution catheter inserted through a percutaneous sidearm sheath have been reported. As the length of the sidearm sheath is 15 cm, it is possible for the RA port of the catheter to open within the sheath rather than in the RA. This would be particularly true with catheters introduced percutaneously into the subclavian or internal jugular veins, in which the in vivo catheter length is shorter. Indications of this occurrence include erroneously high cardiac output values and the appearance of a retrograde surge of blood-tinged fluid through the sidearm of the sheath during injection into the RA port. Correction of this problem consists of proper placement of the proximal port of the catheter within the RA and temporarily turning off the sidearm IV infusion during cardiac output measurements.

Physiologic Considerations

Marked variations in cardiac output values can result from certain physiologic changes. During the ventilatory cycle the temperature of the PA blood varies. This effect can be exaggerated during mechanical ventilation or other irregularities in the ventilatory cycle. These changes in baseline PA temperature, from which the cardiac output is calculated, introduce error in thermodilution cardiac output measurements. Again, visualization of the baseline on a paper writeout should reveal such changes (see Fig. 7-9). When the PA temperature appears to be fluctuating, it might be necessary to use iced injectate (to increase the signal-to-noise ratio), as well as to increase the number of cardiac output determinations to five or six for averaging. Timing of indicator injections relative to the ventilatory phase can also be responsible for wide discrepancies between serial cardiac output measurements. Fig. 7-12 demonstrates the corresponding changes in cardiac output when measurements are made at different times in the respiratory cycle. However, since temperature change and cardic output are measured at some later time (depending on the rate of flow) following injection, no one particular moment of the ventilatory cycle will yield more accurate data. Injections timed to occur at one particular phase of the respiratory cycle will certainly yield more reproducible data but not actually reflect the average or mean flow rate per minute of time. A more accurate

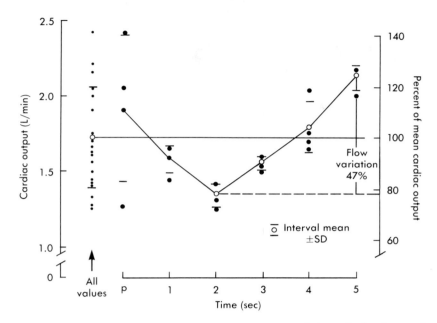

Fig. 7-12. Thermodilution cardiac output measurements at each second of a 6-second ventilation cycle. All measurements are plotted on the left and the same points are grouped by time of the cycle on the right. (From Snyder J, and Powner D: The effects of mechanical ventilation on the measurement of cardiac output by thermodilution, Crit Care Med)

cardiac output measurement would reflect the average of the changes in flow that occur during both inspiration and expiration. Therefore, indicator injections should be timed to occur at various phases of the respiratory cycle. Again, if marked variation occurs, the number of determinations can be increased to five or six.

Changes in stroke volume resulting from arrhythmias or changing heart rates can also produce wide variations in serial cardiac output readings. The patient's heart rate and rhythm should be monitored and, ideally, printed out during each cardiac output measurement. When possible, determinations should be made during a stable, arrhythmia-free period. Since this is often difficult to do, it is again necessary to increase the number of cardiac output determinations in patients with irregular or varying heart rates.

Spurious cardiac output readings can often be checked by obtaining a mixed venous oxygen saturation or by continuously monitoring Svo_2 if an oximeter PA catheter is in place. If low cardiac output readings are obtained in the face of a normal Svo_2, troubleshooting steps should be initiated to determine the cause of error (see Table 7-3). Likewise, high cardiac output readings with low Svo_2 values also indicate an erroneous cardiac output measurement (except in patients with sepsis and inadequate oxygen utilization).

REFERENCES

Barcelona M et al: Cardiac output determination by the thermodilution method: comparison of ice-temperature injectate versus room-temperature injectate contained in prefilled syringes or a closed injectate delivery system, Heart Lung 14:232-235, 1985.

Bearss MG et al: A complication with thermodilution cardiac outputs in centrally-placed pulmonary artery catheters (correspondence). Chest 81:527, 1982.

Carpenter JP, Sreedhar N, and Staw I: Cardiac output determination: thermodilution versus a new computerized Fick method, Crit Care Med 13:576-579, 1985.

Daily EK, and Mersch J: Comparison of Fick method of cardiac output with thermodilution method using two indicators, Heart Lung 16:294-300, 1987.

Elkayan U et al: Cardiac output by thermodilution technique: effect of injectate volume and temperature on accuracy and reproducibility in the critically ill patient, Chest 84:418-422, 1983.

Ehlers KC, Mylrea KC, Waterson CK, and Calkins JM: Cardiac output measurements. A review of current techniques and research, Ann Biomed Engin 14:219-239, 1986.

Fegler G: Measurement of cardiac output in anesthetized animal by a thermodilution method, Q J Exp Physiol 39:153-164, 1954.

Forrester JS, et al: Thermodilution cardiac output determination with a single flow-directed catheter, Am Heart J 83:306-311, 1972.

Gardner PE, and Woods SL: Accuracy of the closed injectate delivery system in measuring thermodilution cardiac output, Heart Lung 16:552-561, 1987.

Hainsworth R: Mixed venous oxygen content and its meaning, Intensive Care Med 7:153-155, 1981.

Haites NE, Mowat DHR, McLennan FM, and Rawles JM: How far is the cardiac output? Lancet 3:1025-1027, 1984.

Hankeln KB, et al: Continuous, on-line, real-time measurement of cardiac output and derived cardiorespiratory variables in the critically ill, Crit Care Med 13:1071, 1985.

Kashtan HI, Salerno TA, Lichtenstein SV, and Byrick RJ: Effects of tricuspid regurgitation on thermodilution cardiac output: studies in an animal model, Can J Anaesth 34:246-251, 1987.

Mintz R, et al: Comparison of cardiac outputs determined by impedance cardiography and thermodilution in cardiac transplant patients, Anesthesiology 67:A213, 1987.

Moxham J, and Armstrong RF: Continuous monitoring of right atrial oxygen tension in patients with myocardial infarction, Intensive Care Med 7:157-164, 1981.

Nelson LD, and Anderson HB: Patient selection for iced versus room-temperature injectate for thermodilution cardiac output determinations, Crit Care Med 13:182-184, 1985.

Nishikawa T, and Nimiki A: Mechanism for slowing of heart rate and associated changes in

pulmonary circulation elicited by cold injectate during thermodilution cardiac output determination in dogs, Anesthesiology 68:221-225, 1988.

Paulsen AW, and Valek TR: Artifactually low cardiac outputs resulting from a communication between the proximal and distal lumens of an Edwards pacing thermodilution catheter, Anesthesiology 68:308-309, 1988.

Pitt B, and Strauss HW: Evaluation of ventricular function by radioisotopic technics, N Engl J Med 296:1097-1099, 1977.

Raffin TA: Technique of thermodilution cardiac output measurements, J Crit Illness 2:73-79, 1987.

Sanmarco ME et al: Measurement of cardiac output by thermal dilution, Am J Cardiol 28:54-58, 1971.

Sedlock S: Cardiac output: physiologic variables and therapeutic interventions, Crit Care Nurse 1:14-22, 1981.

Shellock FG, and Riedinger MS: Reproducibility and accuracy of using room-temperature vs. ice-temperature injectate for thermodilution cardiac output determination, Heart Lung 12:175-176, 1983.

Shellock FG, Riedinger MS, Bateman TM, and Gray RJ: Thermodilution cardiac output determination in hypothermic post cardiac surgical patients: room- vs. ice-temperature injectate, Crit Care Med 11:668-670, 1983.

Siegel LC, et al: Comparison of simultaneous intraoperative measurements of cardiac output by thermodilution, esophageal doppler and electrical impedance in anesthetized patients, Anesthesiology 67:A181, 1987.

Slonim NB, Bell B, and Christensen S: Cardiopulmonary laboratory basic methods and calculations, Springfield, Ill, 1972, Charles C Thomas, Publisher.

Snyder JV, and Powner DJ: Effects of mechanical ventilation on the measurement of cardiac output by thermodilution, Crit Care Med 10:677-682, 1982.

Steele PP et al: Simple and safe bedside method for serial measurement of left ventricular ejection fraction, cardiac output, and pulmonary blood volume, Br Heart J 36:122-131, 1974.

Tahvanainen J, Meretoja O, and Nikki P: Can central venous blood replace mixed venous blood samples? Crit Care Med 10:758-761, 1982.

Van Grondelle A et al: Thermodilution method overestimates low cardiac output in humans, Am J Physiol 245:H690-692, 1983.

Vaughn S, and Puri VK: Cardiac output changes and continuous mixed venous oxygen saturation measurement in the critically ill, Crit Care Med 16:495-498, 1988.

Vennix CV, Nelson DH, and Pierpont GL: Thermodilution cardiac output in critically ill patients: comparison of room temperature and iced injectate, Heart Lung 13:574-578, 1984.

Weisel RD et al: Clinical application of thermodilution cardiac output determination, Am J Surg 129:449-454, 1975.

Wetzel RC, and Larson TW: Major errors in thermodilution cardiac output measurement during rapid volume infusion, Anesthesiology 62:684-687, 1985.

Woog RH, and McWilliam DB: A comparison of methods of cardiac output measurement, Anaesth Intensive Care 11:141-146, 1983.

Yang SS, Bentivoglio L, Maranhao V, and Goldberg H: From cardiac catheterization to hemodynamic parameters, Philadelphia, 1972, FA Davis Co.

Zaret BL, and Cohen LS: Evaluation of cardiac performance, Mod Concepts Cardiovasc Dis 46(7):33-36, 1977.

Zaret BL, and Cohen LS: Evaluation of perfusion and viability, Mod Concepts Cardiovasc Dis 46(8):37-42, 1977.

Chapter 8

Continuous Monitoring of Oxygenation

The function and viability of all mammalian cells depend on a continuing supply of oxygen in amounts equal to or greater than their needs. When oxygen delivery becomes inadequate, cellular metabolism continues anaerobically at the price of critical biochemical changes within the cell. Some of these changes result in increased lactic acid accumulation, which further inhibits normal mitochondrial metabolism and a vicious cycle ensues. For this reason, assessment and monitoring of the adequacy of oxygenation is a primary goal in the care and management of all critically ill patients. Recent technology now permits continuous bedside monitoring of both arterial and mixed venous oxygen saturation to closely assess overall tissue oxygenation. A general understanding of the concepts of oxygen supply and demand are fundamental to the principles of mixed venous and arterial oxygen monitoring.

OXYGEN DELIVERY

Oxygen delivery, the amount of oxygen delivered to the tissues each minute, is the primary function of the cardiopulmonary system. Oxygen delivery is the product of blood flow and the oxygen content of arterial blood (Fig. 8-1). This can be expressed by the formula:

$$\dot{D}o_2 = CO \times Cao_2 \times 10$$

where: $\dot{D}o_2$ = Oxygen delivery (ml/min)
CO = Cardiac output (L/min)
Cao_2 = Oxygen content of arterial blood (ml/dl)
10 = Conversion factoring dl to L

Cardiac Output

Cardiac output, the rate of blood flow from the heart to the lungs and systemic circulation per minute, is a major determinant of oxygen delivery. In general, this rate of blood flow is regulated on a moment-to-moment basis by the metabolic needs of each organ system. However, when cardiac output falls, oxygen delivery also falls. The role of cardiac output in maintaining the balance between oxygen delivery and oxygen demand was discussed in more detail in Chapter 7.

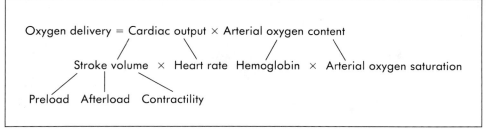

Fig. 8-1. Oxygen delivery (ml/min) is a product of the cardiac output and the oxygen content of arterial blood. In turn, cardiac output is a product of stroke volume and heart rate. The stroke volume is subsequently determined by the preload, afterload, and contractility. The arterial oxygen content is a product of the patient's hemoglobin and oxygen saturation of arterial blood. Alterations in oxygen delivery can be achieved by manipulation of any of these parameters.

Arterial Oxygen Content

The content or total amount of oxygen carried in arterial blood is the sum of the oxygen bound to the hemoglobin and the oxygen that is dissolved in plasma. The amount of oxygen carried by hemoglobin is determined by the total concentration of hemoglobin in blood and the percentage of total hemoglobin that combines with oxygen (arterial oxygen saturation). The content of oxygen can be measured directly or calculated. The calculation can be written:

$$Ca_{O_2} = hemoglobin \times 1.34 \times Sa_{O_2} + Pa_{O_2} \times 0.003$$

where: Ca_{O_2} = Arterial Oxygen Content (ml O_2/100 ml blood)
1.34 = ml oxygen carried by each gram hemoglobin
Sa_{O_2} = Arterial oxygen saturation (%)
Pa_{O_2} = Partial pressure of oxygen in arterial blood (mm Hg)
0.003 = ml oxygen/mm Hg Pa_{O_2}

Hemoglobin

As blood passes through the lungs oxygen is taken up both by the hemoglobin and the plasma portion of the blood. Each heme molecule of hemoglobin can chemically and reversibly combine with four oxygen molecules. (If every heme molecule combines fully with oxygen, the hemoglobin is said to be *fully saturated* or 100% saturated with oxygen). This corresponds to a mean volume of approximately 1.34 ml of oxygen bound to every gram of hemoglobin. (Some confusion exists about the actual oxygen-combining capacity of hemoglobin with reported values ranging from 1.34 ml/g to 1.39 ml/g. Throughout this text, the original value of 1.34 ml O_2/g hemoglobin/100 ml blood will be used.) Thus a patient with a normal hemoglobin of 15 g/dl could carry 20 ml O_2/dl (or 20 ml O_2/100 ml blood) in his hemoglobin, if every heme molecule was fully saturated with oxygen (100% saturation).

Arterial oxygen saturation

The percentage of total hemoglobin that combines or saturates with oxygen is referred to as the oxygen saturation of blood. This is referred to as functional oxygen saturation of arterial blood, in that it only considers those hemoglobin molecules that are capable of binding with and transporting oxygen. The presence of other abnormal or dysfunctional hemoglobin, such as methemoglobin or carboxyhemoglobin, reduces the oxygen carrying capacity of the hemoglobin molecules by either preventing oxygen from binding to hemoglobin, or by interfering with the release of oxygen from hemoglobin. Methemoglobin is formed when the iron ion in the hemoglobin molecule is oxidized from the ferrous (Fe^{++}) to the ferric (Fe^{+++}) form. This may occur in the presence of certain toxic substances such as potassium chlorate, certain intravascular dyes, and nitroprusside, as well as in patients with familial methemoglobinemia. Carboxyhemoglobin is formed when carbon monoxide preferentially binds with hemoglobin displacing oxygen from the hemoglobin molecule. This can occur in patients who are heavy smokers or patients suffering from smoke inhalation or carbon monoxide poisoning. (Increased levels of carboxyhemoglobin can also be seen in persons who are exposed to extended periods of heavy freeway traffic.) Oxygen saturation of hemoglobin can be measured directly via a spectrophotometer, or calculated from the measured Pa_{O_2} using a nomogram or oxyhemoglobin dissociation curve. Normal arterial oxygen saturation is 95% to 100%.

Dissolved oxygen

Oxygen is also carried in the plasma, where it is physically dissolved. The solubility coefficient of oxygen in human plasma is 0.003 ml/mm Hg partial pressure of arterial blood, if the patient is breathing room air. This amounts to approximately 0.25 ml O_2/dl at a normal P_{O_2}. Since this amount is so small, it is generally clinically ignored, particularly when doing trend monitoring. (If oxygen was only carried in plasma, maintenance of normal oxygen delivery would require a flow rate in excess of 100 L/min!) Therefore, the content of oxygen in arterial blood is expressed only as:

$$Ca_{O_2} = \text{Hemoglobin} \times 1.34 \times Sa_{O_2}$$

The actual amount of oxygen delivered to the tissues ($\dot{D}_{O_2}$) each minute can be calculated when the values for cardiac output, hemoglobin, and arterial saturation are known.

EXAMPLE: CO = 5L/min
Hgb = 15g/dl
Sa_{O_2} = 99%
10dl/L = Conversion factor

$$\dot{D}_{O_2} = 5 \text{ L/min} \times 15\text{g/dl} \times .99 \times 1.34 \times 10$$
$$\dot{D}_{O_2} = 5 \times 15 \times .99 \times 1.34 \times 10$$
$$\dot{D}_{O_2} = 995 \text{ ml/min}$$

This represents a normal quantity of oxygen delivered to the tissues each minute and is a commonly used index of the performance of the cardiopulmonary transport system. However, it does not indicate the adequacy of oxygen in relation to tissue oxygen demands. Although low oxygen delivery values are usually associated with tissue hypoxia, normal or even high values do not necessarily ensure that oxygen delivery is adequate.

Oxyhemoglobin Dissociation Curve

Both the uptake and release of oxygen by the hemoglobin molecules are visually represented by the oxyhemoglobin dissociation curve (Fig. 8-2) which relates the partial pressure of oxygen in blood (Po_2) to the saturation of hemoglobin. The S-shape of the curve is a result of the increased affinity of hemoglobin for oxygen as more oxygen molecules combine with it, despite large alveolar Po_2 changes (the flat, upper portion of the curve) and the rapid unloading of oxygen from hemoglobin with little changes in Po_2 (the steep, lower portion of the curve). In this way, the oxygen tension gradient necessary for the diffusion of oxygen from blood into the mitochondria is maintained. A normal uptake and release of oxygen by hemoglobin is characterized by a hemoglobin saturation of 50% when the Po_2 is 26.5 mm Hg. This is known as the P50 (see Fig. 8-2). Certain conditions can change this relationship, resulting in a shift of the oxyhemoglobin curve to the right or to the left, changing the ability of the hemoglobin to either combine with, or release oxygen. Changes in the Po_2 required for a saturation of 50% have become a convenient way to express shifts in the dissociation curve. A right shift is defined by a hemoglobin saturation of 50% at a Pao_2 higher than 26.5 mm Hg, as less tightly bound oxygen is more easily released (see Fig. 8-2). A left shift, then, describes the hemoglobin saturation of 50% at a Pao_2 less than 26 mm Hg, a low pressure gradient of oxygen that prevents diffusion and, thus, tissue oxygenation. These shifts, or changes in affinity, are associated with changes in body temperature, the pH of blood, and the level of 2,3 diphosphoglycerate (2,3 DPG) in blood. Table 8-1 lists factors, which produce these changes or shifts in the oxyhemoglobin dissociation curve.

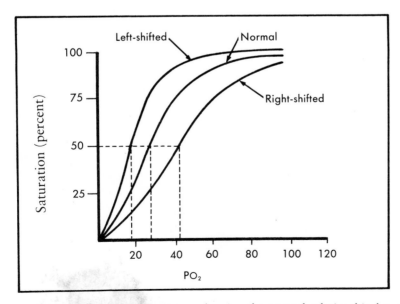

Fig. 8-2. Oxyhemoglobin dissociation curve showing the normal relationship between the Po_2 and oxygen saturation as well as a left and right shift of the curve as defined by either a decreased or increased P_{50}, respectively.

Table 8-1. Factors affecting the position of the oxyhemoglobin dissociation curve

Left shift (increased affinity)	Right shift (decreased affinity)
Alkalosis ($\uparrow$ pH)	Acidosis ($\downarrow$ pH)
Hypocapnia ($\downarrow$ CO_2)	Hypercapnia ($\uparrow$ CO_2)
Decreased temperature	Increased temperature
Decrased 2,3 DPG	Increased 2,3 DPG
Hypophosphatemia	
Carbon monoxide	
Sepsis	

OXYGEN DEMAND

The amount or quantity of oxygen needed or demanded by the tissues to maintain aerobic metabolism is primarily determined by their metabolic rate. This rate of metabolism, in turn, is determined by the rate of cellular activity. Normally, changes in oxygen needs or demands are regulated, in an automatic fashion, by changes in blood flow. When blood flow, or cardiac output, maintains an adequate supply of oxygen, an increase in oxygen demand results in an increase in oxygen consumption.

Oxygen Consumption ($\dot{V}o_2$)

Oxygen consumption ($\dot{V}o_2$) is simply the amount of oxygen actually used by the tissues per minute of time. Normally, at rest, the tissues consume approximately 25% of the available oxygen. During exercise or other forms of stress, oxygen consumption can increase about threefold, using about 75% of the available oxygen. Therefore, if oxygen delivery is normally about 1000 cc/min, oxygen consumption at rest is approximately 25% of this, or 250 cc/min.

Oxygen consumption can be measured directly by analyzing the amount and composition of the patient's inspired and expired air over a known period of time. Other techniques have recently been developed to directly measure oxygen consumption in ventilated patients. However, because of the technical difficulties involved in directly measuring oxygen consumption in critically ill patients, indirect measurement of $\dot{V}o_2$ with the Fick formula is generally used in the critical care setting. Table 8-2 lists mean oxygen consumption values according to age, sex, and heart rate.

Fick Formula

The Fick formula is based on Adolf Fick's equation for cardiac output determination, whereby the difference between the oxygen content of arterial and venous blood in the pulmonary circulation reflects oxygen uptake per unit of blood as it flows through the lungs. This can be expressed as:

$$CO(L/min) = \frac{o_2 \text{ consumption (ml/min)}}{(\text{Arterial } o_2 \text{ content} - \text{Venous } o_2 \text{ content})}$$

Table 8-2. Mean oxygen consumption data grouped by age and heart rate in adults

Age (yr)	Heart rate (bpm)					
	<50	51-60	61-70	71-80	81-90	91-100
FEMALES						
<35			128 ± 2.0	136 ± 5.4	136 ± 18.6	136.5 ± 16.4
36-45		119.7 ± 4.8	124.5 ± 9.5	142.1 ± 9.5	128.4 ± 9.4	
46-55		124.5 ± 8.4	113.1 ± 5.2	117.6 ± 9.2	124.7 ± 6.9	130 ± 12.4
56-65		104.2 ± 4.5	106 ± 7.9	111.4 ± 5.0	124.5 ± 2.9	134.3 ± 15.1
66-75		102.1 ± 6.0	105 ± 9.8	124.3 ± 8.8	117.6 ± 10.3	107.7 ± 8.4
MALES						
<35				158.8 ± 7.3	160 ± 9.4	146 ± 16
36-45		122.9 ± 4.5	135.3 ± 6.3	138.9 ± 11.4	150.9 ± 8.7	134.4 ± 6.4
46-55	119.8 ± 6.8	120.3 ± 2.6	122 ± 3.6	130.6 ± 5.1	134.3 ± 8.6	134.7 ± 5.6
56-65	117.9 ± 8.6	121.6 ± 3.5	121.8 ± 3.8	125 ± 4.4	125.8 ± 7.4	125.4 ± 10.4
66-75	104.8 ± 2.0	113.8 ± 5.7	116.4 ± 6.1	124.1 ± 6.2	124.1 ± 9.2	

From Crocker RH et al: Determinants of total body oxygen consumption in adults undergoing cardic catheterization, Cathet Cardiovasc Diagn 8:363, 1982.

Rearrangement of this formula is used to calculate oxygen consumption when cardiac output and arterial and venous oxygen contents are known.

$$\dot{V}_{O_2} = CO \times \text{Arterial } O_2 \text{ content} - \text{Venous } O_2 \text{ content} \times 10$$

EXAMPLE: CO = 5 L/min
Arterial O_2 content = 20 vol%
Venous O_2 content = 15 vol%

$$\therefore \dot{V}_{O_2} = 5 \times (20 - 15) \times 10$$
or
$$\dot{V}_{O_2} = 250 \text{ ml/min}$$

This estimate of $\dot{V}_{O_2}$ requires simultaneous and precise measurement of cardiac output, and hemoglobin, as well as arterial and venous oxygen saturations. Obviously, this is not always possible in the critical care setting, resulting in estimations of $\dot{V}_{O_2}$ that can vary by as much as 25% or more from direct measurement.

OXYGEN SUPPLY AND DEMAND BALANCE

As previously mentioned, increases in oxygen demand by the tissues are normally met by increases in oxygen supply or delivery. Remembering the three components of oxygen delivery: cardiac output, hemoglobin concentration, and arterial oxygen saturation, it is apparent that there are several ways in which oxygen supply can be increased to meet increased oxygen demands.

Cardiac Output

As tissue demands for oxygen increase, cardiac output automatically increases, primarily via vasoregulatory mechanisms. Normally, blood flow can increase by a factor of at least three (and even higher in exercise). This ability represents the primary compensatory mechanism involved in maintaining the balance between oxygen supply and demand. If, for example, a patient's oxygen needs double (from a normal oxygen consumption of 250 ml to 500 ml), a doubling of the cardiac output (from 5 to 10 L/min) will sufficiently maintain adequate oxygenation:

$$250 \text{ ml} = 5 \times 20 - 15 \times 10$$
$$500 \text{ ml} = 10 \times 20 - 15 \times 10$$

Clearly, increasing cardiac output up to 15 L/min (three times normal) can maintain very high levels of oxygen delivery, if necessary.

Hemoglobin

Compensatory increases in hemoglobin can occur over time (for example, in individuals living at high altitudes) to maintain adequate oxygen delivery, but since this cannot occur quickly in response to acute increases in oxygen demand, it is not applicable to the critically ill patient.

Arterial Oxygen Saturation

Normally, arterial blood becomes fully saturated with oxygen (97% to 100%) as it passes through the lungs. If this does not occur, hypoxemia results. Inherent compensatory mechanisms such as increased depth and frequency of respiration can improve arterial oxygen saturation, but in general, this mechanism is limited, particularly in acutely ill patients.

Venous Oxygen Saturation

If increased oxygen demands are not met with adequate increases in oxygen supply, (with increased cardiac output), the tissues extract more oxygen from the circulating hemoglobin (that is, more than the usual 25%). In fact, oxygen extraction can increase by a factor of three, also. This results in a threefold reduction in the amount of oxygen that returns to the right side of the heart. Therefore, if normally, the tissues extract about 25% of the available oxygen, the result is blood returning to the right side of the heart still being approximately 75% saturated with oxygen. (This is assuming a normal arterial saturation close to 100%.) Increased oxygen needs may result in increased oxygen extraction. However, not all of the remaining 75% of oxygen is able to be extracted by the tissues. When the partial pressure of oxygen in blood reaches approximately 20 mm Hg the diffusion gradient between the cell and capillary blood is insufficient for appropriate transfer of oxygen out of the capillary and into the tissue. In reviewing a normal oxyhemoglobin dissociation curve (see Fig. 8-2), it is apparent that a Pv_{O_2} of 20 mm Hg corresponds to a venous O_2 saturation of 30%. Therefore, oxygen extraction by the tissues can increase until oxygen saturation of blood is approximately 30%, after which point further extraction is limited. However, this still can provide an additional threefold increase in oxygen delivery and, therefore, oxygen extraction or consumption.

EXAMPLE: CO = 15 L/min
Arterial O_2 saturation = 100%
Venous O_2 saturation = 31%
Hemoglobin = 15 g

$$\dot{V}_{O_2} = 15 \text{ L/min} \times (1.00 - .31) \times 15 \text{ g} \times 1.34 \text{ ml} \times 10$$
$$2,080 \text{ ml} = 15 \times (.69 \times 15 \times 1.34 \times 10)$$

In this situation, oxygen consumption can be maintained at almost nine times the normal levels by both high cardiac output and high oxygen extraction rate.

In summary, the first compensatory mechanism to maintain a balance between oxygen demand and supply is an increase in cardiac output. If this still does not supply adequate oxygen delivery relative to demands, *or* if cardiac dysfunction prevents such an increase in cardiac output, then the second compensatory mechanism is evoked. This mechanism is increased oxygen extraction by the tissues, resulting in decreased saturation of venous blood returning to the heart. Tissues can extract about three times more oxygen than usual, until P_{O_2} falls to approximately 20 mm Hg.

Therapeutic Manipulations

The maintenance of a balanced oxygen supply/demand ratio frequently necessitates therapeutic interventions aimed at either increasing one of the three components of oxygen delivery, or decreasing oxygen demands.

Table 8-3 lists some of the therapeutic ways these determinants are manipulated.

Table 8-3. Therapeutic manipulations to increase oxygen delivery

Determinant	Therapeutic Intervention
Cardiac Output	↑ Preload (volume) ↓ Afterload (arterial vasodilators, calcium channel blockers ACE inhibitors, counterpulsation) ↑ Contractility (positive inotropic agents, calcium) Maintain heart rate 50-100 bpm (beta blockers, calcium channel blockers, pacemaker, atropine)
Arterial Oxygen Saturation (Sao₂)	↑ Fio_2 Mechanical ventilation, CPAP, PEEP Hyperbaria Extracorporeal membrane oxygenation (ECMO)
Hemoglobin	Blood or blood products

MONITORING TECHNIQUES
Pulse Oximetry
Principle

The normal loading of oxygen into the arterial blood occurs as blood circulates through the lungs and is exposed to high concentrations of oxygen in the alveoli. The pressure difference between oxygen in the alveoli and the oxygen in the pre-capillary blood causes oxygen to diffuse into the blood where it combines with the hemoglobin molecules. Hypoxemia, inadequate loading of oxygen, results in a reduction in the oxygen saturation of the hemoglobin (less than 95% to 100%). Previously, assessment of arterial oxygenation was available only by blood gas analysis. These measurements require removal of 5 to 10 ml of blood for each analysis. More importantly, analyzed results are often not available for 20 to 30 minutes, at which time appropriate therapy may no longer be appropriate or may be harmfully delayed. Continuous monitoring of the oxygen saturation percentage of arterial blood (SaO_2) provides early and immediate detection of decreases in oxygen saturation and impending hypoxemia.

Technique of continuous SaO_2 monitoring

Continuous measurement of the oxygen saturation of arterial blood is available noninvasively with the use of a pulse oximeter which senses the light absorption differences between nonsaturated and saturated hemoglobin. A special sensor (Fig. 8-3) containing two light-emitting diodes (LEDs) and a light detector is positioned so that the light emitter and light detector are directly across from one another on opposite sides of an arteriolar bed. (For adults, this is either on one of the fingers, or on the bridge of the nose; for infants, a finger, toe, or foot can be used.) The LEDs emit a red light (approximately 660 nm) and an infrared light (approximately 910 nm). The light detector continuously measures the amount of each type of light that passes through the tissue. Saturated or oxyhemoglobin absorbs more infrared light, while unsaturated or deoxyhemoglobin absorbs more red light. When pulsatile blood is not present, the amount of light that is absorbed by tissue, bone, and venous blood remains constant and serves as a baseline for the increase in light absorbancy that occurs as a pulse of arterial blood flows to the tissue. The light absorbance differences between the oxyhemoglobin (saturated) and deoxyhemoglobin (unsaturated) are then described quantitatively according to Beer's law resulting in a determination of the percent saturation of arterial hemoglobin (SaO_2). In addition, the oximeter automatically measures the pulse rate.

Equipment. Fig. 8-3 illustrates the various sensing devices used to measure SaO_2 via pulse oximetry. The sensor is connected directly to a pulse oximeter (Fig. 8-4) which provides visual and auditory data regarding the SaO_2 and the pulse rate. A beep accompanies each heart beat. A change in the tone of the beep occurs when SaO_2 falls. This alerts the clinician to impending hypoxemia even when he or she may not be within view of the monitor.

Preparation. No calibration of equipment is required as the diodes are precalibrated and coded during manufacturing. In addition, frequent and automatic calibration checks are performed internally. Skin preparation for placement of the sensor is not necessary. Skin pigmentation or nail polish do not interfere with accurate oximetry of the arterial pulse. Sensors are best placed on an extremity without an

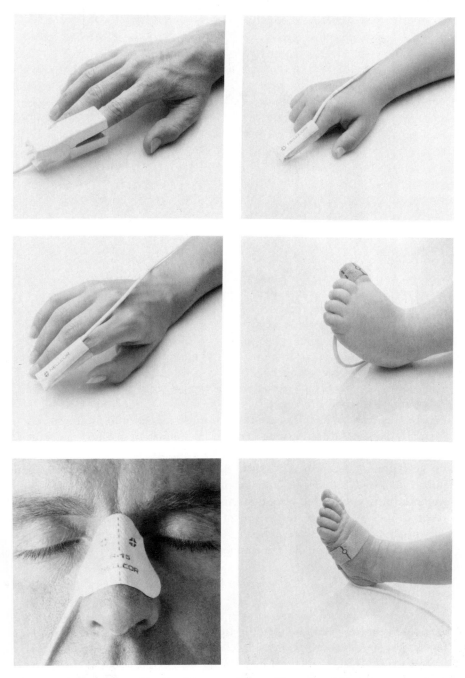

Fig. 8-3. Available adult and pediatric sensors for continous arterial oxygen saturation monitoring using pulse oxymetry. (Courtesy Nellcor, Inc, Hayward Calif.)

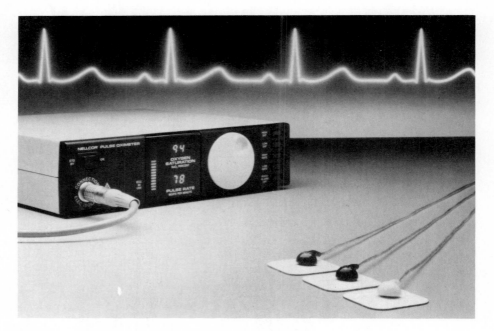

Fig. 8-4. A pulse oximeter displaying the arterial saturation and pulse rate, (Courtesy Nellcor, Inc, Hayward, Calif.)

arterial catheter or blood pressure cuff that would either continuously or intermittently reduce arterial flow distally.

Table 8-4 lists some of the problems as well as causes and recommended actions associated with pulse oximetry.

Clinical application. The use of continuous pulse oximetry to noninvasively monitor arterial oxygen saturation has become an important monitoring tool in the care of all critically ill patients, both adults and children. It is widely used in the operating room, post-anesthesia care units and intensive care units where patients are more likely to experience anticipated or unanticipated periods of hypoxia. Continuous Sao_2 monitoring provides immediate and early warning of impending hypoxemia. It is also useful in assessment of ventilatory management and the effects of other therapeutic interventions. Reductions in arterial saturation to 95% or less should prompt immediate assessment of the patient as well as the adequacy of oxygen delivery.

Continuous Venous Oxymetry (Svo_2)
Principle

The amount of oxygen remaining in the venous blood reflects the oxygen used by the tissues. With a normal oxygen delivery of 1,000 ml, and a normal extraction of about 25%, mixed venous blood remains approximately 75% saturated with oxygen. In fact, when mixed venous blood remains 60% to 80% saturated with oxygen, it is generally assumed that oxygen delivery is adequate for the tissue's needs. On an even broader scale, a normal venous oxygen saturation (Svo_2) usually reflects adequate cardiac output.

Table 8-4. Troubleshooting the pulse oximeter

Problem	Possible cause	Recommended action
? Inaccurate Sa_{O_2}	Excessive patient movement	Quiet patient, if possible. Check security of sensor; replace if necessary. Move sensor to different site. Change type of sensor used. Use ECG signal synchronization. Select a longer (10-15 sec) averaging time, if possible.
	High carboxyhemoglobin or methemoglobin levels	Measure dysfunctional hemoglobin levels. Measure arterial blood gas.
	Reduced arterial blood flow	Do not place sensor on same side as indwelling arterial catheter or blood pressure cuff.
	Electrocautery interference	Move sensor as far as possible from cautery cable; change sites if necessary. Check sensor; replace if damp. Place oximeter plug into a different circuit than cautery unit.
	Excessive ambient light (surgical lamps, heating lamps, bilirubin lights, bright fluorescent lights, direct sunlight)	Cover sensor with opaque material.
Loss of pulse signal	Constriction by sensor	Check sensor; move to a different site or change type of sensor used.
	Reduced arterial blood flow	Same as above.
	Excessive ambient light	Same as above.
	Anemia	Check patient's hemoglobin.
	Hypothermia	Warm monitoring site and replace sensor.
	Shock (hypotension, vasoconstriction)	Check patient's condition including vital signs.
Inaccurate pulse rate	Excessive patient motion	Same as above.
	Pronounced dicrotic notch on arterial waveform	Move sensor to a different site.
	Poor quality ECG signal	Check ECG leads; replace if necessary.
	Electrocautery interference	Same as above.

Svo_2 levels below 60% occur because of increased oxygen extraction by the tissues, most commonly secondary to cardiac decompensation. When Svo_2 continues to fall to 50% or less, lactic acidosis can occur as a result of anaerobic metabolism. The precise Svo_2 level at which anaerobic metabolism and lactic acidosis begin varies, but an Svo_2 of less than 40% likely represents the limits of compensation and impending lactic acidosis. Generally, an Svo_2 of less than 30% (20 mm Hg), indicates insufficient oxygen availability to the tissues. Clinically, this degree of tissue hypoxia is usually accompanied by coma.

The oxygen saturation of venous blood varies, depending on the organ system it serves. Venous blood returning from high flow areas such as the kidney or skin, have higher concentrations of oxygen than venous blood from other areas (for example from the heart). Complete mixing of these varying oxygen saturations occurs in the right ventricle making the PA blood reflective of true *mixed* venous oxygen saturation. The oxygen saturation of PA blood is a flow-weighted average of all the different end-capillary oxygen saturations.

Technique

The combination of fiberoptic technology with a modified 7.5 or 8F thermodilution pulmonary artery catheter was first introduced in 1981 by Oximetrics (Mountain View, California). In addition to the standard features, this catheter has a lumen containing optical fibers that transmit light to and from the blood stream. The light source consists of three diodes that emit alternating pulses of wavelengths of red light through one of the optical fibers. This light is absorbed, refracted by the hemoglobin constituents of the blood, and reflected back through the second optical fiber to the light detector. It is then converted to an electrical signal and transmitted to a remote data processor. The computed oxyhemoglobin saturation is averaged over a 5-second interval, updated every 1 to 2 seconds, and displayed digitally on a monitor as well as on a slow-speed paper recorder. The recorded output also indicates the light intensity at the tip of the catheter. Changes in the light intensity signify a change in catheter position (that is, against the wall of the vessel or spontaneous wedging), inadequate blood flow (thrombus at the tip of the catheter), or damage to the fiberoptic fibers. This light intensity indicator is valuable in troubleshooting problems with either oxygen saturation readings or PA pressure readings.

Equipment

A fiberoptic thermodilution pulmonary artery catheter and a microprocessor with a strip chart recorder or data display and storage system are needed for this procedure (Fig. 8-5).

Preparation

Follow the manufacturer's recommendations for preparation of the fiberoptic catheter before patient insertion. Handle the catheter gently, avoiding any sharp bending of the catheter to prevent damage to the optical fibers. The balloon and thermostat wires of the catheter should also be checked, as discussed on p. 186. Although the fiberoptic pulmonary artery catheter is somewhat stiffer than the standard PA catheter, it compares favorably in both ease of insertion and complication rates.

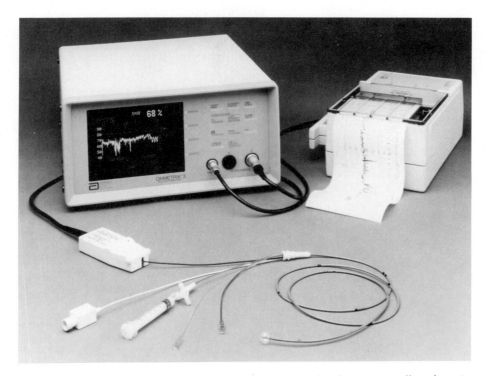

Fig. 8-5. An Svo_2 catheter showing the usual proximal and distal ports as well as thermistor wires and a lumen for balloon inflation. The catheter is connected to an Svo_2 monitor with a digital readout of the current Svo_2 plus a graphic display of the frequently updated Svo_2. A small paper recorder attached to the monitor provides a hard copy of the graphic readings. (Courtesy Abbott Critical Care, Mountain View, Calif.)

Calibration of the oximeter with a blood sample of known oxygen saturation is recommended on a daily basis or whenever there are doubts regarding the displayed Svo_2 reading. Calibration with a known saturation should be carried out at a time when the patient's saturation values are relatively stable, following the specific manufacturer's instructions.

CLINICAL APPLICATIONS OF CONTINUOUS Svo_2 MONITORING

Continuous monitoring of Svo_2 with a fiberoptic catheter provides immediate "real-time" information on changes in cardiopulmonary function and the balance between oxygen demand and supply. A decrease in any of the determinants of oxygen supply (cardiac output, hemoglobin or arterial saturation) is usually associated with a decrease in Svo_2. On the other hand, any change in oxygen consumption is associated with an inverse change in Svo_2. However, it must be pointed out that a "normal" mixed venous oxygen saturation does not ensure adequate oxygen delivery to any one specific organ system, but rather reflects an overall picture of tissue oxygenation.

Normal saturation of mixed venous blood ranges from 65% to 77%. Table 8-5

Table 8-5. Various causes of alterations in Sv_{O_2}

	Sv_{O_2} reading	Physiologic alteration	Clinical causes
(High)	80%-95%	↓ O_2 Consumption	Hypothermia Anesthesia Induced muscular paralysis Sepsis
		↑ O_2 Delivery Mechanical interference	Hyperoxia Catheter wedged Left-to-right shunt
(Normal)	60%-80%	O_2 Supply = O_2 Demand	Adequate perfusion
(Low)	<60%	↑ O_2 Consumption	Shivering Pain Seizures Activity/exercise Hyperthermia Anxiety
		↓ O_2 Delivery	Hypoperfusion (↓ cardiac output) Anemia Hypoxemia

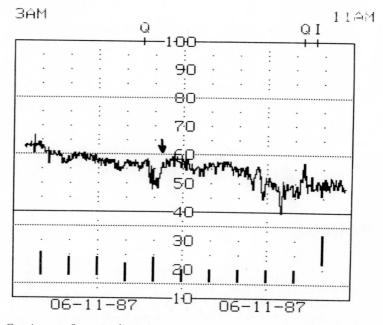

Fig. 8-6. Continuous Sv_{O_2} readings in a patient who had undergone a mitral and aortic valve replacement. On dopamine postoperatively, the patient was hemodynamically stable with a CI of 2.2 L/min/M² and an Sv_{O_2} of approximately 62%. At 3 AM, her Sv_{O_2} began to decline. A drop to 50%, which was associated with hypotension and a CI of 1.5 L/min/M², prompted administration of an epinephrine infusion which resulted in an improved Sv_{O_2} of approximately 58% *(see arrow)*. However, over the next few hours, the Sv_{O_2} further declined despite blood and fluid administration. The patient was subsequently returned to the OR for relief of cardiac tamponade with removal of approximately 400 ml of blood.

lists the probable causes and clinical states associated with high and low Svo_2 readings. A fall in Svo_2 below 60% lasting for 5 minutes or longer indicates a compromise in at least one of the determinants of oxygen transport (cardiac output, hemoglobin, or arterial oxygen saturation) relative to oxygen demands.

Changes in Svo_2 may, and often do, precede hemodynamic changes and events, providing an early warning that should prompt reprofiling of the patient.

Continuous Svo_2 monitoring is also used to immediately assess the effectiveness of therapeutic interventions directed at improving oxygen supply or decreasing oxygen demand. Frequently this results in initiation and/or titration of therapy in a more expedient manner (Figs. 8-6 to 8-8).

Interpretation of Data

Falls in Svo_2 levels (no matter what the value) require immediate assessment to determine the possible cause. The patient should be clinically evaluated to determine whether or not any sudden increases in oxygen demand (and therefore oxygen consumption) have occurred. Increases in patient movement or agitation, pain, shivering, seizure activity, or increased body temperature will increase oxygen demand. This can usually be readily determined. If no apparent increase in oxygen consumption is noted, the determinants of oxygen delivery must then be assessed.

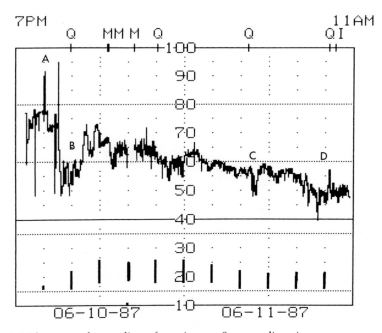

Fig. 8-7. A 16-hour trend recording of continuous Svo_2 readings in an acute trauma victim. The initial high Svo_2 (A) is artifactual and represents distal migration and wedging of the tip of the Svo_2 catheter. This is confirmed by the marked decrease in the light intensity indication at the bottom of the strip. A drop in Svo_2 (B) was associated with increased activity of the patient which was effectively controlled with appropriate sedation. A decline in Svo_2 (C) occurred during turning of the patient which reverted back somewhat, but remained < 60%. The Svo_2 gradually declined over the next 4 hours (D). The measured CO was 9.2 L/min. However the patient's measured hemoglobin had dropped to 7.5 g/dl which severely reduced oxygen delivery.

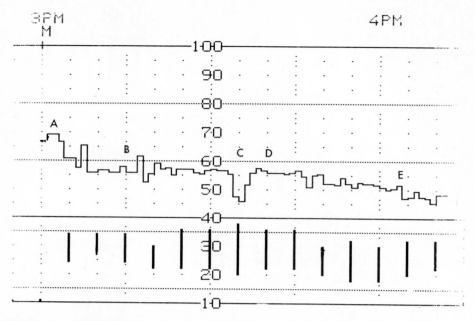

Fig. 8-8. Graph of continuous Svo_2 monitoring in a 64-year-old man admitted to the CCU with severe chest pain associated with dyspnea. Initial Svo_2 readings *(A)* were obtained after administration of oxygen and lasix as well as a nitroglycerin infusion. The patient's chest pain waxed and waned over the next 6 to 8 hours *(B)* despite increases in nitroglycerin administration. Episodes of nonsustained ventricular tachycardia were associated with a drop of Svo_2 to < 50% *(C)*. Lidocaine infusion was begun which resulted in arrhythmia suppression and improved Svo_2 *(D)*. However, the patient's cardiac output as well as Svo_2 continued to decline despite positive inotropic support *(E)*. An IABP was subsequently inserted in this patient in an attempt to improve myocardial and global tissue oxygenation.

A reduction in hemoglobin, unless associated with massive bleeding, is usually a slowly changing determinant and is less frequently responsible for sudden decreases in Svo_2. Hypoxemia, with a low Sao_2 can be evaluated by arterial blood gas determination or continuous pulse oxymetry monitoring Sao_2. While Sao_2 rarely changes more than 10% in most clinical situations, a decrease from 80% to 70% could represent a one-third drop in cardiac output.

Hypoperfusion is by far the most common cause of decreasing Svo_2. To confirm this, cardiac output determination should be performed. In this way cardiac output measurements are made when hemodynamically indicated, rather than at some routine or preset time. Use of continuous Svo_2 monitoring has also reduced the need for *routine* arterial blood gas analysis.

Sustained reductions in Svo_2 of 10% or greater over a 3- to 5-minute period should prompt assessments of the determinations of oxygen delivery as this finding frequently warns of impending deterioration. Therapy should then be directed toward controlling the oxygen demands *or* correcting the decrease in oxygen supply. A rapid improvement in Svo_2 confirms the appropriateness of the chosen therapy. Brief, minor changes in Svo_2 (5% or less) are clinically insignificant and are likely to be caused by some type of interference rather than changes in cardiac output.

Studies to assess correlation between Svo_2 and any one of the individual determinants of oxygen delivery or of oxygen consumption have shown a rather poor relationship. However, correlation of Svo_2 and all the determinants (oxygen extraction or oxygen utilization) is inversely high. This suggests that changes in Svo_2 occur not because of alterations in any one single determinant of oxygen supply/demand balance but rather reflect an overall imbalance. In this way continuous Svo_2 monitoring is used as a "barometer" to reflect overall tissue oxygenation.

REFERENCES

Barker SJ, Tremper KK, Hyatt BS, and Zaccari J: Effects of methemoglobinemia on pulse oximetry and mixed venous oximetry, Anesthesiology 67:A171, 1987.

Blair I et al: Oxygen saturation during transfer from operating room to recovery after anesthesia, Anaesth Intens Care 15:147-150, 1987.

Bryan-Brown CW: Blood flow to organs: parameters for function and survival in critical illness, Crit Care Med 16:170-177, 1988.

Cooper JB, Cullen DJ, and Nemeskal R: Effects of information feedback and pulse oximetry on the incidence of anesthesia complications, Anesth 67:686-694, 1987.

Fahey P: Clinical experience with continuous monitoring of mixed venous oxygen saturation in respiratory failure, Chest 86:748-752, 1984.

Jamieson WRE et al: Continuous monitoring of mixed venous oxygen saturation in cardiac surgery, Can J Surg 25:538-543, 1982.

Jaquith SM: Continuous measurement of Svo_2: clinical applications and advantages for critical care nursing, Crit Care Nurse 5:40-43, 1985.

Kandel G, and Aberman A: Mixed venous oxygen saturation: its role in the assessment of the critically ill patient, Arch Intern Med 143:1400-1402, 1983.

Kao YJ, and Badgwell JM: Reusing the Nellcor pulse probe: clarification, Anesth 67:866-868, 1987.

Krouskop RW, Cabatu EE, and Chelliah BP: Accuracy and clinical utility of an oxygen saturation catheter, Crit Care Med 11:744-749, 1983.

McMichan J: Continuous monitoring of mixed venous oxygen saturation. In Schweiss J, editor: Continuous measurement of blood oxygen saturation in the high risk patient, San Diego, 1983, Beach International.

Mihm FG, and Heperin BD: Noninvasive detection of profound arterial desaturation using a pulse oximetry device, Anesthesiology 62:85-87, 1985.

Neufield GR: Pulse oximetry, Med Instr 20:121, 1986.

Peterson JF: The development of pulse oximetry, Science 232:G135-140, 1987.

Rasanen J, Downs JB, and Oates K: Oxygen tension and oxyhemoglobin saturation to assess pulmonary gas exchange, Anesthesiology 67:A172, 1987.

Shibutani K et al: Critical level of oxygen delivery in anesthetized man, Crit Care Med 11:640-643, 1983.

Snyder JV, and Carroll GC: Tissue oxygenation: a physiologic approach to a clinical problem, Curr Probl Surg 19:652-719, 1982.

Snyder JV, and Pinsky MR: Oxygen transport in the critically ill, Chicago, 1987, Year Book Medical Publishers, Inc.

Strohl KP et al: Comparison of three transmittance oximeters, Med Instr 20:143-149, 1986.

Tremper KK: Monitoring with transcutaneous PO_2 and pulse oximetry devices, Can J Anaesth 35:61-63, 1987.

Tremper KK, et al: Accuracy of a pulse oximeter in critically ill adults: effect of temperature and hemodynamics, Anesthesiology 63:A175, 1985.

Turnbull KW: Mixed venous oxygen saturation, Can J Anaesth 34:59-61, 1987.

vanLanschot JJB, Feenstra BWA, Vermeij CG, and Bruining HA: Outcome prediction in critically ill patients by means of oxygen consumption index and simplified acute physiology score, Intensive Care Med 14:44-49, 1988.

White KM: Completing the hemodynamic picture: Svo_2, Heart Lung 14:272-280, 1985.

White KM: Continuous monitoring of mixed venous oxygen saturation (Svo_2): a new assessment tool in critical care nursing—Part II, Cardiovasc Nurs 23:7-12, 1987.

Yelderman M, and New W: Evaluation of pulse oximetry, Anesthesiology 59:349-352, 1983.

Chapter 9

Circulatory Assist

$\mathbf{N}$umerous methods of assisting the patient's circulation during periods of transient myocardial depression have been attempted. Of these methods, counterpulsation has been the most successful in improving circulation while causing the lowest incidence of complications. The principles and use of counterpulsation devices are discussed in this chapter.

PHYSIOLOGIC BASIS FOR COUNTERPULSATION DEVICES

The two primary goals for the clinical use of circulatory assist devices are to provide temporary assistance to the patient's circulation until the underlying pathophysiologic condition is corrected and to afford optimal conditions for repair of the heart until it can provide adequate circulation unaided. The intra-aortic balloon pump employs the principles of counterpulsation as a means of achieving these goals.

The intra-aortic balloon consists of a polyurethane balloon (40 to 60 cc capacity for adults) mounted on a vascular catheter, inserted into the femoral artery, and positioned in the descending aorta just distal to the left subclavian artery (Fig. 9-1). The balloon catheter is connected to a pump console that shuttles helium or carbon dioxide into the balloon during diastole to inflate it. During isovolumetric contaction, the gas is rapidly withdrawn to deflate the balloon (counterpulsation). The hemodynamic results of this action are to augment intra-aortic pressure during diastole and to lower intra-aortic pressure during systole. In this section the physiologic basis for circulatory assist devices and its application to patient care are discussed.

Diastolic Augmentation

Diastolic augmentation occurs as the direct result of the pumping of the assist device during diastole. The primary effect of this pumping action is to displace blood and force it back into the aortic root. This increase in ascending aortic blood volume is accompanied by a rise in diastolic pressure (diastolic augmentation). Augmenting diastolic pressure is particularly beneficial for the patient with coronary occlusive disease, since approximately 70% of arterial perfusion to the myocardium occurs during the diastolic phase of the cardiac cycle. By augmenting the intra-aortic pressure during diastole, the counterpulsation device mechanically increases coronary perfusion of the failing myocardium without increasing myocar-

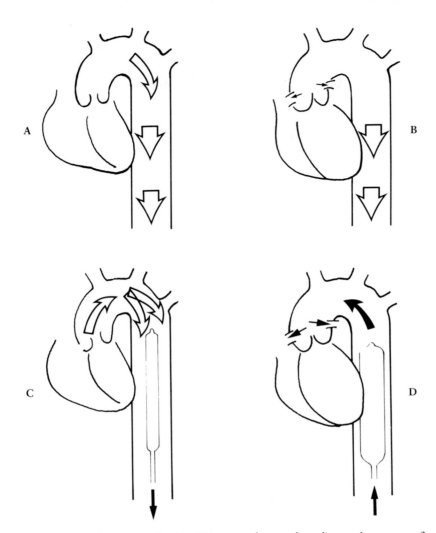

Fig. 9-1. Physiology of counterpulsation. Diagram of normal cardiac cycle pressure flow sequence as compared with the counterpulsed pressure flow sequence. **A,** Normal systole characterized by antegrade volume flow and peak intra-aortic pressure; **B,** normal diastole showing continued antegrade volume flow and adequate intra-aortic pressure for coronary perfusion; **C,** balloon deflation before systole allowing antegrade volume flow from the aortic arch (systolic unloading); **D,** courterpulsed diastole mechanically boosting volume flow retrograde to the aortic arch, heightening diastolic pressure and coronary perfusion.

dial work or oxygen demands. Thus the additional coronary perfusion, at no oxygen expense to the myocardium, may potentially limit the infarction size or reverse the cardiac ischemic dysfunction.

Whereas the systolic pressure usually decreases, the augmentation in diastolic pressure results in an increase in the mean arterial pressure, which acts as an in-line boost to the general circulation, improving perfusion to other vital organs as well.

Afterload Reduction

The second effect of counterpulsation is to reduce the afterload of the heart. Afterload, or resistance to LV ejection, is determined by the residual aortic blood volume and pressure met during LV systole. Afterload reduction is accomplished by the relaxing motion of the counterpulsation device at the end of diastole, just before ventricular ejection. With the intra-aortic balloon pump, the balloon collapses; with the noninvasive assist device, the positive pressure applied to the patient's lower extremities is released. Blood volume leaves the aortic arch to fill the space previously occupied by the inflated balloon or positive pressure. Less effort or work is then required for the left ventricle to empty into the area of lower blood volume. Since blood in the aorta is already moving forward and there is less resistance to flow, afterload reduction can occur with small decreases in systolic pressure.

There are three beneficial effects of afterload reduction by the use of circulatory assist devices. First, myocardial oxygen requirements are reduced because less work is required to eject stroke volume. Second, systolic ejection time is shortened; the duration of diastole is thereby increased, allowing more time for coronary perfusion. Third, the heart can eject more blood per beat because of the decreased resistance (systolic unloading) to forward flow. Thus stroke volume increases while diastolic filling pressure remains the same or decreases.

Counterpulsation meets the primary goals of circulatory assist by its combined actions of diastolic augmentation and afterload reduction. The overall effect of counterpulsation is to improve both coronary and systemic circulation until the heart can maintain circulation without assistance.

APPLICATION TO PATIENT CARE
Indications

The effectiveness of counterpulsation in assisting the circulation provides the basis for many applications of counterpulsation devices (Table 9-1). Some of the applications listed are based on theoretic or experimental data and have not as yet been shown to be clinically effective. This is particularly true of the more recent use of counterpulsation in children.

Contraindications

The two primary contraindications to counterpulsation circulatory assist are aortic valve incompetency and a dissecting thoracic aortic aneurysm. Diastolic augmentation may aggravate aortic insufficiency and further compromise LV function. Diastolic augmentation is also contraindicated in the presence of an aneurysm of the descending thoracic aorta, because additional stress would be applied to an already weakened aortic wall. Counterpulsation is also contraindicated in patients with underlying brain death or advanced or terminal disease states.

INTRA-AORTIC BALLOON PUMP

The intra-aortic balloon pump has been one of the most effective methods of counterpulsation used in the clinical setting. Moulopoulos, Topaz, and Kolff first introduced the basic principles of the intra-aortic balloon pump in 1962 and

Table 9-1. Potential uses of counterpulsation devices

Use	Rationale
For cardiogenic shock resulting from an acute myocardial infarction	To maintain circulatory perfusion until the heart can maintain adequate perfusion without assistance To provide optimal conditions for maintenance and repair of the ischemic myocardium
For low cardiac output states	To maintain adequate perfusion until the underlying cause of the condition is corrected
During emergency diagnostic procedures (ventriculograms, arteriograms, and cardiac catheterization)	To provide optimal coronary and peripheral perfusion during study
In the critically ill patient before emergency cardiovascular surgery for papillary muscle rupture, ventricular aneurysms, and VSD resulting from myocardial infarction	To maintain optimal perfusion until surgery
To assist in removing patients from cardiopulmonary bypass	To support patients who become hypotensive when removed from bypass until transient myocardial depression is resolved
For drug-resistant, life-threatening arrhythmias	To increase myocardial perfusion if arrhythmias are caused by ischemia
For unstable angina pectoris	To increase myocardial perfusion and possibly avoid irreversible ischemia leading to infarction
For acute myocardial infarction	To increase myocardial perfusion and thus limit or reduce the infarction size

Kantrowitz et al had further developed these principles by 1967. The device itself consists of a balloon-tipped catheter that is positioned in the descending thoracic aorta via the femoral artery. This catheter is then attached to the gas-driving unit. Counterpulsation is achieved by alternate inflation of the balloon during distole and rapid deflation of the balloon just before systole.

Equipment

Balloon models available for clinical use include the single-chambered balloon and the dual-chambered balloon. The single-chambered balloon, by far the most widely used, is assembled on a 12 Fr double-lumen catheter. One lumen opens into the balloon and is used to deliver gas (either carbon dioxide or helium), whereas the other lumen opens at the catheter tip and is used to monitor the aortic pressure. The *single-chambered balloon* consists of a single, sausage-shaped cylinder. When inflated, this device displaces blood volume, both retrograde to the aortic arch and antegrade, perfusing those areas distal to the balloon. The *dual-chambered balloon* has a small round chamber located distally and a larger second cylinder more proximal to the aortic root. The smaller chamber is timed to inflate slightly before the larger one, thus providing resistance to the antegrade boost caused by inflation of the second chamber. This addition of resistance downstream in the aorta results in an even greater volume of retrograde flow to perfuse the coronary arteries. Table 9-2 lists types and sizes of various adult IABs.

Selection of the correct balloon size is an important consideration when therapy is being initiated. Balloon capacities vary from 20 to 40 cc. The more blood volume displaced, the better the intra-aortic balloon pump functions. However, total occlusion of the aorta may injure the aortic intima and cause hemolysis of red blood cells. To avoid these complications, the balloon should fill at least 85% of the diameter of the aorta and yet be nonocclusive. Estimating the aortic diameter is an uncertain process, because the diameter varies with the individual patient and with the mean arterial pressure. Hence the aortic diameter must be estimated from the size of the femoral artery and the patient's body surface area.

Additional equipment needed to insert an intra-aortic balloon include:
1. Supplies for skin preparation
2. Cutdown or percutaneous catheter insertion tray
3. Resuscitation equipment including crash cart and defibrillator
4. ECG and pressure monitoring equipment
5. Gas-driving pump with emergency power source

Patient Preparation

The following steps should be taken to prepare the patient for IAB insertion:
1. Explain the procedure to the patient and/or to the family, if appropriate.
2. Obtain informed consent.
3. Obtain and review current lab values, including hemogram, platelets, prothrombin time (PT), partial thromboplastin time (PTT), and bleeding time.
4. Secure and maintain an IV line if a PA catheter is not in place.
5. Secure and maintain an intra-arterial line. (This may not be necessary if intra-aortic pressure is monitored through the central lumen of the percutaneous IAB catheter.)

Table 9-2. Types, sizes, and balloon volumes of various adult IABs

Manufacturer	Catheter size	Insertion mode	Balloon volume (ml)
Datascope	12 Fr adult, 117 cm	Surgical	30-40
	8.5, 9.5 & 10.5 Fr Percor and Percor STAT-DL, 117 cm	Percutaneous or surgical	40-50
Kontron	12 Fr adult, 110 cm	Surgical	20-40
	10.5 & 12 Fr adult, 110 cm	Percutaneous	40
SMEC	12 Fr adult, 79 cm	Surgical	30-60
	10.5, 11, & 11.5 Fr adult, 79 cm	Percutaneous	30-60

Insertion

The introduction of the percutaneous IAB catheter in 1979 greatly increased the overall use of counterpulsation. Because the percutaneous route can be performed more rapidly than the surgical approach and is not dependent on the availability of a cardiac or vascular surgeon, therapy can be initiated sooner, with better long-term results.

The percutaneous balloon catheter with a central lumen permits insertion of a guidewire through the lumen and facilitates passage of the balloon through atherosclerotic and tortuous vessels. In addition, contrast medium can be injected through the lumen and intra-aortic pressure monitoring can be performed.

Percutaneous balloon insertion. Before insertion, the percutaneous intra-aortic balloon should be prepared under sterile conditions. The balloon is prepared by testing the balloon integrity with the injection of 20 cc of air and by wrapping the balloon snugly around the catheter by turning the catheter's wrap handle in a clockwise direction (Fig. 9-2). If the catheter is wrapped while negative pressure is applied to the chamber with the use of a syringe, all the air will be removed and the balloon will wrap more compactly. To facilitate unwrapping when positioned in the aorta, it is important that the balloon catheter be moistened with saline before wrapping. The pressure lumen of the balloon catheter should be flushed with sterile, heparinized IV fluid. The appropriate length of catheter required for optimal placement in the descending aorta can be estimated by placing the tip of the catheter approximately 1 cm below the sternal angle of Louis before insertion.

After appropriate skin preparation and the administration of a local anesthetic,

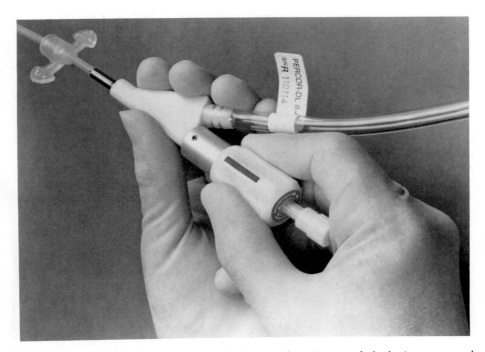

Fig. 9-2. The handle on the percutaneous balloon catheter is turned clockwise to wrap the balloon snugly around the catheter to facilitate percutaneous insertion. (Courtesy Datascope Corporation, Peramus, N.J.)

either the right or left common femoral artery is punctured approximately one fingerbreadth below the inguinal crease with an 18-gauge arterial needle. A 0.038-inch J-tip guidewire is advanced through the needle into the abdominal aorta. The needle is removed and an 8 Fr Teflon dilator is inserted over the guidewire to enlarge the puncture site. This dilator is removed and a 12 Fr Teflon dilator is inserted over the guidewire into the femoral artery. After removal of the guidewire, the prepared balloon-catheter is inserted through the 12 Fr dilator and positioned with the tip just distal to the takeoff of the left subclavian artery (see Fig. 9-3). Correct positioning is confirmed by fluoroscopy or chest x-ray. The balloon is then unwrapped by turning the wrap handle in a counterclockwise position until it reaches a stop. The balloon-sheath system is sutured to the skin with several sutures to ensure stability.

The catheter-balloon is now ready for the connection of one lumen to a prepared transducer for intra-arterial pressure monitoring and attachment of the other lumen to a gas-pumping system for inflation and deflation of the balloon.

Arteriotomy. The balloon can be inserted into either common femoral artery. The artery with the strongest pulse is chosen to permit easier insertion of the balloon and better perfusion to the limb once the balloon catheter is in position.

With the use of local anesthesia, an arterial cutdown is performed. A Dacron graft is sewn to the side of the artery (Fig. 9-3). The balloon is inserted through the side graft and rapidly advanced to its position in the descending thoracic aorta. Heparin is administered intravenously (maintenance doses are then given every 4 to 6 hours for the duration of counterpulsation). A tie is placed around the Dacron side graft (as opposed to the artery itself) to secure the catheter. This method secures the catheter and affords the best opportunity for adequate distal perfusion to the leg.

The percutaneous IAB catheter can also be inserted directly into an exposed

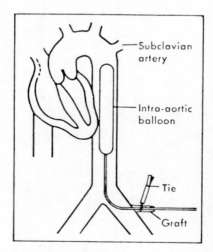

Fig. 9-3. Placement of the intra-aortic balloon. Insertion is made through a sidearm graft via a cutdown on the common femoral artery. The balloon position is just distal to the left subclavian artery. Ties around the graft secure the catheter in place without jeopardizing perfusion to the leg distal to the insertion site.

femoral artery. This may be performed after cardiopulmonary bypass or if difficulty is encountered with percutaneous insertion. The balloon catheter is prepared in the routine fashion and inserted through the arteriotomy or with the optional use of a Dacron graft. Use of a guidewire through the central lumen of the IAB can aid in passage through tortuous vessels.

The optimal position for the balloon is just distal to the left subclavian artery. This position should be confirmed by fluoroscopic examination after insertion. In this position the balloon is close enough to the aortic valve to optimize diastolic augmentation yet far enough away to reduce the risk of cerebral embolism. This position also decreases the potential for balloon-tip perforation of the aortic arch during catheter insertion or patient movement.

Operation

Once the balloon is positioned properly, the catheter is attached to the gas-pumping apparatus and therapy is initiated. Several different types of IAB pumps are available for use in counterpulsation. It is recommended that all personnel involved in the care of a patient undergoing counterpulsation receive detailed instruction and carefully follow the specific manufacturer's recommendations and procedures for proper usage. Basic pump setup consists of establishing power, establishing gas pressure, setting controls, and establishing ECG and arterial pressure signals. The two types of gases used to drive the balloon pump are helium and carbon dioxide. Because helium is more light-weight and has a more rapid delivery time, balloon function at faster heart rates and during arrhythmias is facilitated. Carbon dioxide, on the other hand, is more soluble in blood; therefore the seriousness of gas embolization if the balloon ruptures is reduced.

Display the patient's arterial pressure and observe the appearance of the waveform with a distinct dicrotic notch.

Obtain a reliable, artifact-free ECG with a tall (0.2 mV) positive R wave. This is essential for safe, effective intra-aortic balloon pumping. Obtaining such a signal depends on properly preparing the skin (shave the electrode site if necessary and rub the site briskly with a dry gauze pad); avoid electrode placement on bony prominences, joints, or skin folds, and securely attach pre-jelled electrodes to the skin. If 60-cycle electric interference is present in the ECG, isolate and remove the interference. Antiarrhythmic therapy may be necessary to reduce or eliminate premature beats (atrial or ventricular) that would prevent proper timing of counterpulsation.

Timing

Timing of inflation and deflation should not be set solely according to the ECG. Effective timing of counterpulsation is achieved through utilization of the arterial pressure waveform. Although the R wave of the ECG serves as the reference point for inflation and deflation, the normal physiologic electric-mechanical delay necessitates use of the intra-arterial waveform for more accurate timing of inflation and deflation. Inflation of the balloon can safely occur immediately after closure and before opening of the aortic valve (Fig. 9-4).

Balloon deflation should occur just before the aortic valve opens. Optimal augmentation occurs when (1) the assisted diastolic arterial pressure exceeds the pa-

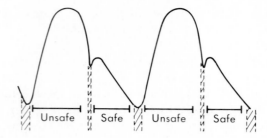

Fig. 9-4. Functional range of safe timing for counterpulsation. (From Quaal SJ: Comprehensive intra-aortic balloon pumping, St Louis, 1984, The CV Mosby Co.)

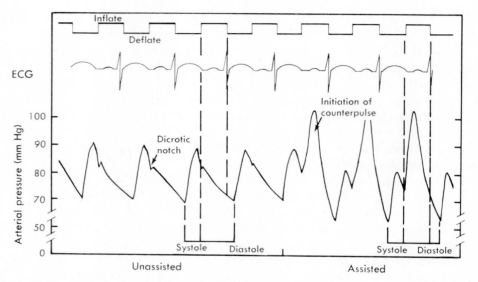

Fig. 9-5. Timing and effect of the counterpulsation sequence by the ECG and arterial pressure waveform. With initiation of counterpulsation, diastolic pressure is heightened and systolic and end-diastolic pressures are lowered.

tients' unassisted systolic arterial pressure and (2) the assisted aortic end-diastolic pressure is 5 to 15 mm Hg lower than the patient's unassisted end-diastolic pressure (Fig. 9-5).

Proper timing can best be achieved when inflation occurs with every other beat (1:2 frequency) so as to compare the augmented with the nonaugmented arterial waveform. Fine adjustments in inflation control should be made to time the occurrence of inflation with the dicrotic notch of arterial waveform, creating a V configuration of the dicrotic notch. Adjustments in the deflation control should result in a balloon-assisted systolic pressure that is lower than the patient's unassisted systolic pressure. In addition, the balloon-assisted aortic end-diastolic pressure should be 10 to 15 mm Hg lower than the patient's unassisted aortic end-diastolic pressure. Inflation should be set and adjusted first, then deflation should be optimized.

Additional timing adjustments may be necessary if the heart rate changes more than 10 beats/min. The newest computerized IAB pump automatically and instantaneously adjusts timing for changes in heart rate and rhythm. Balloon pumping is most effective if the heart rate is greater than 80 beats/min and less than 110 beats/min in normal sinus rhythm.

Tachycardia. Heart rates above 120 beats/min compromise the duration of diastole and therefore diastolic augmentation. Tachycardia may also pose mechanical problems in the pump's ability to track higher heart rates resulting in reduced carbon dioxide gas flow and volume. Use of helium, rather than carbon dioxide, as a driving gas is suggested for patients with higher heart rates. For heart rates greater than 120 beats/min, decrease the pumping frequency rate to 1:2 and institute appropriate therapy to lower the heart rate.

Atrial fibrillation. Irregularity of the R-R interval poses a severe timing problem, particularly if the R wave appears early. Overall effects of augmentation are best achieved by adjusting the augmentation sequence to the shortest R-R interval. It is also prudent to adjust the deflation control bar, causing the balloon to deflate on the peak of the R wave. This prevents inflation during any systolic event, regardless of timing. Digoxin may be used to slow the heart rate; verapamil may also be used unless there is severe left ventricular dysfunction. Antiarrhythmic therapy or cardioversion may be used to achieve a sinus rhythm and improve augmentation.

Ventricular tachycardia. Ventricular tachycardia can usually trigger the balloon pump if the timing frequency is decreased to 1:3. Balloon fill time can be reduced so that balloon inflation and deflation require less time. Antiarrhythmic therapy or cardioversion is used to correct the arrhythmia.

Ventricular fibrillation. Defibrillation can be carried out in the usual manner, with discontinuation of counterpulsation for a few seconds during delivery of the current. Because the system is not completely isolated from the patient, there is the danger of damaging the unit during defibrillation.

Cardiac arrest. The IAB does not interfere with cardiopulmonary resuscitation (CPR); in fact, balloon inflation during the diastolic phrase of CPR would be beneficial. If chest compressions are regular, the balloon pump will be triggered with each compression (or systole). If compressions are not regular, the balloon will automatically deflate. Balloon fill time should be reduced. The IAB catheter can be inserted percutaneously during resuscitation to provide immediate circulatory assistance. Fig. 9-6 depicts various examples of correct and incorrect timing of counterpulsation.

Aortic pressure monitoring with the IAB catheter

Monitoring of the aortic pressure rather than peripheral arterial pressure provides a more accurate basis for timing of counterpulsation. Direct aortic pressure monitoring can be performed through the central lumen of the IAB catheter in the following way:
1. After insertion of the percutaneous IAB catheter, and following removal of the stylet or guidewire from the central lumen, aspirate 3 ml of blood from the central lumen and flush with 3 ml sterile heparinized saline.
2. Attach a three-way stopcock with a continuous flush device, transducer, tubing, and heparinized IV solution to the hub of the inner lumen of the IAB catheter (Fig. 9-7). Carefully ensure that all air bubbles are removed from any of the attached equipment.

A
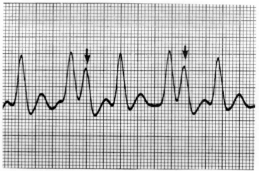

Early deflation 1:2 assist

B

Late deflation 1:2 assist

C
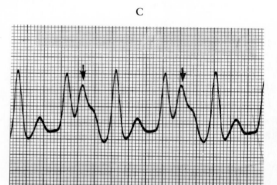

Early inflation 1:2 assist

D

Late inflation 1:2 assist

E
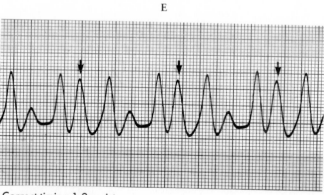

Correct timing 1:2 assist

Fig 9-6. Examples of arterial pressure waveforms with correct and incorrect timing of the inflation-deflation sequence in a patient on 1:2 assist ratio counterpulsation. Arrows indicate augmentation. **A,** Early balloon deflation evidenced by rapid equilibration of the augmented end-diastolic pressure to the nonaugmented end-diastolic pressure. **B,** Slight delay in balloon deflation. Note the similarity between the nonaugmented end-diastolic pressure and the augmented end-diastolic pressure. **C,** Early balloon inflation producing shortened systolic ejection time and stroke volume with augmentation. **D,** Late balloon inflation evidence by small augmented waveform following the dicrotic notch. **E,** Correct timing.

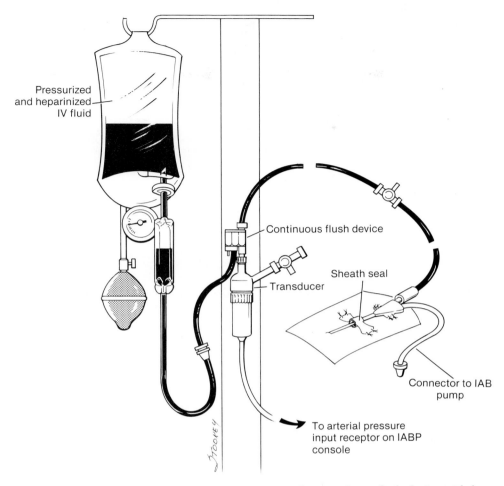

Fig. 9-7. Central lumen of the IAB catheter connected to continous-flush device with heparinized solution and a transducer for monitoring of the intra-aortic pressure.

3. Maintain a continuous infusion of heparinized solution through the catheter lumen and activate the "fast flush" on an hourly basis to maintain catheter patency. Always discontinue balloon pulsation before fast flushing or blood sampling to reduce the risk of retrograde embolus.

Associated Therapy

When balloon pumping is initiated, other supportive therapies are begun to enhance the effect of counterpulsation. These therapies include the following:
1. Discontinuation of inotropic and vasopressor agents as soon as possible, because their therapeutic action may oppose the effect of the balloon pump
2. Fluid administration to maintain adequate filling pressures in the face of reduced vasoconstriction as peripheral vasoconstriction lessens and diastolic filling pressures fall
3. Administration of small doses of peripheral vasodilators (sodium nitroprusside)

to further decrease the afterload and increase peripheral perfusion, particularly to the kidneys

4. Intravenous administration of heparin for the duration of balloon placement to prevent thrombus formation on the balloon catheter
5. Administration of prophylactic, broad-spectrum antibiotics

Patients require close monitoring if optimal counterpulsation is to be realized. Parameters to be monitored include the following:

1. Vital signs
2. Hemodynamic pressures, including CVP or, preferably, PA pressure (systolic, diastolic, mean), PAW mean pressure, and arterial pressure
3. Oxygenation (SaO_2 and SvO_2)
4. Renal function (monitored by urinary flow, specific gravity, and blood chemistries; frequent monitoring is facilitated by the insertion of a urinary catheter)
5. Blood flow to the catheterized limb (monitored for signs of circulatory insufficiency such as cyanosis or decreased pulses and temperature)
6. Anticoagulation (monitored by a Lee-White clotting time or partial thromboplastin test)

Table 9-3 lists suggested monitoring parameters during counterpulsation.

Complications

Complications associated with intra-aortic balloon pumping occur frequently and many relate to the problem of passing a large catheter into an atherosclerotic vessel. Approximately half of the 20% to 25% of complications reported are major and include aortic dissection, perforation of the common iliac artery, and thrombotic complications, particularly of the renal artery. Death related to one of these complications occurs in 1% of patients. The use of heparin minimizes but does not prevent peripheral embolic complications. In addition, the prolonged use of heparin is associated with bleeding from the insertion site and frequently requires surgical exploration. Septic complications including septicemia or an infected wound site require early removal of the balloon and appropriate antibiotic therapy.

The single most frequently occurring complication of balloon pumping has been vascular insufficiency of the catheterized limb (5% to 47%). Although this complication is usually transient, Fogarty catheterization to restore circulation may be necessary.

The enhanced ease and speed of insertion of the percutaneous intra-aortic balloon has not decreased the incidence of complications that occur with balloon pumping. Additionally, failure to insert the percutaneous balloon-catheter is not uncommon in patients with arteriosclerotic disease. Occasionally, the introduction of a longer, 15-inch 12 Fr dilator will facilitate insertion, whereas at other times an arteriotomy is necessary for balloon insertion.

Table 9-4 lists possible complications of the intra-aortic balloon pump and suggestions for their prevention.

Improved Hemodynamics and Removal

Hemodynamic improvement with the intra-aortic balloon pump is rapidly observed within the first hour or two of the therapy. Mean arterial pressure rises, and both coronary and peripheral perfusion improve. Mental confusion decreases, and

Table 9-3. Suggested monitoring schedule of hemodynamic, laboratory, and clinical parameters in patients with IABP

Parameters	Monitoring frequency
HEMODYNAMICS	
RA, PA, PAW or LA pressures	Every 30 min until stable (and during weaning), every 2 hr thereafter
Intra-arterial pressure (systolic, diastolic, and augmented diastolic)	
CI, SVR, SWI	Every 1 hr until stable, every 4 hr thereafter
PERIPHERAL CIRCULATION	
Quality of dorsalis pedis, posterior tibial pulses	Every 15 min the first hr, every 30 min the next 2 hr, every 2 hr and as needed thereafter
Color, temperature, movement, and sensation of legs	
Doppler flowmeter	
RENAL CIRCULATION	
Urine output	Every 1 hr
CEREBRAL CIRCULATION	
Mental status	Every 1 hr and as needed
HEMATOLOGIC ASSESSMENT	
Hemogram	Daily and as needed
Platelet count, PTT	Every 8 to 12 hr and as needed after therapeutic anticoagulation is obtained
OXYGENATION	
Arterial blood gases	Every 8 hr and as needed
Mixed venous oxygen saturation	Continuously (via fiberoptic catheter) or every 8 hr and as needed
VITAL SIGNS	
Heart rate, respiratory rate, temperature	Every hr until stable, then every 2 to 4 hr and as needed
AUSCULTATORY EXAMINATION	
Heart sounds	Every 2 hr and as needed
Breath sounds	

urinary flow improves. Because of afterload reduction, cardiac output increases and preload or LV end-diastolic volume decreases. This is evidenced by a decrease in PAW mean and PA diastolic pressures.

The optimal duration for balloon pumping has not been established. Some investigators believe that pumping should be terminated within 48 hours, even though longer assistance is possible. This early termination time is recommended

Table 9-4. Complications of the intra-aortic balloon pump

Complication	Incidence	Prevention
Circulatory insufficiency of the catheterized limb distal to the insertion site	Most frequent	Use the largest femoral artery with the best pulse for balloon insertion. Administer heparin for anticoagulation. Frequently check the limb for signs of decreased circulation (temperature, color, pulses, movement, and sensation). When the balloon is removed, explore the femoral artery with a Fogarty catheter to remove clots.
Aortic or arterial damage (dissection, intimal laceration, or hematoma)	Occasional	Position the balloon catheter in the descending aorta just distal to the left subclavian artery. Select the correct balloon size, so that the inflated balloon does not occlude the aorta. Never advance the balloon-catheter if resistance is felt. Do not elevate head of bed >30 degrees; limit patient movement (leg flexion can move the balloon tip up in the aorta, resulting in possible puncture of the arch).
Emboli from the balloon, catheter, sheath, or graft	Occasional	Administer heparin therapy. Do not leave the balloon in place if it is collapsed and motionless. Remove percutaneous sheath and catheter together. Allow wound to bleed vigorously 1 to 2 sec after removal of percutaneous balloon catheter.
Infection	Occasional	Use aseptic technique. Care for wound daily. Use prophylactic antibiotics. Change IV tubing every 24 to 48 hr.
Hemolysis	Minimal	Select the correct balloon size, so that the inflated balloon does not occlude aorta.
Platelet reduction	Frequent	Unknown; heparin may help.
Balloon leak or rupture with gas embolism	Rare	Use careful insertion technique to prevent damage to the balloon. Use carbon dioxide as the inflation gas since it is more soluble in blood. Choose the largest femoral artery for insertion.
Pseudoaneurysm or hematoma	Rare	Direct mechanical pressure at puncture site for 30 to 60 min after balloon removal.
Bleeding at puncture site	Occasional	Same as above.

Table 9-5. Clinical and hemodynamic criteria for discontinuation of IABP

Clinical criteria	Hemodynamic criteria
Evidence of adequate perfusion	Cardiac index >2.0 L/min/m²
Urine output >30 ml/hr	
Improved mental status	MAP >70 mm Hg with minimal or no
Skin temperature warm	pressors
No evidence of congestive heart failure	PAEDP/PAWP or LAP <18 mm Hg
Rales absent	
S3 absent	
No life-threatening dysrhythmias	Heart rate <110 beats/min without
	complex ventricular arrhythmias

to prevent balloon dependence. Dependence on the intra-aortic balloon pump is indicated by a reversion to a previous shock state when balloon assistance is discontinued. Table 9-5 lists hemodynamic and clinical criteria for cessation of counterpulsation.

Once it has been established that a patient is to be removed from circulatory assist, a systematic weaning process is begun. One method of weaning the patient from circulatory assist is to alternate the amount of time on the balloon with an equal time off the balloon. Another method is to gradually decrease the volume of the balloon inflation, allowing it to displace less blood each time. A third method is to pump every other heartbeat, then every third or fourth beat, and so on, until the patient is finally weaned. The weaning process may take hours to days, depending on the hemodynamic status of the patient.

The use of the intra-aortic balloon pump to improve cardiac output and blood pressure during cardiogenic shock has been well documented. Also, it appears to be of particular value in the treatment of cardiogenic shock that is transient, such as after cardiac surgery, and in the maintenance of the circulatory assist during diagnostic studies.

REFERENCES

Alcan KE et al: Comparison of wire-guided percutaneous insertion and conventional surgical insertion of intra-aortic balloon pumps in 115 patients, Am J Med 75:24-28, 1983.

Alcan KE et al: Current status of intra-aortic balloon counterpulsation in critical care cardiology, Crit Care Med 12:489-495, 1984.

Alderman JD et al: Incidence and management of limb ischemia with percutaneous wire-guided intraaortic balloon catheters, J Am Coll Cardiol 9:524-530, 1987.

Bicking M: The patient on the intra-aortic balloon pump, Crit Care Nurse 2:50-52, 1982.

Bolooki H: Clinical application of intra-aortic balloon pump, New York, 1984, Futura Publishing Co Inc.

Bolooki H; Current status of circulatory support

with an intra-aortic balloon pump, Med Instrum 20:266-275, 1986.

Bregman D, and Cohen SR: Mechanical support of the circulation: current status, Contemp Surg 18:71-88, 1981.

Bregman D et al: Percutaneous intraaortic balloon insertion, Am J Cardiol 46:261-264, 1980.

Bullas JB: Care of the patient on the percutaneous intra-aortic counterpulsation balloon, Crit Care Nurse 2:40-49, 1982.

Dunkman WB et al: Clinical and hemodynamic results of the intra-aortic balloon pumping and surgery for cardiogenic shock, Circulation 46:465-477, 1972.

Flaherty JT et al: Results of a randomized prospective trial of intra-aortic balloon counterpulsation and intravenous nitroglycerin in patients with acute myocardial infarction, J Am Coll Cardiol 6:434-446, 1985.

Goldberg MJ et al: Intra-aortic balloon pump insertion: a randomized study comparing percutaneous and surgical techniques, J Am Coll Cardiol 9:515-523, 1987.

Goldberger M, Tabak SW, and Shah PK: Clinical experience with intra-aortic balloon counterpulsation in 112 consecutive patients, Am Heart J 111:497-502, 1986.

Harvey JC et al: Complications of percutaneous intra-aortic balloon pumping, Circulation 64(part 2):114-117, 1981.

Kantrowitz A et al: Initial clinical experience with intra-aortic balloon pumping in cardiogenic shock, JAMA 203:135-140, 1968.

McEnany MT et al: Clinical experience with intra-aortic balloon support in 728 patients, Cardiovasc Surg 58(suppl. 1):124-132, 1978.

Moulopoulos SD, Topaz S, and Kolff WJ: Diastolic balloon pumping (with carbon dioxide) in the aorta: mechanical assistance to the failing circulation, Am Heart J 63:669, 1962.

Mueller H et al: Effect of isoproterenol, l-norepinephrine and intra-aortic counterpulsation on hemodynamics and myocardial metabolism in shock following acute myocardial infarction, Circulation 45:335-351, 1975.

Mundth ED, Buckley MJ, and Austen WG: Myocardial revascularization during postinfarction shock, Hosp Prac 8:113-123, 1973.

Quaal SJ: Comprehensive intra-aortic balloon pumping, St Louis, 1984, The CV Mosby Co.

Resnekov L: Mechanical assistance for the failing ventricle, Mod Concepts Cardiovasc Dis 43(4):81-85, 1974.

Sanders CA et al: Mechanical circulatory assistance: current status and experience with combining circulatory assistance, emergency coronary angiography, and acute myocardial revascularization, Circulation 45:1292-1313, 1974.

Scheidt S et al: Intra-aortic balloon counterpulsation in cardiogenic shock: report of a cooperative clinical trial, N Engl J Med 288:979-984, 1973.

Subramanian VA: Preliminary clinical experience with percutaneous intraaortic balloon pumping, Circulation 62(part 2):123-129, 1980.

Vignola PA, Swaye PS, and Gosselin AJ: Guidelines for effective and safe percutaneous intra-aortic balloon pump insertion and removal, Am J Cardiol 48:660-664, 1981.

Willerson JT et al: Intraaortic balloon counterpulsation in patients in cardiogenic shock, medically refractory left ventricular failure and/or recurrent ventricular tachycardia, Am J Med 58:183-191, 1975.

Yahr WZ et al: Cardiogenic shock: dynamics of coronary blood flow with intra-aortic phase-shift balloon pumping, Surg Forum 19:142-143, 1968.

Chapter 10

Clinical Management Based on Hemodynamic Parameters

The care and management of cirtically ill patients has been enhanced with the advent of bedside hemodynamic monitoring. Knowledge of the patient's individual cardiopulmonary profile gives the clinician the ability to not only direct appropriate therapy to specific deranged parameters, but also to immediately assess the patient's response to such therapy.

A primary goal in the clinical management of all critically ill patients is the maintenance of adequate tissue oxygenation. Fig. 10-1 depicts the determinants of oxygen delivery or transport to the tissues, namely: cardiac output, hemoglobin, and arterial oxygen saturation. Furthermore, cardic output can be broken down into the determinants of preload, afterload, contractility, and heart rate. When viewed in this way it becomes clear that with the use of invasive monitoring of all the determinants of oxygen delivery can be either measured directly or calculated from direct measurements. Preload is measured by RA, PAW or LA pressures. Afterload is measured as PVR or SVR. Contractility is calculated as left ventricular stroke index (LVSWI) or right ventricular stroke work index (RVSWI). Heart rate is measured continuously. Arterial saturation can also be measured continuously with a pulse oximeter, and hemoglobin concentration can be measured intermittently. Monitoring of all these determinants allows the capability of intervening to effectively alter whichever of these determinants is deranged to bring them into normal or preferably supernormal range for effective delivery and maintenance of tissue oxygenation. Additionally, continuous hemodynamic monitoring permits the clinician to ssess the effectiveness of a chosen intervention and to titrate or perhaps discontinue it, depending on the patient's response. Frequently, these decisions are left to critical care nurses, who often practice with standing orders to maintain certain hemodynamic parameters at specific levels. Thus it is imperative that there be a clear understanding of how certain thera-

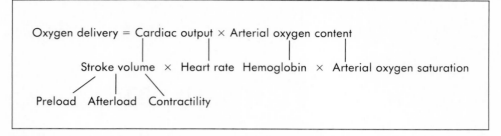

Fig. 10-1. Oxygen delivery ($\dot{D}o_2$) is a product of cardiac output and arterial oxygen content. Cardiac output is a product of stroke volume and heart rate, with preload, afterload, and contractility being the determinants of stroke volume. Arterial oxygen content is the product of the hemoglobin concentration and the oxygen saturation of arterial blood. Monitoring of these parameters along with the appropriate interventions are used clinically to increase oxygen delivery to the tissues.

peutic agents are used to alter various hemodynamic parameters, all for the purpose of maintaining a balance between oxygen supply and demand.

PRELOAD

Preload, the diastolic stretch or filling of the ventricle, is an important determinant of stroke volume. Adequate stroke volume requires sufficient myocardial fiber stretch, or preload, according to the Starling law. Inadequate preload of the normal left ventricle, as reflected by left ventricular end-diastolic pressure of <12 mm Hg, may be associated with reduced stroke volume. Patients with ventricular dysfunction or decreased compliance of the ventricle usually require a higher filling pressure of 18 to 20 mm Hg. However, left ventricular filling pressures higher than 20 or 22 mm Hg are often associated with pulmonary congestion secondary to transudation of fluid from the vascular network into interstitial, or even intraalveolar spaces. This results in reduced oxygen uptake and overall decreased tissue oxygenation.

Low Preload

If signs of hypoperfusion occur in the face of the low preload pressures (that is, <6 mm Hg RAP/CVP on the right side, <8 mm Hg PAW or LAp in patients without cardiac dysfunction, or <18 mm Hg PAWP or LAp in patients with cardiac dysfunction), efforts are directed towards increasing preload levels. This is best achieved by the administration of fluid in an attempt to increase circulating volume. In general, patients who do not have cardiac disease usually do not require a filling pressure >10 to 16 mm Hg (as measured by the PAWP) to obtain optimal stroke volume. Patients with cardiac disease usually require a higher filling pressure (16 to 22 mm Hg PAWP) and more judicious fluid administration. Most commonly this is achieved with IV fluid challenges of 100 to 250 cc of crystalloid solution over 10 minutes until evidence of improved perfusion occurs. Plotting ventricular function curves during this time is helpful to define the optimal filling pressure for the individual patient (that is, that filling pressure which produces the best stroke volume).

High Preload

When left-sided filling pressures become excessively high, pulmonary venous pressure becomes higher than the colloid osmotic pressure surrounding the vasculature. This causes fluid to be driven from the vasculature and into surrounding interstitial or intraalveolar spaces. This backward congestion is often manifested clinically by dyspnea and rales, in addition to signs of hypoperfusion. This can occur when the PAWP pressure acutely increases to >20 to 22 mm Hg. Cardiogenic pulmonary edema usually occurs with a PAWP higher than 30 mm Hg. (However, in patients with chronic heart failure, PAWP of >30 mm Hg may be seen without evidence of congestion or pulmonary edema.) Fluid in the interstitial or alveolar spaces interferes with oxygen uptake in the lung and hypoxemia with decreased oxygen delivery results. Reductions in preload to the lowest level compatible with adequate stroke volume can be obtained with the following means.

Diuretics

Furosemide, bumetanide, and ethacrynic acid, the three IV diuretics most commonly used in the critical care setting, are called *loop diuretics* because they inhibit the reabsorption of sodium in Henle's loop. This results in diuresis (usually about 30 minutes after administration) with resultant decreases in circulating blood volume and decreased preload (PAWP). Additionally, these agents have a venodilatory effect that occurs within 5 minutes of administration and lasts about 1 hour. This venodilation results in venous pooling, decreased venous return and, therefore, preload (PAW) pressures. The effect on cardiac output following IV diuretic administration depends on the individual patient's ventricular function. Excessive reductions of preload can result in reduced cardiac output. This can be avoided with careful monitoring of the PAWP and construction of ventricular function curves to determine the patient's optimal filling pressure (see Fig. 10-2).

Venodilators

Venodilators redistribute blood volume in the capacitance vessels and, thus, reduce ventricular filling. Nitrate preparations (nitroglycerin) are predominantly venous vasodilators, although they also cause some arteriovasodilation. This reduces venous return and preload (PAWP) and therefore relieves pulmonary congeston. (In addition, nitroglycerin dilates the epicardial coronary arteries and improves collateral coronary blood flow.) Because of its rapid action and short half-life, IV nitroglycerin can be quickly titrated to obtain optimal filling pressure as determined by ventricular function curves. Careful monitoring of arterial blood pressure should be done to avoid significant hypotension, which can occur as preload and, to a certain extent, afterload are reduced.

If direct manipulation of preload with the above measures does not produce an improvement in cardiac output and therefore oxygen delivery to the tissues, therapeutic alterations of the other determinants of cardic output may be necessary.

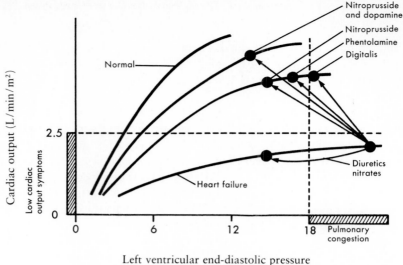

Fig. 10-2. Effects of various agents used for treating heart failure on the ventricular function curve. Diuretics and nitrates lower atrial pressure along the same curve and have little action on forward cardiac output. Positive inotropic agents and arterial vasodilators shift the ventricular function curve upward and to the left, increasing cardiac output for any left ventricular end-diastolic pressure. The combination of an arterial vasodilator and a positive inotropic agent (for example, nitroprusside and dopamine) can augment cardiac output and lower filling pressure to a greater extent than either agent alone. (Adapted from Mason DT, editor: Congestive heart failure, New York, 1976, Yorke Medical Books).

AFTERLOAD

True ventricular afterload is a complex measurement of the total force opposing left ventricular ejection. Clinically, afterload refers to the resistance to ventricular ejection which is primarily determined by systemic arterial resistance. A clinical reflection of the afterload of the left ventricle is the calculated SVR while afterload of the right ventricle is the calculated PVR (Table 10-1). Normally, the reserve capacity maintains stroke volume fairly constant despite changes in resistance with either vasoconstriction or vasodilation. In the failing heart, however, afterload or impedance is inversely related to cardiac output or stroke volume (Fig. 10-3).

Low Afterload

Arterial vasodilation results in decreased resistance (decreased afterload) and increased blood flow. However, since BP= CO × SVR, excessive reduction in SVR can result in severe hypotesion and consequently inadequate coronary artery perfusion. In this situation vasopressor agents may be used to increase resistance and establish an adequate perfusion pressure. Vasopressors cause vasoconstriction secondary to stimulation of alpha receptors in vascular smooth muscle. This produces an increase in both systolic and diastolic blood pressure. These agents include phenylephrine, metaraminol, epinephrine, norepinephrine, ephedrine, and dopamine (>10 to 20 mcg/kg/min). Of these agents, epinephrine, norepinephrine, ephedrine, and dopamine also possess beta$_1$ stimulating properties that cause an increase in cardiac contractility and ejection. The secondary effects of increased resistance to ejection, or afterload, with the use of vasopressor agents are an accompanying in-

Table 10-1. Derived hemodynamic parameters

Parameter	Abbreviation	Formula	Units	Normal values
Cardiac index	CI	$\dfrac{\text{Cardic output}}{\text{Body surface area}}$	L/min/M^2	2.5-4.0
Coronary perfusion pressure	CPP	Dias BP − PAWm	mm Hg	60-80
Left ventricular stroke work index	LVSWI	SVI × (MAP − PAWm) × .0136	g·m/m^2/beat	40-75
Oxygen delivery	$\dot{D}o_2$	Cardiac output × Arterial oxygen content	ml/min	750-1000
Pulmonary vascular resistance	PVR	$\dfrac{\text{PAm} - \text{PAWm}}{\text{Cardiac output}} \times 80$	dynes·sec·cm^{-5}	100-250
Pulmonary vascular resistance index	PVRI	$\dfrac{\text{PAm} - \text{PAWm}}{\text{Cardiac index}} \times 80$	dynes·sec·cm^{-5}·M^2	200-450
Rate pressure product	RPP	Syst BP × HR	mm Hg/min	12000
Right ventricular stroke work index	RVSWI	SVI × (PAm − RAm) × .0136	g·m/m^2/beat	4-8
Stroke volume	SV	$\dfrac{\text{Cardiac output}}{\text{Heart rate}} \times 1000$	ml/beat	60-120
Stroke volume index	SVI	$\dfrac{\text{Stroke volume}}{\text{Body surface area}}$	ml/beat/M^2	30-60
Systemic vascular resistance	SVR	$\dfrac{(\text{MAP} - \text{RAm})}{\text{Cardiac output}} \times 80$	dynes·sec·cm^{-5}	900-1400
Systemic vascular resistance index	SVRI	$\dfrac{(\text{MAP} - \text{RAm})}{\text{Cardiac index}} \times 80$	dynes·sec·cm^{-5}·M^2	1700-2600

crease in stroke work and $M\dot{V}o_2$. However, when adequate coronary perfusion pressure must be established, vasopressors are used to effectively increase blood pressure by increasing resistance. In general, a diastolic blood pressure of 60 mm Hg is necessary to maintain coronary artery perfusion, while a mean arterial pressure of 65 to 70 mm Hg is required to adequately perfuse the brain, kidney, and splanchnic organs. Reductions in peripheral perfusion may also occur with the use of vasopressors. However, increasing coronary perfusion pressure, and, therefore, perfusion to the myocardium becomes the primary goal.

High Afterload

When cardiac output and blood pressure fall, sympathetic stimulation causes arterial vasoconstriction to maintain blood pressure. However, arterial vasoconstriction increases the resistance and forward blood flow is reduced. In addition, increased afterload increases the work of the heart and, therefore, $M\dot{V}o_2$. In such situations pharmacologic afterload reducing agents are employed to increase stroke volume and reduce $M\dot{V}o_2$. This favors a better balance between oxygen supply and

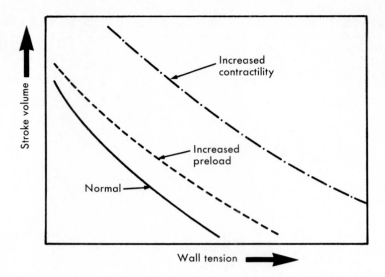

Fig. 10-3. Relationship between stroke volume and wall tension (that is, afterload) for the intact left ventricle. At constant preload, increases in wall tension result in decline in stroke volume. Increased preload or increased contractility shifts the curve upward and to the right, resulting in a greater stroke volume for any given afterload.

demand and thus has become a cornerstone of management of patients with cardiac failure.

Decreases in SVR usually result in increases in cardiac output with little or no reduction in BP (BP = CO× SVR). However, careful monitoring of both preload (PAW) and blood pressure are necessary to prevent severe hypotension. Maintaining adequate PAW pressures through concomitant volume administration is frequently necessary during afterload reduction.

Arteriovasodilators

Smooth muscle relaxants. Agents that directly activate beta$_2$ receptors in the smooth muscle of the arterioles causing vasodilatation include hydralazine, sodium nitroprusside and nitroglycerin. Hydralazine is solely an arteriovasodilator while nitroprusside dilates the smooth muscle in both veins and arteries. Thus, nitroprusside reduces both afterload and preload. Because of this, careful attention must be paid to the maintenance of adequate preload levels with sufficient volume administration when nitroprusside is given. The use of nitroprusside in patients with a normal PAWP can result in relative hypovolemia and a consequent fall in cardiac output. Nitroglycerin is, primarily, a peripheral venous dilator that also dilates epicardial coronary arteries and increases collateral coronary blood flow. It does, however, cause some arteriovasodilation, particularly at higher doses, and therefore can also reduce afterload. The associated increase in cardiac output is usually small.

Calcium channel blockers

Agents that reduce or block the influx of calcium into arterial smooth muscle result in coronary and peripheral vasodilation and therefore afterload reduction. In addition extracellular calcium influx into myocardial fibers is inhibited, to a certain extent, resulting in a negative inotropic effect with decreased contractility. Certain calcium channel blockers (diltiazem and verapamil) also reduce extracellular calcium influx into AV nodal cells resulting in slower conduction. All of these effects decrease $M\dot{V}O_2$, whereas coronary vasodilation increases oxygen delivery to the myocardium and thus, strikes a more favorable balance between oxygen supply and demand. Use of calcium channel blockers in patients to reduce a high preload or afterload should be done with caution, since these agents also possess negative inotropic effects, which could worsen heart failure.

Alpha blockers

Inhibition of stimulation of the alpha adrenergic receptors in the peripheral vasculature results in vasodilation of both arteries and veins and, therefore, afterload reduction. Prazosin and phentolamine are both alpha blockers that can produce peripheral vasodilation and, thus, afterload reduction.

Angiotensin converting enzymes (ACE) inhibitors

An angiotensin converting enzyme converts angiotensin I to angiotensin II, which is a potent vasoconstrictor. Agents that inhibit this enzyme prevent the conversion from angiotensin I to angiotensin II and, thus, produce vasodilation and afterload reduction. In addition, preload pressures are reduced and cardiac output is improved, with variable change in arterial blood pressure. Severe hypotension may occur, particularly in patients who are overdiuresed and hyponatremic. If it occurs, it is usually observed following the first dose. Currently available angiotensin converting enzyme inhibitors include captopril and enalopril.

Counterpulsation

Intra-aortic balloon pumping with sudden balloon deflation during systole creates a vacuum space in the ascending aorta, which aids in ventricular ejection and therefore reduces ventricular afterload as well as $M\dot{V}O_2$. In addition, balloon inflation during diastole increases coronary blood flow and oxygen delivery to the myocardium (see Chapter 9).

CONTRACTILITY

Contractility refers to the inotropic state of the myocardium or, more specifically, the velocity of fiber shortening during systole. Since contractility cannot be directly measured or even approximated in the clinical setting, an index of ventricular work (stroke work index) is used to assess changes in contractility. Decreased contractility associated with reduced ejection can occur with myocardial ischemia or infarction or following the use of certain anesthetic agents. In such cases, increases in inotropism may be necessary to maintain adequate stroke volume and, more importantly, oxygen delivery. However, in patients with ischemic heart disease this benefit must be carefully weighed against the associated increase in $M\dot{V}O_2$ that accompanies increased contractility. In fact, decreases in oxygen demands of the myocardium may be necessary in such patients and agents that reduce contractility might be required.

Decreased Contractility

Studies by Shoemaker et al have shown that maintenance of a stroke work index of the left ventricle >55 g/meter/beat is associated with improved survival in shock patients. Improvement in myocardial contractility can be obtained with the use of positive inotropic agents which increase the amount of intracellular calcium available for actin and myosin crossbridging. The catecholamines (dopamine, dobutamine, isoproterenol, and epinephrine) increase cyclic AMP and thus calcium entry while the phosphodiesterase inhibitors (amrinone and milrinone) inhibit the breakdown of cyclic AMP into its inactive form. Increases in contractility are accompanied by increases in stroke volume, and therefore end-diastolic volume usually falls. However, increases in contractility usually are associated with an increase in $M\dot{V}O_2$, although other determinants of $M\dot{V}O_2$ (systolic wall stress and heart rate) also affect this response. For example, the use of positive inotropic agents in a patient with a dilated and failing ventricle can produce an increase in stroke volume (secondary to increased contractility) with a decrease in both end-diastolic and end-systolic chamber size and, thus, wall stress. In such a case the increase in contractility may be offset by a decrease in LV chamber size effecting no change in $M\dot{V}O_2$. On the other hand, the use of positive inotropic agents in patients with a normal-sized ventricle are likely to increase $M\dot{V}O_2$ and negatively affect the myocardium oxygen supply/demand balance.

In addition to the positive inotropic effects of isoproterenol and the phosphodiesterase inhibitors amrinone and milrinone, these agents produce systemic vasodilation through stimulation of beta$_2$ receptors in vascular smooth muscle. Hemodynamically, this results in a reduction in SVR (afterload) in addition to the increased contractility.

Certain other positive inotropic drugs possess vasoconstrictor properties (such as epinephrine, norepinephrine and high dose dopamine). Thus these agents can increase perfusion pressure as well as augment contractility (Table 10-2).

Increased Contractility

Because of the increase in oxygen demands that occur with increased myocardial contractility, patients with myocardial ischemia may benefit from reductions in contractility as well as heart rate and blood pressure. This can be obtained with the use of beta blockers, which inhibit stimulation of beta$_1$ receptors in the myocardium (cardioselective) and beta$_2$ receptors in the smooth muscle in the arterioles of the lungs (nonselective). Blockage of beta$_1$ stimulation results in decreased inotropic and chronotropic response to catecholamine stimulation with consequent reductions in contractility, heart rate, and cardiac output. Blockage of stimulation to beta$_2$ receptors results in vasoconstriction.

HEART RATE

Heart rate is a major determinant of cardiac output, coronary perfusion and $M\dot{V}O_2$. Within limits, increases in heart rate can increase cardiac output (CO = SV × HR). However, heart rates greater than 120 to 125 bpm may be associated with decreases in stroke volume and cardiac output because of decreased diastolic filling time of the left ventricle. Fast heart rates with shortened diastolic duration also decrease left ventricular coronary perfusion time and increase myocardial oxygen consumption causing an imbalance between myocardial oxygen supply and demand. High heart rates markedly increase MVo_2 in two ways: (1) by increasing the frequency of work per minute, and (2) by an accompanying increase in contractility (the Bowditch effect). Pharmacologic agents that are used to decrease heart rate include beta blockers to reduce chronotropism and calcium channel blockers to decrease conduction. In general, heart rates greater than 100 to 110 bpm are not hemodynamically advantageous.

Bradycardia with heart rates of <50 bpm results in reductions in cardiac output and overall tissue perfusion. Agents used to increase the heart rate depend on

Table 10-2. Hemodynamic effects of commonly used cardiovascular drugs

Drug	Heart rate	Afterload	Contractility	Preload	Comments
INOTROPIC AGENTS					
Digoxin	− or ↓	±	↑	−	↓ Ventricular rate in AF
Dopamine	± or ↑	− or ↑	↑ ↑	↑ or ↓	Effect on SVR is dose dependent; ↑ renal blood flow
Dobutamine	− or ↑	±	↑ ↑	↓	
Isoproterenol	↑ ↑	↓ ↓	↑ ↑	↓	Can cause arrhythmias
Norepinephrine	↑ or ↓	↑ ↑	↑	↑	Can cause arrhythmias
Epinephrine	↑ ↑	↑ or ↓	↑ ↑	↑	Can cause arrhythmias
Methoxamine	−	↑ ↑	−	↑	
Amrinone	− or ↑	↓	↑	↓	
ANALGESIC AGENTS					
Morphine	−	↓	−	↓	
DIURETICS					
(Furosemide, ethacrynic acid, bumetanide)	−	↓	−	↓	May ↓ cardiac output if diuresis excessive
ANTIARRHYTHMIC AGENTS					
Lidocaine	−	−	± ↓	−	
Procainamide	−	−	± ↓	−	
Quinidine	−	−	± ↓	−	
Atropine	↑	−	−	− or ↓	
CALCIUM CHANNEL BLOCKERS					
Nifedipine	↑	↓	↓ or −	↓	
Diltiazem	↑	↓	− or ↓	−	
Verapamil	± ↓	± ↓	↓	−	
BETA BLOCKERS	↓ ↓	− or ↑	↓	↑	

Continued.

Table 10-2. Hemodynamic effects of commonly used cardiovascular drugs—cont'd

Drug	Heart rate	Afterload	Contractility	Preload	Comments
VASODILATORS					
Nitroprusside	− or ↑	↓ ↓	−	↓	↑ cardiac output by ↓ peripheral resistance
Nitroglycerin	− or ↑	↓	−	↓ ↓	↑ cardic output by ↓ peripheral resistance
Hydralazine	−	↓	−	−	↑ cardiac output by ↓ peripheral resistance
ALPHA BLOCKERS					
Phentolamine	− or ↑	↓	−	− or ↓	↑ cardic output by ↓ peripheral resistance
Prazosin	−	↓	−	↓	↑ cardic output by ↓ peripheral resistance
ACE INHIBITORS					
Captopril, enalapril	− or ↓	↓	−	↓	May cause hypotension, particularly if urine Na ↓
OXYGEN	−	↑	−	± ↑	

the underlying cause of the bradycardia. Vasovagal responses are usually managed with atropine and volume administration. A pacemaker (temporary or permanent) may be necessary if heart block is present.

Hemoglobin

Abnormal reductions of hemoglobin can impose a significant threat to tissue oxygenation, since approximately 98% of the oxygen is carried by the hemoglobin molecules. Maintenance of hemoglobin at normal levels is usually obtained with administration of whole blood products. On the other hand, abnormal elevation in hemoglobin can decrease cardiac output secondary to increased viscosity, again compromising overall oxygen delivery. Hemodilution may be necessary in such situations.

Arterial Oxygen Saturation

Oxygen saturation of arterial blood can be maintained at normal levels (>97%) with increases in Fio_2, with PEEP, CPAP, hyperbaria or, when all of the above fail, extracorporeal membrane oxygenation (ECMO). While a Pao_2 of 60 mm Hg can be considered within normal limits, it is associated with an arterial saturation of only 92% to 93%, if the oxyhemoglobin dissociation curve is normal. However, consideration must be given to those interventions that can also decrease cardiac output (such as PEEP). If cardiac output is compromised, oxygen delivery can be reduced despite increases in Pao_2. Maintenance of Pao_2 levels at above 100 mm Hg usually ensures adequate oxygen uptake with complete saturation of the hemoglobin with oxygen.

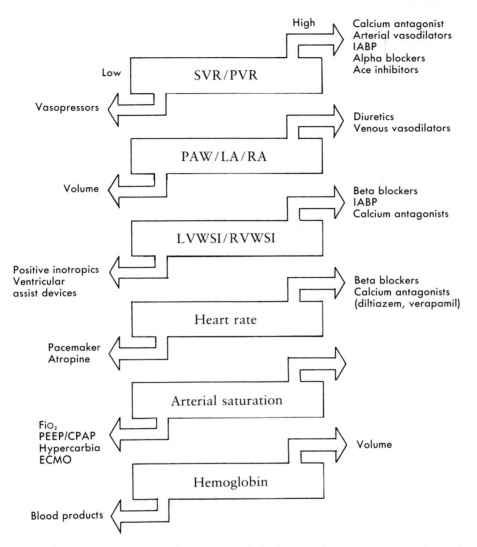

Fig. 10-4. Schematic diagram outlining some of the interventions more commonly used to appropriately affect the hemodynamic parameters that reflect the determinants of oxygen delivery. (See text for complete discussion.)

Summary

Fig. 10-4 is a schematic illustration depicting the interventions used to manipulate the major determinants of oxygen delivery. In general, critically ill patients suffer from multiple hemodynamic derangements, and a variety of agents are used simultaneously to alter them. In addition, a number of therapies can effect more than one hemodynamic parameter. Thus the critical care nurse must possess a sound knowledge of the pharmacologic and hemodynamic effects of agents that are commonly used in critical care. For example, the use of nitroprusside to reduce afterload in a patient with a normal preload may have a deleterious effect on cardiac output secondary to its venodilatory effect. Therefore, this agent must be used cautiously with adequate volume administration to maintain preload and thus cardiac output and oxygen delivery. This is only one example of the myriad of interactions that necessitate a clear understanding of the goal of all therapies, which is the maintenance of adequate oxygen delivery to all tissues.

REFERENCES

Alpert MA: Pharmacotherapy of congestive heart failure, Postgrad Med 81:257-267, 1987.

Braunwald E: The myocardium: failure and infarction, New York, 1974, HP Publishing.

Braunwald E: Heart disease, Philadelphia, 1980, WB Saunders Co.

Cohn J: Vasodilator therapy: implications of acute myocardial infarction and congestive heart failure, Am Heart J 49:45-59, 1982.

Cohn JN: Treatment by modification of circulatory dynamics, Hosp Prac Aug 19:37-52, 1984.

Crexells C et al: Optimal level of left ventricular filling pressures in acute myocardial infarction, N Engl J Med 289:1263-1266, 1974.

Dalen JE, Goldberg RJ, Gore JM, and Struckus J: Therapeutic interventions in acute myocardial infarction: survey of the ACCP section on clinical cardiology, Chest 86:257-262, 1984.

Deepak V et al: A simplified concept of complete physiological monitoring of the critically ill patient, Heart Lung 10:75-82, 1981.

Dracup K et al: The physiologic basis for combined nitroprusside-dopamine therapy in postmyocardial infarction heart failure, Heart Lung 10:114-117, 1981.

Foster S and Canty R: Pump failure following myocardial infarction: an overview, Heart Lung 9:293-297, 1980.

Giles D: Principles of vasodilator therapy for left ventricular congestive heart failure, Heart Lung 9:2-5, 1980.

Harvey WP et al: The year book of cardiology, Chicago, 1986, Year Book Medical Publishers, Inc.

Karliner J, and Gregoratos G: Coronary care, New York, 1981, Churchill-Livingstone.

Keung E et al: Effects of combined dopamine and nitroprusside therapy in patients with severe pump failure and hypotension complicating acute myocardial infarction, J Cardiovasc Pharmacol 2:113-119, 1980.

LeJemtel TH, Katz SD, and Sonnenblick EH: Newer inotropic agents for managing patients with congestive heart failure, J Appl Cardiol 2:361-377, 1987.

Low R et al: The effects of calcium channel blocking agents on cardiovascular function, Am J Cardiol 49:547-552, 1982.

Mason DT: Congestive heart failure, New York, 1976, Yorke Medical Books.

Mason J: Symposium on vasodilator and inotropic therapy of heart failure, Am J Med 65:101-106, 1978.

Murray A: Haemodynamic measurements: a comment on units used, Eur Heart J 6:812-814, 1985.

Parmley W, and Rouleau J: Vasodilators in heart failure secondary to coronary artery disease, Am Heart J 103:625-631, 1982.

Rahimtoola S: Treatment of pump failure in acute myocardial infarction, JAMA 245:2093-2096, 1981.

Shoemaker, WC et al: Clinical trial of survivors' cardiorespiratory patterns as therapeutic goals in critically ill postoperative patients, Crit Care Med 10:398, 1982.

Siegl PKS: Overview of cardiac inotropic mechanisms, J Appl Pharmacol 8:S1-S10, 1986.

Weber K, and Andrews V: Cardiotonic agents in the management of chronic failure, Am Heart J 103:639, 1982.

Weber KT, Sundram P, and Reddy HK: Managing heart failure with positive inotropic drugs, J Crit Illness June 2:14-23, 1987.

Chapter 11

Hemodynamic Monitoring of Children

MARY FRAN HAZINSKI

The critically ill child is both physically and physiologically immature and differs from the critically ill adult in several important ways. As a result, hemodynamic monitoring in children requires special equipment and skills. The equipment used must be available in several small sizes and often requires more careful calibration and maintenance than similar equipment used with adult patients. In addition, the pediatric patient may be unable to understand or cooperate with invasive monitoring procedures, so it can be difficult to insert and to secure monitoring lines in the child. Careful explanations and use of restraints will be needed. Finally, as with any monitoring technique, the data obtained are only as reliable as the professional at the bedside; pediatric monitoring equipment must be carefully calibrated and operated, and the clinician must be able to validate and evaluate the data obtained in light of patient appearance and progress.

PHYSIOLOGIC DIFFERENCES BETWEEN CHILDREN AND ADULTS
Cardiovascular Differences

The child's cardiovascular system continues to mature after birth. Changes in the child's cardiac output and myocardial function accompany the child's growth. At birth, cardiac output is higher *per kilogram body weight* than during any other time in life, and averages approximately 200 ml/kg/min; cardiac output per kilogram body weight ultimately decreases to 100 ml/kg/min in the adolescent. Since the child's body weight is small, the child's *absolute cardiac output* at birth is only approximately 0.6 L/min, but it increases to approximately 6 L/min in the large adolescent male. *Cardiac index* throughout childhood is slightly higher than the cardiac index of the adult and is normally 3.5 to 4.5 L/min/m^2 body surface area.

Cardiac output is a product of heart rate and stroke volume. Heart rate is nor-

Table 11-1. Normal pediatric vital signs

Normal heart rates and respiratory rates		
AGE	HEART RATE	RESPIRATORY RATE
Infants	120-160/min	30-60/min
Toddlers	90-140/min	24-40/min
Preschoolers	80-110/min	22-34/min
School-aged children	75-100/min	18-30 min
Adolescents	60-90/min	12-16/min
NORMAL BLOOD PRESSURE RANGES*		
AGE	SYSTOLIC PRESSURE	DIASTOLIC PRESSURE
Neonate (1 month)	85-100	51-65
Infant (6 months)	87-105	53-66
Toddler (2 years)	95-105	53-66
School age (7 years)	97-112	57-71
Adolescent (15 years)	112-128	66-80

Heart rate and respiratory rate tables reproduced with permission from: Hazinski MF: Children are different. In Hazinski MF, editor: Nursing care of the critically ill child, St Louis, 1984, The CV Mosby Co.
*Blood pressure tables taken from the 50th to 90th percentile ranges, extrapolated from graphs published by Horan, MJ, chairman, Task Force on Blood Pressure Control in Children, Report of the second task force on blood pressure in children, Pediatrics 79:1, 1987. These blood pressure ranges were derived by the Task Force from a sampling of more than 70,000 children.

mally more rapid than during adult years, and stroke volume averages 1.5 ml/kg. During childhood, cardiac output is very heart rate–dependent (see Table 11-1 for normal pediatric vital signs). Neonatal myocardium contains less contractile elements, and the neonatal ventricle may be slightly less compliant and less able to increase tension and contractility than adult myocardium. For these reasons, the infant's ventricle may have limited ability to increase stroke volume, particularly during episodes of hypoxemia, shock, or heart failure.

At birth, pulmonary and systemic vascular resistances are approximately equal, and the right and left ventricles have equal thickness. During the first weeks of life pulmonary vascular resistance normally falls from 8 to 10 units/m^2 BSA to 1 to 3 units/m^2 BSA as a result of pulmonary vasodilation and regression of the medial muscle layer in the pulmonary arteries. When pulmonary vascular resistance falls, right ventricular muscle mass decreases, and its compliance increases. Systemic vascular resistance gradually rises during childhood, and normally ranges between 15 and 30 units/m^2 BSA; left ventricular muscle mass increases in a corresponding fashion, and the left ventricle becomes less compliant than the right ventricle (see the box on p. 249 for other normal resting values).

Bradycardia is the most common pediatric arrhythmia, and it most often occurs as the result of vagal stimulation or hypoxia. Profound or persistent bradycardia in the absence of reversible hypoxia is an ominous finding in the pediatric patient and often indicates impending arrest.[15] In fact, bradycardia (progressing to asystole) is the most common terminal cardiac rhythm in children. Whenever bradycardia is observed, the child's oxygenation, airway, and gas exchange must be carefully evaluated.

Supraventricular tachyarrhythmias may also be observed in the critically ill

Normal resting values in children

A. Normal cardiac index in children: 3.5 to 4.5 L/min/m^2

B. Normal cardiac output in children

Age	Cardiac output (L/min)	Heart rate	Normal stroke volume
Newborn	0.8-1.0	145	5 ml
6 mo	1.0-1.3	120	10 ml
1 yr	1.3-1.5	115	13 ml
2 yr	1.5-2.0	115	18 ml
4 yr	2.3-2.75	105	27 ml
5 ur	2.5-3.0	95	31 ml
8 yr	3.4-3.6	83	42 ml
10 yr	3.8-4.0	75	50 ml
15 yr	6.0	70	85 ml

Reproduced with permission from Hazinski, MF: Cardiovascular disorders. In Hazinski MF, editor: Nursing care of the critically ill child, St Louis, 1984, The CV Mosby Co. Modified from extrapolation of normal postnatal changes in cardiac output, heart rate, and stroke volume from Rudolph AM: Changes in the circulation after birth. In Congenital diseases of the heart, Chicago, 1974, Year Book Medical Publishers, Inc.

C. Calculation of systemic vascular resistance

$$\text{SVR (in units)} = \frac{\text{Mean arterial pressure} - \text{Mean right atrial pressure}}{\text{Cardiac index}}$$

Normal SVR in neonates: 10-15 units/m^2 BSA
Normal SVR in children: 15-30 units/m^2 BSA
NOTE: To convert units to dynes-sec cm^{-5}, change cardiac index to cardiac output in denominator of equation, and multiply equation by 80.

D. Calculation of pulmonary vascular resistance

$$\text{PVR (in units)} = \frac{\text{Mean pulmonary artery pressure} - \text{Mean left atrial pressure}}{\text{Cardiac index}}$$

Normal PVR in neonates: 8-10 units/m^2 BSA
Normal PVR in children: 1-3 units/m^2 BSA
NOTE: To convert units to dynes-sec cm^{-5}, change cardiac index to cardiac output in denominator of equation and multiply the entire equation by 80.

E. Normal oxygen consumption
Infants < 2-3 weeks of age: 120-130 ml/min/m^2 BSA
Children > 2-3 weeks of age: 150-160 ml/min/m^2 BSA
Or: 5-8 ml/kg/min

F. Normal arterial oxygen content: 18-20 ml oxygen/dl blood

child. Although tachycardia is an expected response to fever, stress, pain, and critical illness and may help to maintain cardiac output, excessively high heart rates may compromise cardiac output. If the ventricular rate exceeds 180 to 230 per minute, ventricular diastolic filling time and coronary artery perfusion time will be reduced, and cardiac output may fall dramatically. Brief episodes of SVT may be tolerated without clinical signs in the normal infant, but can be expected to produce significant compromise of systemic perfusion in the child with underlying heart disease.

Whenever the nurse cares for the child with an alteration in heart rate or rhythm, attempts should be made to correlate clinical appearance and hemodynamic measurements and calculations with varying heart rates. The nurse should attempt to determine the heart rate at which the child's cardiac output and systemic perfusion are best, and attempt to maintain that heart rate, if possible.

The normal pediatric myocardium is less likely to develop malignant ventricular arrhythmias, even during stimulation (such as may occur during placement of a pulmonary artery catheter), than adult myocardium. Malignant ventricular arrhythmias are almost exclusively seen in children with complex heart disease, left ventricular outflow tract obstruction, myocarditis, or cardiomyopathy.

Pulmonary edema in any patient can result from either high pulmonary capillary pressures or from increased pulmonary capillary permeability. Even when congestive heart failure results in increased pulmonary capillary pressures, however, rales may not be appreciated during clinical examination if the child breathes shallowly. There is evidence that the infant is more likely than the older child or adult to develop increased pulmonary capillary permeability and pulmonary edema during episodes of respiratory dysfunction, so evaluation of pulmonary arterial wedge pressure in young children often reveals normal pressures despite evidence of pulmonary edema.

It is thought that biventricular failure is more common in children than univentricular failure. While this may be true in the presence of some congenital heart defects, it may not be true of the pediatric patient with shock, myocarditis, or pulmonary hypertension. In these patients, significant discrepancies may exist between right and left ventricular end-diastolic pressures. Therefore, central venous pressure measurements should be used only to evaluate right ventricular end-diastolic (or right atrial) pressure; pulmonary artery catheterization should be undertaken if measurement of left ventricular end-diastolic (or left atrial) pressure is necessary.

The child's circulating blood volume averages approximately 75 to 80 ml/kg and is smaller than the blood volume of the adult. Unreplaced blood loss of 25 ml

Table 11-2. Calculation of circulating blood volume in children

Age	ml/kg body wt
Neonates	85-90
Infants	75-80
Children	70-75
Adults	65-70

Reproduced with permission from Hazinski MF: Children are different. In Hazinski, MF, editor: Nursing care of the critically ill child, St Louis, 1984, The CV Mosby Co.

will result in a 12% hemorrhage in the 3 kg infant. Therefore, it is extremely important to consider any blood lost during procedures or blood drawn for laboratory analysis as a percentage of the child's circulating blood volume (Table 11-2). If acute unreplaced blood loss totals more than 5% to 7% of the child's circulating blood volume, transfusion should be considered. *When intravascular or intracardiac monitoring lines are in place, scrupulous attention should be paid to securing all tubing connections.* Loose connections or stopcocks inadvertently turned to allow blood loss may result in significant hemorrhage within a few moments. *All monitoring lines should be connected to monitors with adjustable low pressure alarms, so that line separation or pressure loss will be detected immediately.*

If the child has unrepaired cyanotic congenital heart disease, systemic venous blood is allowed to enter the systemic arterial circulation without passing through the lungs. Thus *when the child has unrepaired cyanotic heart disease absolutely no air can be allowed to enter any intravenous or central venous line,* because it may be shunted into the left heart and ultimately produce a cerebral air embolus. All venous lines should be inspected frequently and thoroughly, and all air must be eliminated.

Maintenance Fluid Requirements

The child's metabolic rate is higher than that of the adult, so the child's maintenance fluid requirements are higher per kilogram than the adult. However, the child's body weight is small, so the child's total fluid needs are less than those of an adult (see Table 11-3 for maintenance fluid requirements in children). For this reason, it is imperative that all sources of the critically ill child's fluid intake and fluid loss be recorded on an hourly basis. Fluids used to flush monitoring lines and catheters may be a source of unrecognized fluid overload in the small child.

The infant or young child has high glucose and caloric needs and low glycogen stores. As a result, the critically ill infant requires a virtually constant source of glucose intake, and attempts should be made to ensure that most fluid administered to the child contains glucose or other sources of nutrition. Since most monitoring lines are flushed with glucose-free solution, to reduce risk of bacterial growth, the "flush" fluid will be a source of increased fluid intake of no nutritional value to the child. Therefore, the rate of fluid administered to flush the monitoring lines should be no greater than the minimal amount necessary to maintain catheter patency (usually 2 to 5 ml/hr). The use of heparinized flush solutions (in concentration of 1 to 5 units/ml) may contribute to the longevity of monitoring lines.

Since small catheters must be inserted into the small vessels of the child, these catheters can quickly become obstructed if they are not flushed appropriately. It is

Table 11-3. Calculation of maintenance fluid requirements in children

Body weight increments	ml/hr fluid requirements
First 10 kg	4 ml/kg/hr
Second 10 kg	2 ml/kg/hr (plus 40 ml/hr for kg 1-10)
Third 10 kg	1 ml/kg/hr (plus 60 ml/hr for kg 1-20)
If m^2 body surface area (BSA) used:	60 ml/m^2 BSA/hr

imperative that careful attention be paid to the tubing and flush system, to guarantee uninterrupted delivery of fluids through the catheter lumen. If intermittent (rather than continuous) hemodynamic measurements are required, heparin (in concentrations of 20 to 100 units/ml) may be instilled in some catheters to maintain catheter patency between measurements without the need for constant fluid infusion.

Thermoregulatory Differences

Infants and small children have large surface area-to-volume ratios, and they can lose a great deal of heat to the environment through evaporation. In addition, the infant cannot shiver to generate heat and must break down brown fat in an energy-requiring process called "nonshivering thermogenesis." If the infant is exposed to a cold environment, oxygen consumption will increase for the purpose of nonshivering thermogenesis; this is clearly undesirable when cardiorespiratory distress or failure is present.[15,16] For these reasons, it is very important to keep young children warm. Incubators are usually impractical thermoregulatory devices in the critical care unit, since they are only large enough for young infants, and the inside temperature will fall if the incubator is entered frequently. In addition, the infant must be removed from the incubator during procedures. Overbed warmers are ideal thermoregulatory devices in the critical care unit, since they will maintain a warm ambient temperature by heating the air surrounding the child; these warmers enable constant observation of the child and immediate access to the child, while preventing cold stress. Such warmers should particularly be used during procedures that require that the child be uncovered for prolonged periods of time.

NONINVASIVE MONITORING
General Assessment

Anyone caring for the critically ill patient of any age should develop the ability to determine at a glance whether that patient "looks good" or "looks bad." The ability to recognize when the patient "looks bad" is one of the most important observation skills required in the intensive care unit. When hymodynamic monitoring is performed, it is essential to correlate values obtained with the appearance of the child, so that the monitoring serves as an adjunct to thorough clinical assessment.[15,16]

To determine the degree of distress that the child is demonstrating, the child's color, level of activity, responsiveness, position of comfort, and feeding behavior should be assessed. The healthy child will have pink mucous membranes and nailbeds, with consistent skin tones. The child with cardiorespiratory distress will develop a mottled appearance to the skin, and the nailbeds and lips may be pale. Untimately, the child may demonstrate a grey pallor, consistent with hypoxemia and poor systemic perfusion.[15,16]

The well-oxygenated, well-perfused child should have warm extremities, with strong peripheral pulses and brisk (instantaneous) capillary refill. Keep in mind that *"normal" vital signs are not always "appropriate" vital signs for the critically ill child* (refer again to Table 11-1 for normal vital signs). An early sign of cardiorespiratory distress, pain, or fear will be tachycardia, and tachycardia is nearly always more appropriate than "normocardia" when the child is seriously ill or injured. Bradycardia is usually an ominous clinical sign in the critically ill child.

The healthy infant or child will be alert and active, and will move all four extremities. The normal infant or child will demonstrate good eye contact with parents and health care professionals. The healthy toddler should protest vigorously when separated from parents or touched by strangers and will resist placement in the supine position. The typical preschooler should be able to converse and may ask questions about treatment or caregivers. The normal school-aged child and adolescent may tolerate examinations if prior explanation is provided and should be able to voice complaints and be able to recall where he or she is hospitalized.

The moderately ill infant or child will probably not demonstrate good eye contact, may be irritable when aroused, and often is unable to find a comfortable position. The extremely ill child will be unresponsive to most stimulation, and usually demonstrates flaccid muscle tone. *If the child is unresponsive to pain (such as a venipuncture), severe cardiorespiratory or neurologic compromise should be suspected.*[15,16] The child's responsiveness should be evaluated during all aspects of critical care, particularly during invasive and noninvasive procedures.

While approaching the child, it is important to perform a thorough visual inspection, noting all vascular pressures and counting respiratory rate before touching the child. Resting values should be compared to those obtained after the child is stimulated. Then tactile and auscultatory examination may be performed, and the child's vascular pressures during stimulation may be noted.

As noted earlier, signs of poor systemic perfusion in children include nonspecific signs of distress, including tachycardia, irritability, and tachypnea. If the child deteriorates further, the child will be lethargic, with decreased response to painful stimulus. Early signs of cardiorespiratory failure include mottling of the skin, peripheral vasoconstriction and cooling of extremities, prolonged capillary refill, diminished intensity of peripheral pulses, and decreased urine volume (less than 1 to 2 ml/kg/hr). If an arterial line is in place, narrowing of the pulse pressure and dampening of the waveform may be noted before hypotension develops. The child may maintain a "normal" blood pressure despite the presence of shock or significant (up to 20% to 25%) hemorrhage. *Hypotension is only a very late sign of cardiorespiratory distress in children* and indicates that cardiorespiratory arrest is imminent.[15,16]

Signs of congestive heart failure in the child are similar to those observed in the adult, including signs of adrenergic stimulation and systemic and/or pulmonary venous congestion. In children, however, jugular venous distension cannot be appreciated, so the most reliable sign of elevated right ventricular end-diastolic pressure and central venous pressure will be hepatomegaly. When central venous pressure is monitored, attempts should be made to correlate the degree of hepatomegaly with the child's CVP, so that the CVP can be estimated even after the central venous catheter has been removed.

In adult patients, changes in cardiac output, right atrial pressure, and systemic vascular resistance may be predicted approximately 50% of the time on the basis of clinical examination. Prediction of pulmonary artery occlusive (wedge) pressure on the basis of clinical examination is much less accurate. Although the relationship between clinical examination and documented pulmonary artery occlusive

Table 11-4. Normal blood pressure cuff sizes for use in children

Cuff name*	Bladder width (cm)	Bladder length (cm)
COMMONLY AVAILABLE BLOOD PRESSURE CUFFS		
Newborn	2.5-4.0	5.0-9.0
Infant	4.0-6.0	11.5-18.0
Child	7.5-9.0	17.0-19.0
Adult	11.5-13.0	22.0-26.0
Large arm	14.0-15.0	30.5-33.0
Thigh	18.0-19.0	36.0-38.0

*Cuff name does not guarantee that the cuff will be appropriate size for a child within that age range.
Reproduced from Horan MJ, chairman, Task Force on Blood Pressure Control in Children, Report of the second task force on blood pressure control in children, Pediatrics, 79:1, 1979.

pressure has not been studied in the pediatric population, it is generally thought that clinical appearance does not provide reliable indication of pulmonary artery occlusive pressure. Hence, if such measurements are needed to determine or evaluate therapy, insertion of a balloon-tipped, flow-directed pulmonary artery catheter will be necessary.

Arterial pressure monitoring can be performed through use of cuff pressure (automatic or manual), or through use of an indwelling arterial catheter, monitoring system, and transducer. If intermittent cuff pressures are obtained, the nurse must frequently evaluate the child's clinical appearance, tissue perfusion, and quality of peripheral pulses to promptly recognize changes in the child's condition that indicate a change in arterial pressure. It is imperative that the blood pressure cuff used be of appropriate size—the width should cover two thirds the length of the upper arm, and the bladder of the cuff should not wrap more than once around the upper arm. (Appropriate blood pressure cuff sizes are listed in Table 11-4.)

Pulse Oximetry
Hemoglobin saturation

The saturation of hemoglobin in arterial blood may be continously monitored using a pulse oximeter placed on the child's finger, toe, hand, foot, or ear lobe. Pulse oximeters correlate well with measured and calculated arterial oxygen saturations in children over a wide range of clinical conditions.[12] In addition, continous monitoring of oxygenation has been shown to allow recognition and treatment of acute episodes of hypoxemia that may not be detected with intermittent blood sampling alone.[12] Such continuous monitoring will enable modification of nursing care based on the child's response and may allow more prompt confirmation of deterioration (which may result from pneumothorax, endotracheal tube displacement, or airway obstruction) than is possible with intermittent blood sampling.

The pulse oximeter indicates *hemoglobin saturation*, rather than partial pressure of oxygen. To determine the child's approximate PaO_2 from the hemoglobin saturation, the nurse must be familiar with (or consult) the oxyhemoglobin dissociation curve (refer to Fig. 8-2) in Chapter 8. Under normal conditions, the child's PaO_2 will be adequate once the hemoglobin saturation exceeds 90% to 95%, and hypoxemia is present if the hemoglobin saturation is less than 90%.

To evaluate the effectiveness of the child's oxygenation, the arterial oxygen content (volume of oxygen carried per liter or deciliter of blood) should be calculated. Oxygen content is determined by multiplying the child's hemoglobin concentration (in g/dl) times 1.34 ml oxygen/g of hemoglobin (this is the amount of oxygen carried by saturated hemoglobin), times the hemoglobin saturation. Normal arterial oxygen content is approximately 18 to 20 ml oxygen/dl of blood. The patient may have a normal hemoglobin saturation, but may have a low oxygen content if anemia is present.

Oxygen delivery to the tissues is the product of arterial oxygen content and cardiac output. If cardiac output is inadequate, oxygen delivery to the tissues will be inadequate even if arterial oxygen content is normal. During pulse oximetry, the nurse should monitor not only the patient's hemoglobin saturation, but also the hemoglobin concentration and signs of systemic perfusion and cardiac output.

Principles of oximetry

Pulse oximeters use two light-emitting diodes that direct a red and an infrared light through the tissue to a photodetector. The diodes and photodetector must be carefully placed so the light is transmitted through tissue perfused by a pulsatile artery to the photodetector. The amount of red light absorbed by the tissue will be inversely related to the saturation of the hemoglobin passing through the pulsatile arterial circulation; hemoglobin that is well-saturated with oxygen will absorb little of the red light, and poorly saturated hemoglobin will absorb a great deal of the red light before it reaches the photodetector (refer to Chapter 8 for further information).

Pulse oximeters provide reliable evaluation of the child's hemoglobin saturation unless profound anemia (Hct is less than 20%) or hypotension is present. Several pulse oximeters are commercially available, and include portable and bedside monitors, and those with hard-copy print-out of heart rate and hemoglobin saturations. It is important that the nurse be aware of individual differences between brands of pulse oximeters; some oximeters (for example, the Nellcor oximeter) may demonstrate more delay in signals with lower heart rates, while others demonstrate more delay with higher heart rates.[38] In addition, the cost, accuracy, and reliability of disposable and reusable probes should be considered when selecting a pulse oximeter.

Differences in the reliability of pulse oximetry may be seen when different types of oximeter probes are used. The oximeter probes are most commonly mounted on a disposable adhesive strip or a spring-loaded plastic clip. With either device, it is important to secure the device so that the light transmitters are directly aligned with the photosensors, separated only by well-perfused tissue. Accurate pulse oximetry can only be achieved if the probes are placed and maintained properly.

Clinical use

In infants, the disposable probes are used most commonly; these probes consist of the light diodes and photosensors mounted a few centimeters apart on an adhesive strip. The strip is placed on the infant's hand, foot, thumb, or great toe. A well-perfused, warm extremity should always be used. Once the site is selected, positioning of the probe and sensor should be attempted while the oximeter unit is turned on, and the strength of the pulse signal is displayed. Once a strong, reliable pulse signal is obtained, the adhesive strip is used to secure the light and photosensor in place. The adhesive strip is wrapped around the infant's palm, foot, thumb, or toe in such a way that the red light is directly aligned with the photosensor, separated by the monitored tissue (Figure 11-1, A). When the probe is correctly positioned, the light will be able to pass directly through the tissue to the photosensor.

A reusable probe may be contained in a hard plastic, spring-loaded clip that can be clamped on the thumb or great toe of a small child, or on the middle finger of a large child or adolescent. It is important that the child's digit be large enough so that the clip remains in place, clamped firmly on the digit, or excessive artifact will result. In addition, when any reusable probe is used, the photosensor should be regularly but gently cleansed with an alcohol wipe before use, to remove any oils that may have accumulated during previous use.

Excessive amounts of ambient light can interfere with the accurate detection of light absorption by the photosensor. Therefore, if the infant or child is placed under warming or phototherapy lights, it is often helpful to loosely wrap the child's monitored extremity and the pulse oximeter probe in gauze to block ambient light from the photosensor.

If the pulse oximeter probe is placed over a finger or thumb tip, all nail polish must be removed from the digit, since the nail polish will interfere with light transmission and detection. In addition, the digit should be wiped with alcohol to remove excess dirt or oil.

Movement artifact is one of the most common causes of inaccurate pulse oximetry results in children. It is often very difficult to secure the pulse oximeter probe properly and to eliminate movement artifact when monitoring an active infant. Such artifact will be reduced if a proximal portion of the infant's extremity is used

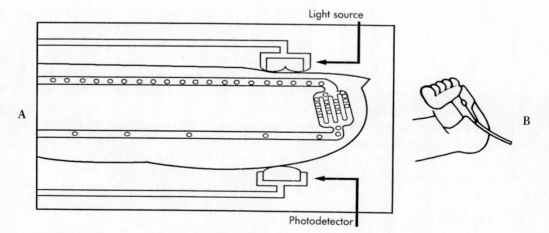

Fig. 11-1. Use of the pulse oximeter probe. **A,** Proper alignment of the light source and photodetector. **B,** Placement of the disposable probe on infant's foot—note that light source and photodetector should still be in direct alignment. (Illustrations courtesy of Nellcor Inc, Hayward, Calif.)

(for example, place the disposable probe around a wrist, hand, ankle, or foot, rather than the thumb or toe— Figure 11-1, *B*). If one extremity is restrained with an intravenous line in place, that extremity should also be used for probe placement for pulse oximetry. This will eliminate the need for restraint of more than one extremity, and will reduce movement artifact. The pulse oximetry probe should not be placed distal to an arterial line, if that arterial line has produced any compromise in distal extremity perfusion.

Cautions

Once the hemoglobin is fully saturated, the child's partial pressure of oxygen can be any number *above* 70 to 100 mm Hg. When the neonate's hemoglobin is fully saturated, the PaO_2 may exceed 100 mm Hg, introducing a risk of retrolental fibroplasia. Therefore, if a hemoglobin saturation of 95% to 97% is observed during supplemental oxygen therapy, the arterial oxygen tension should be checked, and the neonate's inspired oxygen concentration adjusted to prevent the PaO_2 from exceeding 80 to 100 mm Hg.

When pulse oximetry is monitored in a neonate with a right-to-left (pulmonary artery-to-aorta) *ductal* shunt, the pulse oximeter probe should be placed on an upper extremity if monitoring of ascending aortic hemoglobin saturation is desired. If the probe is placed on a lower extremity, the hemoglobin saturation monitored will reflect that in the right ventricle, pulmonary artery, and descending aorta. Excellent correlation between arterial oxygen saturation and pulse oximetry in children with cyanotic congenital heart disease has been documented.[2]

Pulse oximeters should be used with caution in patients with acute or significant changes in arterial pH, pCO_2, or temperature, since these variables will affect the relationship between hemoglobin saturation and arterial oxygen tension. In patients with such variables, caution should be used when attempting to derive PaO_2 from hemoglobin saturation.[36] Frequently, critically ill children with head injury or pulmonary hypertension are maintained in the alkalotic state. *In alkalotic patients, the oxyhemoglobin dissociation curve shifts to the left*, so the hemoglobin is better saturated at even low arterial oxygen tensions. Thus, while a hemoglobin saturation of 85% may be associated with an arterial oxygen tension of 50 mm Hg in the patient with normal pH, it will probably be associated with an arterial oxygen tension of 40 mm Hg or less in the alkalotic patient. Unless the nurse is responsive to even mild reduction in hemoglobin saturation in the alkalotic patient, the detection of severe hypoxemia (and institution of therapy to improve ventilation and alveolar oxygenation) may be delayed.

(Skin Surface) Transcutaneous Blood Gas Monitoring
Principles of transcutaneous monitoring

Under normal conditions, the oxygen tension measured across the skin is much lower than the arterial oxygen tension. In 1969, Huch, Huch, and Lubbers demonstrated that an approximation of the arterial partial pressure of oxygen could be measured on the surface of the skin if hyperemia was produced in the skin beneath the electrode.[19] This discovery led to the development of the modified heated Clark electrode which may be mounted to the skin. When the electrode heats the skin to

43 to 45 degrees centigrade, oxygen diffuses rapidly through the skin, and blood flow through the dermal capillary bed is stabilized; as a result, as long as cardiac output (and skin blood perfusion) is adequate, there is good correlation between skin surface (or transcutaneous) oxygen tension ($Ptco_2$) and arterial oxygen tension (Pao_2). If blood flow to the tissues is significantly compromised, however, $Ptco_2$ will be much lower than Pao_2; such a discrepancy is commonly seen during periods of low cardiac output.

When a Stowe-Sevringhaus electrode is added to the Clark electrode, monitoring of the child's skin surface (transcutaneous) carbon dioxide may be performed. In neonates, there is good correlation between $PtcCo_2$ and $PaCo_2$, although the skin surface carbon dioxide tension tends to be approximately 2 to 11 torr higher than the arterial carbon dioxide tension.[14] If skin blood flow is compromised (such as in low cardiac output), the $PtcCo_2$ may become significantly higher than the Pao_2. Since the Stowe-Sevringhaus electrode is pH-sensitive, the $PtcCo_2$ may correlate poorly with the $PaCo_2$ when the child is acidotic (pH is less than 7.3) or profoundly hypoxemic (Pao_2 is less than 40 mm Hg).

Clinical use

Transcutaneous blood gas monitoring may be used in a variety of clinical settings; however, it has only been used to any great extent in the newborn intensive care unit. When any transcutaneous monitor is used, adequate electrode warm-up time must be allowed, and the unit must be appropriately calibrated, according to the manufacturer's specifications. *Careless or irregular calibration of the transcutaneous blood gas machine and electrode will result in inaccurate monitoring results.*

The electrode should be placed over a well-perfused area of the skin; placement over the trunk or proximal portion of an extremity is preferred, because these areas should remain well perfused even if mild reductions in cardiac output develop. Placement over bony prominences or over large blood vessels should be avoided, because these areas do not have consistent capillary density. The electrode should never be placed on the child's face because a burn may develop.

Once the monitor has been warmed up, and appropriate calibration performed, the skin at the selected monitoring site is wiped with alcohol to remove oil and dead tissue. The electrode is secured on the skin, using the adhesive mounting ring. After the electrode is in place, adequate skin warming time (up to 25 minutes) should be allowed before $Ptco_2$ or $PtcCo_2$ values are recorded. Unit policy should indicate the frequency of correlation of arterial blood gas values with transcutaneous blood gas values.

Warming of the skin by the electrode results in a circular erythematous area, similar to a sunburn. For this reason, heated electrodes should be moved to new skin sites every 2 to 4 hours (see manufacturer's recommendations). The erythema usually becomes most noticeable several hours after electrode removal, and will usually fade within 12 to 24 hours.

Correlation between the arterial and transcutaneous oxygen tensions is reduced when cardiac output and systemic and skin perfusion are compromised. As a result, transcutaneous blood gas monitoring may provide an indication of poor systemic perfusion (for example, during trauma resuscitation) if $Ptco_2$ is less than 80% of the Pao_2. Correlation between transcutaneous and arterial oxygen tension should improve when perfusion improves.

Cautions

The popularity of transcutaneous monitoring devices has decreased dramatically in recent years as the result of consumer frustration with the meticulous and frequent calibration required, and the tendency of some monitors to drift. In many institutions, the pulse oximeter has replaced the $Ptco_2$ monitor for noninvasive monitoring of patient systemic arterial oxygenation. Transcutaneous monitors may still provide useful monitoring of trends in infant carbon dioxide levels, particularly when monitoring infants with respiratory failure.

There is no question that these devices require proper care to ensure maximal performance and reliability. In addition, the correlation of arterial blood gases to transcutaneous gases varies with the specific brand and model of monitor used. Therefore, it is imperative that personnel be familiar with proper operation of the monitor and electrode and interpretation of the transcutaneous blood gas results obtained with each model used.

Reported correlation of $Ptco_2$ with Pao_2 is definitely best when used in neonatal care. Older patients or patients with thick skin often demonstrate poor correlation between $Ptco_2$ and Pao_2 values, and machine drift in these patients is significant.[13] Pao_2 will also be affected by capillary density in the skin below the transducer.

If the infant's cardiac output is significantly reduced, or if vasoactive drugs result in increased or diminished skin blood flow, transcutaneous blood gas values may vary significantly from arterial blood gases, despite careful monitor calibration and electrode placement. Halothane anesthesia and hypothermia will also interfere with accurate transcutaneous blood gas monitoring.

The heated electrode may produce blisters and second degree burns in infants with extremely sensitive skin. The purposes of the transcutaneous monitoring should be explained to the parents, and the possible development of a reddened area (not unlike a sunburn) should be discussed. The heated electrode should not be applied over the skin of the hypothermic infant, because burns may result, and reliable monitoring will not be possible.

If the monitored neonate has a right-to-left shunt at the level of the ductus arteriosus (such as may occur in the presence of some congenital heart defects, or persistent pulmonary hypertension of the newborn), it is advisable to place the electrode over the upper portion of the child's trunk (above the nipple line) or on the proximal portion of either arm. With this electrode placement, the $Ptco_2$ should reflect ascending aortic Pao_2.

Some electrodes must be wrapped if they are used under phototherapy lights. Throughout the use of the transcutaneous monitor, regular correlation between arterial blood gases and monitored blood gases should be documented.

Automatic Oscillometric Monitoring of Blood Pressure

Oscillometric blood pressure monitoring devices use standard sizes of blood pressure cuffs joined by cables to a monitor unit. The unit inflates and deflates the cuff, and documents cuff inflation pressures and oscillations in cuff pressure, which are related to systolic, diastolic, and mean arterial pressure.

Principles of use

The cuff is inflated to a systolic pressure of approximately 200 mm Hg, although this maximal inflation pressure is modified based on previous cycled readings of the patient's systolic pressure. As the cuff is deflated, oscillations in cuff pressure are detected as the patient's arterial pressure exceeds cuff pressure, and pulsatile flow occurs in the artery under the cuff. Small but recognizable oscillations will correspond to the systolic blood pressure, maximal oscillations correspond approximately to the mean arterial pressure, and recurrence of small oscillations is recognized as corresponding to the patient's diastolic blood pressure.[6]

The accuracy of the blood pressures obtained depends on the programmed characteristics of the monitor—each monitor must recognize oscillations that are caused by arterial pulsations rather than movement or muscle artifact. Yet if small oscillations are discarded, the monitor may be unreliable when monitoring the hypotensive or very young patient. Furthermore, the magnitude of the oscillations will be related to the patient's systolic, diastolic, and mean arterial blood pressure. If the patient has a narrow pulse pressure, very low cardiac output, or arterial pulsations that are not classic in configuration, inaccurate blood pressure readings may result.

Clinical use

To begin monitoring the patient's blood pressure by oscillometry, one must select a cuff of the proper size. (see Table 11-4). The cuff should be wrapped securely around the extremity selected, then the monitor is turned on. The monitor can obtain the blood pressure immediately or can be programmed to automatically and regularly document the blood pressure at a specified interval (for example, every 3 minutes, or at selected intervals between 1 and 90 minutes). Average elapsed time to display of systolic, diastolic, and mean blood pressure and heart rate will be approximately 20 to 30 seconds, although a longer time may be required if the patient is hypotensive. If characteristic oscillations are not recognized, a monitor alarm usually sounds and flashing numbers appear on the screen to indicate that the cuff must be repositioned or that the blood pressure is undetectable.

Alarm limits may be set to activate audible and visual alarms for low and high blood pressures (for systolic, diastolic, and mean pressures), and for low or high heart rate. Flashing numbers in any of the display panels usually indicate an alarm condition.

The clinical use of the Dinamap monitor (manufactured by the Critikon Company of Johnson and Johnson) in the pediatric setting has been most extensively documented in the literature. Excellent correlation between auscultatory blood pressures ($r = 0.97$ for systolic pressure, and $r = 0.90$ for diastolic pressure) and oscillometrically derived blood pressures have been established in normotensive pediatric patients,[27] and in normotensive neonates.[37] However, oscillometric determination of blood pressure may correlate poorly with direct blood pressure measurement or with auscultatory measurement when the patient is hypotensive or when the blood pressure is falling. Such discrepancies have been documented in hypotensive neonates[9] and are currently being studied in hypotensive children.[17]

Cautions

When automatic, oscillometric blood pressure monitors are used in the care of critically ill children, it is essential that unit policies dictate comparison with intra-arterial or auscultatory pressure measurements at specified intervals. If the patient is extremely unstable, direct monitoring will provide a continuous display of the patient's blood pressure and arterial waveform, and will also provide intra-arterial access for blood sampling. When intra-arterial pressures are available with a properly flushed system and a transducer that is properly zeroed, levelled, and calibrated, direct pressure measurements should be used instead of indirect oscillometric pressures.

When oscillometric pressure measurements are used as the primary source of blood pressure measurements in critically ill children, the pressures recorded should be verified by auscultatory technique at least once every shift, and during any change in patient condition. On the basis of the correlation studies published to date, *oscillometric pressure measurements can only be used with confidence in the stable, normotensive neonatal or pediatric patient.*

Movement artifact or seizure activity may produce inaccurate oscillometric pressure measurements in the child with an otherwise stable blood pressure. If movement artifact is suspected, the nurse should wrap the cuff around the child's extremity and hold the extremity in position while the cuff inflates and deflates. Oscillometric blood pressure measurements should not be attempted during seizure activity.

INVASIVE MONITORING
Basic Monitoring Technique

Invasive hemodynamic monitoring in the pediatric patient must be undertaken only by practitioners skilled in establishing and maintaining intravascular access and in interpreting the measurements obtained. It is important to remember that invasive measurements are usually more useful in trending changes in patient conditons and responses to therapy than in determining a single measurement in time. Therefore, it is imperative that each measurement by any member of the health care team be made under the same conditions; if error cannot be eliminated, it must at least be standardized.

Because arterial blood pressure measurements and cardiac output calculations are smaller in children than in adults, a small error in measurement technique can result in a proportionally more significant error in data. Monitoring system tubing length should be kept to a minimum so that excellent transmission of pressure waves will occur. All air bubbles, tubing kinks, and loose connections must be eliminated from the system. The number of stopcocks in a monitoring line should be kept to a minimum (preferably less than three stopcocks) and the stopcock must be turned to perfectly align stopcock ports with catheter lumens; this will minimize changes in the radius of the tubing system.

Finally, the transducer must be properly zeroed and mechanically calibrated, and the monitor digital display and waveform must also be zeroed and electronically calibrated. Although the transducer may be placed at any level and zeroed, it is easiest to consistently place the transducer at the level of the right atrium (also called the phlebostatic axis). The level is commonly considered to be at the junction of the nipple line and the anterior axillary line. The transducer should be placed at the phlebostatic axis and zeroing and calibration should be accomplished (refer to the box on p. 263). Once the transducer is zeroed, the relationship between the patient's right atrium and the transducer must always remain constant; if the relationship changes, the transducer must be rezeroed. Effects of transducer movement on invasive monitoring measurements are summarized in the box on p. 264.

Proper maintenance of intravascular monitoring must consider anatomic and physiologic differences between children and adults. Particular differences that will affect invasive monitoring are listed here.

Basic Pediatric Considerations

1. The child will have small vessels. These vessels may be difficult to cannulate, and small catheters (and introducers and guidewires) will be needed. The lumen of a small catheter can become occluded by small kinks, or with small accumulation of fibrin or blood products. It is imperative that the catheter be continuously flushed with 1 to 5 ml/hr of the desired flush solution, and that regular assessment be made of the patency of the catheter. Use of heparinized continuous flush solution (1 to 5 units heparin/ml) has been shown to increase the patency of these small catheters.[4] If the catheter is used for only intermittent pressure measurements, concentrated heparinized flush solution (containing 20 to 100 units of heparin/ml) may be instilled into the catheter to ensure patency. This heparin should be withdrawn, however, before fluid is instilled into the catheter.

2. Even apparently small amounts of blood loss during catheter insertion may represent significant blood loss for the child. As a result, the child's circulating blood volume should be calculated, and blood replacement planned if acute blood loss totals 3.5 to 5.0 ml/kg body weight (2.5% to 5% of the child's total circulating blood volume). Following catheter insertion, the nurse should monitor the child closely for evidence of bleeding, or evidence of hypovolemia (including tachycardia with compromise of systemic perfusion). All blood withdrawn for laboratory analysis should be totaled if the patient is an infant, and blood replacement should be considered if the hematocrit falls or blood drawn totals 5% to 7% of the circulating blood volume.

3. Fluid overload can result from excessive fluid administration through monitoring lines. It is imperative that this source of fluid intake be meticulously totaled each hour, and added to the child's total fluid intake for that hour. Fluids used to flush monitoring lines should be infused only through a volume infusion pump with a buretrol, so that the exact volume of fluids administered may be calculated. Intermittent flushing of the catheter and monitoring tubing should be performed with a syringe, rather than through a valved flow-limiting device, so that the exact volume of such "flushes" can be added to the child's recorded fluid intake (refer to discussion of central venous pressure monitoring). The health care team should be aware of the heparin and electrolyte content of all fluids instilled through monitoring lines.

4. Most children will move all extremities vigorously. Therefore, all tubing con-

Procedure for mechanical calibration of transducer

NOTE: This procedure uses the principle that a column of water 27 cm high exerts a pressure equal to 27 cm H_2O pressure; 27 cm H_2O = 20 mm Hg.

1. Assemble and flush transducer, tubing (with appropriate stopcocks and syringes), monitor cable, and tape measure. Be sure that a 12-inch piece of flushed, noncompliant tubing is attached to transducer. Prepare monitor printer.
2. Plug transducer into monitoring cable and cable into bedside monitor.
3. Turn bedside monitor on, and select appropriate pressure monitoring scale.
4. Place transducer at level of phlebostatic axis.
5. Open transducer stopcock port to AIR, and depress "O" button on bedside monitor (this will zero the transducer and monitor to atmospheric pressure).
6. If monitor has an electronic calibration button, depress that after transducer is zeroed—this will electronically calibrate monitor digital display and waveform.
7. Begin printing pressure display.
8. Turn transducer stopcock off to air port, and close this port with sterile dead-end plug. Turn transducer stopcock open to 12-inch noncompliant tubing.
9. When free end of the 12-inch tubing is open to air, and tip is at level of phlebostatic axis, digital display and waveform should correspond to "O" reading.
10. Elevate the tip of the free end of the noncompliant tubing 27 cm above transducer (and phlebostatic axis); this applies a pressure equal to 20 mm Hg on the transducer, and the monitor digital display and pressure waveform should read "20 mm Hg."
11. Return tubing tip to level of phlebostatic axis and ensure that digital display and waveform return to "O" level.
12. Depress graphic calibration signal.
13. Examine graphic recording of this calibration, and ensure that graphic recording is calibrated with mechanical (27 cm H_2O) calibration and with electronic calibration.
14. Adjust monitor or printer as needed to ensure appropriate calibration. If transducer faulty, change it.

For further information refer to Civetta, JM: Pulmonary artery catheter insertion. In Sprung, CL, editor: The pulmonary artery catheter, methodology and clinical applications, Baltimore, 1983, University Park Press.

nections should be luer-locked, to reduce the possibility of inadvertent disconnections. In addition, all tubing connections should be taped securely, and catheters should be taped or sutured into place. Whenever possible, the nurse should tape an additional loop of tubing to the patient so that vigorous movement will be more likely to place tension on the loop of tubing rather than on the catheter itself. The transducer, catheter insertion site, and all tubing and connections should be visible at all times. "High" and "low" pressure monitoring alarms should be set so that sudden changes in patient condition or tubing separation will immediately trigger an audible alarm. The bedside nurse should carefully check the entire monitoring

---

Common causes of error in vascular monitoring systems

Transducer leveled incorrectly
  Transducer placed above right atrium will result in falsely low vascular pressure readings
  Transducer placed below right atrium will result in falsely high vascular pressure readings
Dampening of signal (usually will produce falsely low results)
  Kink in monitoring tubing or catheter
  Air in monitoring line or transducer
  Clot in tip of catheter
  Clamp or stopcock obstructing waveform transmission
  Catheter wedged against vessel wall
  Leak or loose connection in monitoring tubing/system
  Blood backup in tubing or transducer
  Faulty transducer (check calibration)
Signal artifact
  Catheter fling may result in erroneously high digital pressure readings
  60-cycle interference may introduce error in readings
  High fluid infusion rate may dampen waveform signal or result in increased pressure within monitoring system (reduce flow rate in monitoring line and ensure that flow-limiting valve is in place)

---

system and all connections at least every hour to ensure that loose connections will be detected.

5. The child's arterial blood pressure is usually much lower than the blood pressure of the adult. Therefore, small errors in blood pressure measurement may be relatively more significant in the child. For this reason, it is imperative that transducers used in children be carefully zeroed, levelled, and calibrated before use, so that the data obtained with the transducer will be reliable (see the box on p. 263).

6. There is a general conception that the child is immunologically immature and is at greater risk for infection than the adult. Certainly, the critically ill child is susceptible to infection. However, extensive studies of invasive hemodynamic monitoring in children have failed to document a higher incidence of catheter-related septicemia in children than that reported for adults.[33] There is no question that the combination of a prolonged ICU stay and multiple invasive monitoring lines will make any patient's risk of nosocomial infection extremely high.[23] It is, therefore, imperative that these lines be established under strict sterile conditions, and maintained under strict aseptic conditions.

7. Children are often frightened and unable to cooperate with invasive procedures. Careful explanations should be given to the child (at an age-appropriate level) before initiation of any procedure. Children often interpret intentional pain as punishment, so the child should be reassured that he or she is "good." In addition, adequate analgesia must be provided during any painful procedure.

The child should be securely restrained to prevent the child from dislodging or separating essential therapeutic or monitoring equipment. The parents should be allowed to remain with the child once the sterile insertion procedure has been completed, because they will provide a critical source of comfort to the child.

Central Venous Pressure Monitoring

Insertion of a central venous catheter may be performed to enable fluid or drug infusion, or to allow measurement of central venous pressures. Central venous pressure (CVP) monitoring will reflect right atrial pressure, unless superior or inferior vena caval obstruction is present. Right atrial pressure will, in turn, reflect right ventricular end-diastolic pressure (RVEDP), unless tricuspid valve stenosis is present.

Very often, if myocardial function and vascular resistances are normal, the child's right and left ventricular end-diastolic pressures will be equal. Then, the CVP will be approximately equal to the pulmonary artery wedge and left atrial (and LVED) pressures. However, this equality should not be assumed when the child is critically ill. Sepsis, septic shock, respiratory disease, cardiomyopathy, myocarditis, and congenital heart disease can all depress right *or* left ventricular contractility and function, and may result in a discrepancy between right and left ventricular end-diastolic pressures. For this reason, the central venous pressure should only be interpreted as reflecting right ventricular end-diastolic pressure. Indirect assessment of left ventricular end-diastolic pressure (LVEDP) may be made through echocardiography, and further assessment of LVEDP may be obtained through use of a flow-directed balloon-tipped pulmonary artery catheter (refer to Chapter 5 for further information about central venous and pulmonary artery pressure monitoring).

The CVP will be low if the child demonstrates inadequate intravascular volume relative to the vascular space. Such low pressures may be observed as the result of absolute volume loss, such as may occur with hemorrhage, dehydration, capillary leak, or other causes of hypovolemia. In addition, a low CVP may result from expansion of the vascular space, such as may occur with early septic shock, or administration of vasodilatory agents.

An elevated CVP reflects an increase in RVEDP. This may result from an absolute gain in intravascular volume, such as occurs with excessive intravenous fluid administration and hypervolemia. However, an elevation in CVP more commonly occurs when there is right ventricular failure, with a decrease in right ventricular compliance, contractility, and ejection fraction. Such right ventricular failure may occur as the result of congenital heart disease, myocarditis, cardiomyopathy, sepsis, or increased pulmonary vascular resistance (for example, pulmonary hypertension).

The CVP measurement will aid in titration of fluid administration for the pediatric or adult patient in shock (see Chapter 10 for further information). During fluid administration, the nurse should attempt to identify the CVP associated with optimal systemic perfusion (including blood pressure, capillary refill, and urine output). This optimal CVP may then be maintained through careful fluid administration.

As noted above, the critically ill child's pulmonary artery wedge and LVEDP may be normal, low, or elevated in the presence of a high, normal, or decreased CVP. Therefore, when the nurse monitors the CVP during shock resuscitation, attempts should be made to evaluate left ventricular function and systemic perfusion. The two-dimensional echocardiogram may reveal dilation of the left ventricle if significant left ventricular failure is present. The development of pulmonary edema can also indicate the presence of elevated (greater than 20 to 25 mm Hg) LVEDP, but this clinical sign may also occur as the result of increased capillary permeability and a normal or low LVEDP. If assessment of LVEDP is necessary, a flow-directed, balloon-tipped pulmonary artery catheter should be inserted.

The appearance of the CVP pressure tracing will be identical in the child and the adult. The normal mean CVP in the infant is 0 to 4 mm Hg, and the normal mean CVP in the child is 2 to 6 mm Hg.[31]

CVP measurements may be affected by positive pressure ventilation and high levels of positive end-expiratory pressure. The effects observed will be dependent on the compliance of the child's lungs, and the amount of positive pressure provided. If the child's lungs are extremely compliant, intrapleural pressure created by the ventilator is likely to be transmitted to the pleural space and vessels, including any vessels in the chest. Thus, the CVP may rise during the inspiratory phase of positive pressure ventilation. If the child's lungs are noncompliant (that is, they are very stiff), the intrapleural pressure created by the ventilator may not affect the CVP. Higher peak inspiratory pressures and end-expiratory pressures are more likely to affect the CVP than are lower pressures (effects of respiratory disease on hemodynamic monitoring are also discussed in Chapter 13).

Indications

Indications for use of CVP catheters in children include the following:
1. Rapid infusion and delivery of intravenous fluids
2. Measurement of central venous pressures for the purposes of determining:
   a. Intravascular volume status (and venous return)
   b. Right ventricular end-diastolic pressure
   c. Ideal RVEDP (and CVP) necessary to optimize systemic perfusion
3. Rapid delivery of resuscitative and vasoactive drugs to the right atrium
4. Administration of hypertonic fluids (such as parenteral alimentation)
5. Venous access for blood sampling

CVP catheters may be inserted percutaneously or by cutdown through several sites (Fig 11-2): umbilical vein, external or internal jugular vein, femoral vein, basilic vein, or subclavian vein. The choice of sites will be determined by the experience of the clinician, the age the child, and the acuity of the child's condition. Umbilical venous, subclavian vein, external and internal jugular venous, and femoral venous catheterization will be discussed in detail in subsequent sections.

Umbilical venous catheterization is only possible during the first weeks of life. External jugular venous cannulation is relatively easy, but this site is often impractical to use during resuscitative efforts. Internal jugular or subclavian vein catheterization should be attempted only by a clinician experienced in the technique, because these procedures may result in bleeding or pneumothorax, respectively.

Femoral vein catheterization may be most appropriate during resuscitative efforts, because this site is distant from the child's airway and chest. However, resuscitative drugs administered into the inferior vena cava may pool below the diaphragm during cardiac compression, unless the catheter is sufficiently long to allow

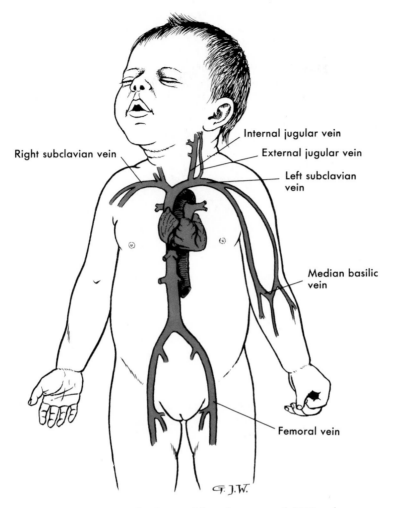

Fig. 11-2. Location of veins used for placement of CVP catheters.

the tip to pass above the diaphragm. In addition, a femoral venous line may easily become contaminated by urine or stool, so it is usually removed as quickly as possible.

Before insertion of any central venous catheter, the nurse should explain the procedure to the child (if the child is conscious) and the parents, and informed consent should be obtained from the parents or legal guardian (unless the procedure is performed under emergent conditions). Adequate analgesia should be provided, and the child should be restrained before the procedure.

Many clinicians use the Seldinger technique to pass a catheter percutaneously into the child's vein. This technique involves insertion of a large-bore hollow needle into the desired vein. A small-gauge guidewire is then threaded through the needle, until several centimeters of the wire are within the large vein. Once the guidewire has been inserted, the needle is withdrawn over the guidewire. Finally, the central venous catheter is threaded over the guidewire, into the vein, until it lies

---

Equipment needed for umbilical venous or artery catheterization

Appropriate catheter and blunt needle
Povidone-iodine solution
Sterile hat, mask, gown, and gloves for clinician
Sterile towels
Gauze sponges
Sterile container (for povidone-iodine)
A #11 surgical blade
Scalpel handle
4-0 or 5-0 silk suture on cutting needle
Needle holder
Two small (5-inch) delicately curved mosquito hemostats
Small toothed forceps
4-inch curved forceps
4-inch straight forceps
Small scissors
Sterile umbilical tape (several 6-inch lengths)
Sterile measuring tape
Several syringes
Flush solution for catheter
Monitoring system (with calibrated transducer)

---

in proper position. The guidewire is then withdrawn, intravenous fluids are attached to the catheter, and the catheter is sutured into place. This technique is especially effective for percutaneous insertion of catheters of relatively large size into infants and young children.

Umbilical venous catheterization (UVC)

Umbilical venous catheters may provide immediate intravascular access during neonatal resuscitation and will allow central venous access for blood sampling and monitoring. The equipment needed for umbilical venous or arterial catheterization is listed in the box above.

Before catheter insertion, the neonate is securely restrained. Electrocardiographic monitoring is provided throughout the procedure. The proper depth of catheter insertion is estimated by adding 4 cm to the distance (in centimeters) between the distal ends of the infant's clavicles and the umbilicus. A sterile piece of cord tape should be tied around the catheter at the calculated insertion depth. The sterile catheter is then irrigated with the desired flush solution and attached to a fluid-filled transducer and monitoring system to enable monitoring of the umbilical venous waveform during catheter insertion. The umbilical area is draped with sterile towels, and scrubbed with a povidone-iodine solution.

Using sterile technique, the clinician will examine the umbilical stump, and identify the umbilical vein as the largest vessel in the umbilical cord (the two smaller umbilical arteries will have thicker walls). The vein is usually located on the superior portion of the umbilicus.

Sterile umbilical cord tape is placed around the umbilicus and tied loosely; this tie should prevent bleeding during the procedure, although it may be necessary to loosen it as the catheter is inserted. The cord should be pulled upright, with slight tension, and a scalpel should be used to cut the cord horizontally. This cut enables catheterization of nondistorted, uncontaminated umbilical vessels.

Sterile forceps should be used to remove any fibrin or clots from the lumen of the vein, then the forceps should guide the catheter into the umbilical vein. As the catheter is advanced into the vein, the pressure waveform should be displayed on the monitor oscilloscope.

As the umbilical catheter is passed into the subdiaphragmatic portion of the umbilical vein and portal vein, only respiratory pressure variations will be visible on the oscilloscope. As the catheter enters the inferior vena cava, a characteristic central venous pressure waveform will be visible on the oscilloscope. The appearance of a CVP waveform should coincide with insertion of the catheter to the measured (and marked) maximal insertion point. The catheter should be marked with indelible ink at this insertion point, and the catheter should be carefully taped in position.

Proper location of the distal tip of the umbilical venous catheter in the IVC should be verified by chest radiograph. It is essential that proper placement of the catheter be confirmed before any drugs or fluids are infused through the catheter. Once proper placement is ensured, the catheter is sutured and firmly taped in place.

The tape used to secure an umbilical artery or venous catheter should hold the catheter in a straight line from the umbilicus, perpendicular to the anterior plane of the infant's body. This requires creation of a tape "bridge." Two pieces of tape (one on either side of the umbilicus) are placed vertically, anchored at each end to the infant's abdomen. These two pieces of tape are used to brace a third, horizontal piece of tape which suspends the catheter upright between the vertical tapes (the horizontal piece of tape creates the appearance of the crossbar of football goalposts, or the letter H).

The neonate may be placed in the prone position while umbilical artery or venous catheters are in place as long as the nurse is able to constantly observe the umbilicus for evidence of bleeding. Care must be taken to avoid tension on the catheter or the insertion site.

When the umbilical venous catheter is removed, pressure is applied over the umbilicus for at least 5 minutes, or until bleeding stops. A sterile gauze pad is then taped over the umbilical site. The nurse should monitor for bleeding from the vein for several hours following catheter removal.

Subclavian vein catheterization

Pediatric subclavian vein catheterization is gaining in popularity, because the catheter may be taped securely in place on the child's chest, and it will not interfere with positioning of the child or movement of the child's extremities. Placement of this catheter should only be attempted by clinicians skilled in the technique, or tension pneumothorax or hemothorax may result.

When a subclavian vein catheterization is performed, the child should be placed in the Trendelenburg position, with the head 20 to 30 degrees lower than the

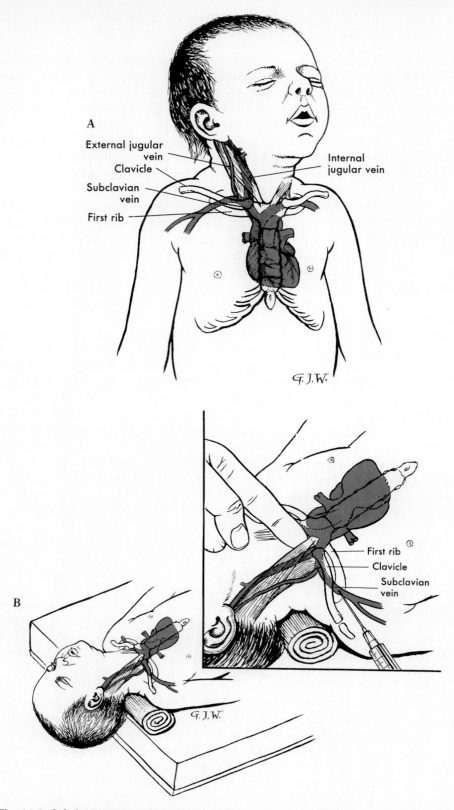

Fig. 11-3. Subclavian vein catheterization. **A,** Anatomy. **B,** Technique. (Modified from Chameides, L: Textbook of pediatric advanced life support, Dallas, 1988, American Heart Association.)

heart, and the head turned away from the site. This position will distend the sub-clavian vein, and make air embolus during catheterization unlikely. The site should be draped with sterile towels, and scrubbed with povidone-iodine solution. Local anesthetic (1% xylocaine) should be instilled subcutaneously.

The subclavian vein is cannulated at the point where it crosses over the first rib, just before it passes under the clavicle. The clinician's index fingertip is placed in the suprasternal notch to provide a reference point. A needle attached to a syringe will be inserted just under the clavicle at the distal margin of the medial third of the clavicle (a distance equal to one third of the length of the clavicle, measured from the junction of the clavicle and the sternum). The syringe and needle should be held parallel to the frontal plane of the body, and the needle is inserted in a medial, cephalad direction, pointing toward the suprasternal notch and the reference fingertip (Fig 11-3). The syringe plunger should be aspirated as the needle is advanced, and insertion should stop when blood is aspirated freely into the syringe, since this will indicate entrance into the subclavian vein.[7]

Once the needle is in the subclavian vein, it should be rotated so that the bevel of the needle faces downward. The syringe is detached from the needle, and the needle hub is covered with the clinician's (gloved) thumb, to prevent entry of air into the central venous system. During patient spontaneous exhalation or positive pressure ventilation, a guidewire will be passed through the needle, and advanced to the approximate length required to enter the superior vena cava. Once the guidewire is successfully passed, the needle is withdrawn over the guidewire. Finally, the catheter is passed over the guidewire and into the subclavian vein, and ultimately into the superior vena cava (and right atrium, if desired). The guidewire may then be withdrawn and the catheter sutured into place. A sterile dressing is applied to the site. The catheter should be intermittently flushed to maintain patency, but it should not be attached to infusion fluids until appropriate placement is verified by chest radiograph.

External jugular venous catheterization

External jugular venous catheterization is generally popular for children over 5 years of age. Since the vein is superficial and visible, this vessel may be used when emergency venous access must be rapidly achieved.

Placement of the child for external jugular venous catheterization is identical to the recommended position for subclavian catheterization (30–degree head-down position, with the head turned away from the catheterization site—see previous discussion). The child must be properly restrained and 1% xylocaine should be injected to anesthetize the insertion site. The right external jugular vein is preferred over the left for initial approach.

After the insertion site is draped with sterile towels and scrubbed with a povidone-iodine solution, the external jugular vein is visualized—visualization may be enhanced if the vein is occluded proximally (just above the clavicle). The skin over the insertion site should be broken using a large (16- to 18-gauge) needle. Then a catheter with stylette, or a large hollow catheter attached to a syringe is inserted directly into the external jugular vein, several centimeters above the clavicle (Fig. 11-4). As soon as free flow of blood appears in the syringe, insertion of the needle should stop. If a catheter with stylette is used, the stylette is withdrawn, and the

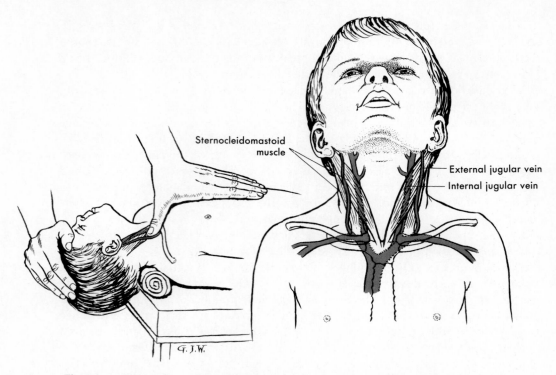

Sternocleidomastoid muscle

External jugular vein
Internal jugular vein

Fig. 11-4. External jugular venous catheterization. (Modified from Chameides, L: Textbook of pediatric advanced life support, Dallas, 1988, American Heart Association.)

catheter is advanced and sutured into place, and hand irrigation of the catheter is provided. If a hollow needle has been inserted into the vein, the needle is held carefully in place (with the clinician's thumb covering the needle hub), and a guidewire is threaded through the needle, and inserted several centimeters into the vein. There may be some difficulty threading the guidewire below the clavicle. If resistance is encountered, it may be helpful to keep the needle in place, remove the initial guidewire, and substitute a small J-wire.[7]

Once the guidewire has been successfully passed well into the jugular vein, the needle is withdrawn over the guidewire, and a catheter is then threaded over the guidewire, into the vein. Once the catheter is in place, the guidewire is withdrawn, and the catheter is sewn into place. The catheter should be only gently flushed by hand, and no medications should be infused through the catheter until proper position is verified by radiograph. Reported success rate of external jugular venous catheterization in children is approximately 60% to 75%, and the success rate is highest in children beyond 5 years of age. Failure of proper external jugular venous catheter placement most often results in advancement of the catheter up into the neck.[26]

Internal jugular venous catheterization

Catheterization of the internal jugular vein should not be attempted by unskilled clinicians, because faulty technique may result in puncture of the right carotid artery and hemorrhage. The incidence of this complication in children is approximately 8%—the risk is apparently higher than during catheterization of adults because the internal jugular vein and the carotid artery are virtually side by side in the neck of the child.[26]

The child is positioned with the head 15 to 45 degrees below the trunk, with the head turned to the left—this will facilitate right jugular venous catheterization. The right internal jugular vein is preferred because it joins the right subclavian vein and enters the right atrium in a direct path. In addition, the apex of the right lung is lower below the clavicle than the apex of the left lung, and the right approach prevents injury to the thoracic duct.

The internal jugular vein courses between the sternal and clavicular heads of the sternocleidomastoid muscle, above the medial end of the clavicle. The major landmarks to be identified before the procedure include the sternal and clavicular heads of the sternocleidomastoid muscle, the external jugular vein, the right nipple, and the suprasternal notch. Once the landmarks have been identified, the area is draped (leaving the landmarks visible), and scrubbed with povidone-iodine solution. The skin entrance site is anesthetized with a 1% xylocaine solution.

If a *posterior* approach is used, the internal jugular vein will be cannulated from a needle directed under and behind the external jugular vein. A hollow needle attached to a syringe is inserted at a 30 to 45 degree angle from the skin, just above the point where the external jugular vein crosses the sternocleidomastoid muscle (Fig. 11-5, *A*). The needle should be pointed toward the suprasternal notch during insertion. Once the vein is entered, the Seldinger technique is used to thread the catheter.[7]

If the *anterior* route of insertion is used, the needle enters between the sternocleidomastoid muscle and the right common carotid artery. It will be necessary to retract the artery medially so that it is not punctured. The needle is introduced just lateral to the right common carotid artery, but medial to the sternocleidomastoid muscle. It is inserted at a 30- to 45-degree angle from the skin, directed toward the right nipple (Fig. 11-5, *B*). Once free flow of blood is observed in the syringe, the needle is held carefully in place and the syringe is removed. The clinician's thumb should cover the needle hub if the patient is breathing spontaneously. The Seldinger technique is then used to thread a guidewire, then the catheter, into the internal jugular vein.

If the catheter threads freely, it will almost certainly thread into the superior vena cava (and, if desired, into the right atrium). Proper placement is verified by radiograph, and by the appearance of a central venous pressure tracing when the catheter is connected to a monitor.

A *central* route of internal jugular venous catheterization requires insertion of a needle at the apex of the triangle formed by the sternal and clavicular heads of the sternocleidomastoid muscle and the clavicle. The needle is inserted just medial to the clavicular head of the sternocleidomastoid, angled 15 to 30 degrees above the skin, and aimed at the right nipple (Fig. 11-5, *C*). If immediate blood return does not occur, the needle should be aimed more laterally, toward the right shoulder. The needle should not be directed medially from this approach, since the right common carotid artery may easily be punctured (it courses just medial to the internal jugular vein).

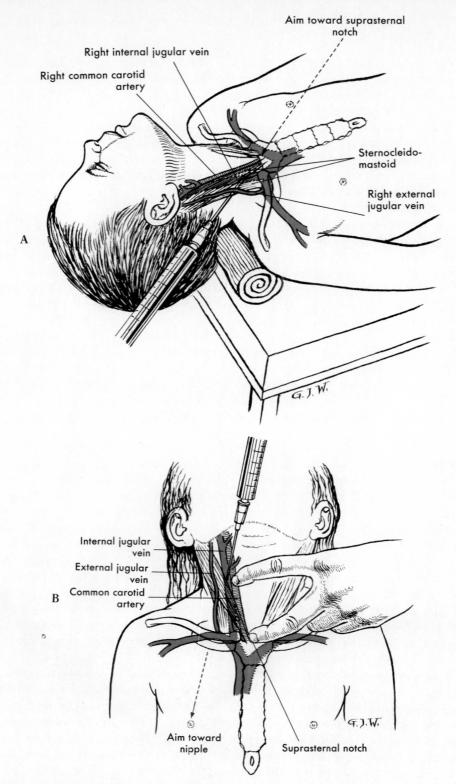

Fig. 11-5. Internal jugular venous catheterization. **A,** Posterior route. **B,** Anterior route.

Continued.

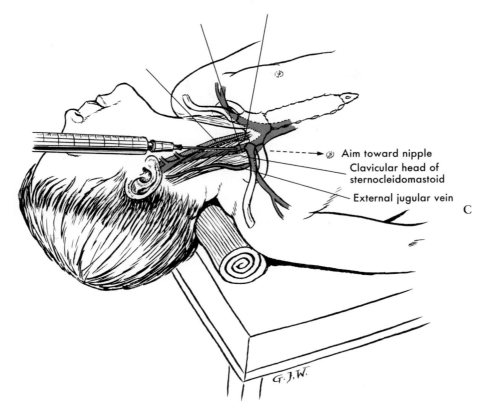

Aim toward nipple
Clavicular head of
sternocleidomastoid
External jugular vein

C

Fig. 11-5, cont'd. C, Central route. (Modified from Chameides, L: Textbook of pediatric advanced life support, Dallas, 1988, American Heart Association.)

Once free blood return into the syringe is observed, the needle is held in place and the syringe is removed. The needle hub is covered until the patient exhales spontaneously, or until delivery of a positive pressure inspiration; then the Seldinger technique is used to thread the guidewire, then the catheter into the vein. The catheter should thread easily, directly into the internal jugular vein, the superior vena cava, and toward the right atrium.

If the catheter advances easily, and free blood return occurs whenever the catheter is aspirated, the catheter is almost certainly in place. In addition, a typical central venous pressure waveform should be observed when the catheter is joined to a monitoring system. However, radiographic confirmation will be necessary before infusion of large volumes of fluids or medications.

During internal jugular venous cannulation, everyone at the bedside should observe the patient closely for signs of carotid artery puncture. This complication should be immediately recognized by the appearance of bright red blood into the syringe when the needle is initially inserted. However, if unrecognized carotid arterial catheterization is performed, the arterial waveform should be recognizable when the vascular waveform is displayed on the monitor. Occasionally, the carotid artery is inadvertently nicked as the internal jugular vein is catheterized—this would result in an immediate hematoma. Whenever the carotid artery is punctured, the needle should be withdrawn immediately, and pressure should be applied over the artery for 10 minutes or until bleeding has stopped.

Femoral venous catheterization

The child's leg should be rotated externally and restrained. The upper portion of the leg is draped with sterile towels and scrubbed with an iodine solution. Using sterile technique, the clinician locates the inguinal ligament, then palpates femoral arterial pulsations, in the area approximately midway between the anterior superior iliac spine and the symphysis pubis. A large needle attached to a syringe is inserted one finger-breadth below the inguinal ligament, just medial to the femoral arterial pulsations. The needle is directed cephalad, and in a 45-degree angle downward (Fig. 11-6). As the needle is inserted, the plunger is withdrawn until blood flows freely into the syringe—at this point, insertion should stop. The syringe is detached from the needle, while the needle is held carefully in place. The Seldinger technique is then used to insert a guidewire, and then the catheter into the femoral vein and into the inferior vena cava. The catheter is sutured in place, and a sterile dressing is applied. Infusion of fluid and drugs may begin once the proper placement of the catheter is confirmed radiographically.

Maintenance

Any central venous line must be inserted under sterile conditions, and it should be covered with a sterile dressing. The simple monitoring catheter should be continuously flushed with heparinized saline. The addition of 0.5 to 2 units of heparin/ml flush solution will reduce the incidence of catheter thrombus occlusion. If the catheter is inserted to allow intermittent access for daily blood sampling, it may be "heparin-locked," with instillation of 1 to 2 ml of higher concentrations of heparin (20 to 100 units/ml). However, this heparin should always be withdrawn from the catheter and tubing (rather than "flushed" into the patient) whenever the catheter is entered.

Continuous irrigation of central venous and arterial catheters in children should be accomplished only through use of volume-controlled pumps and syringes (Fig. 11-7). The use of pressurized irrigation bags for pediatric monitoring is discouraged, because it is impossible to verify the exact quantity of fluids delivered to the child on a continuous basis (although approximately 3 ml/hr will be delivered through standard flow-limiting devices, if they are functioning properly). In addition, any rapid "flushing" of lines with the flow-limiting devices will deliver an unknown quantity of fluid under extremely high pressure. This can result in fluid overload as well as in damage to the catheterized vessel. Monitoring catheters should only be flushed with gentle irrigation from a syringe. This enables documentation of the exact quantity of fluids delivered to the child and will reduce trauma to the catheterized vessel.

If the CVP catheter is used for monitoring and for infusion of intravenous fluids, the fluids and transducer may be joined to the catheter at a 3-way stopcock. With this tubing configuration, pressure measurements may be made intermittently, when the stopcock is turned off to the fluid infusion and on to the trans-

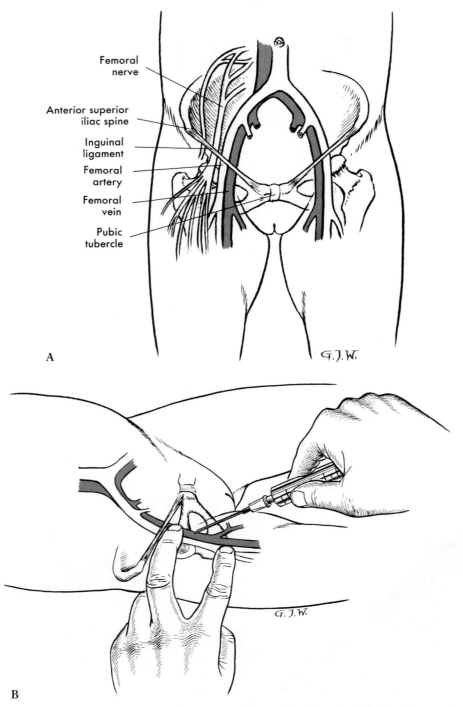

Fig. 11-6. Femoral venous catheterization. **A,** Anatomy. **B,** Technique. (Modified from Chameides, L: Textbook of pediatric advanced life support, Dallas, 1988, American Heart Association.)

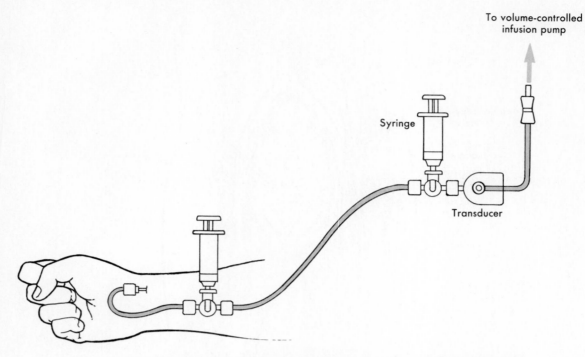

Fig. 11-7. Use of syringes and volume-controlled infusion pumps for flushing of monitoring lines.

ducer (Fig. 11-8, *A*). If such intermittent measurements are made, it is advisable that the transducer be attached to the stopcock port that is in direct alignment with the monitoring catheter (the infusion fluid may be joined to the stopcock port at a 90-degree angle from the catheter); this will provide the best conduction of pressure waveforms to the transducer.

If large-volume (up to 30 ml/hr) fluid infusion is required while central venous pressure measurements are made, it will be necessary to administer the fluid with a volume-controlled pump through a 30-ml/hr flow-limiting device. Such a device will prevent the fluid infusion from interfering with pressure measurements (Fig. 11-8, *B*). The central venous fluid and monitoring (flush) line fluid and tubing should be changed every 48 to 72 hours.[21,34] More frequent tubing and fluid changes will be required if parenteral alimentation is administered through the CVP line.

Central venous catheters are often used for administration of drugs and parenteral alimentation. When parenteral alimentation is administered, attempts should be made to avoid entry into that alimentation line. Several small (4, 5.5, and 7 French) multilumen catheters are now commercially available for central venous insertion (made by Arrow, Cook, and Deseret, among others) in the pediatric patient. These lines are often preferable to single-lumen catheters, in that they allow uninterrupted delivery of parenteral alimentation through one lumen, while a second (or even third) lumen remains available for blood sampling, monitoring, and drug administration. It is important to consider the complete monitoring and intra-

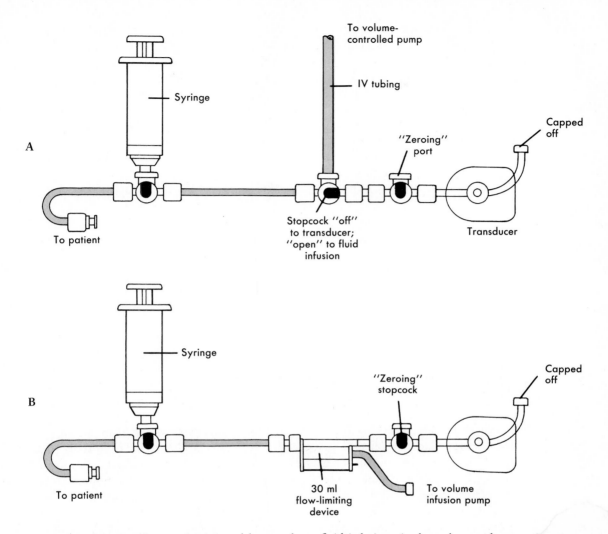

Fig. 11-8. System for monitoring and large volume fluid infusion, **A**, through use of stopcock with intermittent pressure measurements and **B**, through continuous monitoring and infusion using flow-limiting device.

venous access needs of the child before a central venous catheter is inserted, to enable placement of the most suitable catheter in the most logical site.

Complications

The most common complications following central venous catheterization in children include infection, bleeding, ventricular arrhythmias (if the catheter enters the right ventricle), and thromboembolus formation. Additional complications include those of insertion: pneumothorax and hemothorax are possible complications of subclavian vein catheterization, and bleeding may complicate internal or external jugular venous, umbilical venous, or femoral venous catherization.

Infection of central venous lines can be prevented with the use of good handwashing technique before and after patient contact, prevention of catheter contamination, and minimization of duration of catheterization. The use of transparent vapor-permeable occlusive dressings may also reduce the risk of catheter sepsis. It is imperative that everyone responsible for placing these catheters adhere to the use of strict sterile technique and that flawless aseptic technique be used when the catheter, tubing, or stopcock is handled.

The risk of catheter-related nosocomial infections is associated with duration of central venous catheterization—the risk increases most notably in association with catheter duration beyond 3 to 5 days. Risk of infection is also increased if the catheter is used for blood sampling.[23,30]

Early signs of sepsis in children include a mild respiratory alkalosis (if the child is breathing spontaneously), or an unexplained metabolic acidosis. In addition, the child may develop thrombocytopenia (or other early signs of disseminated intravascular coagulation), leukocytosis, or leukopenia. Fever may also be present (although temperature instability is a common sign of sepsis in the neonate).

The catheterization site should be observed daily, and evidence of inflammation reported to a physician. Use of vapor-permeable, occlusive, transparent dressings may facilitate continuous observation of the entrance site without interruption of the occlusive dressing.

Bleeding is an unusual complication following central venous catheterization in children. It occurs most frequently in critically ill children with preexisting coagulopathies. If the CVP line is used for pressure measurements, it should be joined to a monitor with a high-and low-pressure audible alarm. This alarm should be activated if the patient's CVP falls by 10% or more. This will ensure rapid detection of changes in patient condition or tubing separation.

The entire CVP monitoring system should be joined with only luer-lock connections, so that inadvertent tubing separation is unlikely. The catheter entrance site and all tubing connections should be visible at all times, so that tubing separation or blood loss will be immediately detected.

Central venous catheter migration may result in vascular perforation and resultant hydrothorax or hemothorax. This complication should be apparent by the disappearance of the characteristic central venous pressure waveform on oscilloscope. In addition, evidence of free fluid in the thorax should be apparent on clinical examination. If extravascular catheter migration is suspected, fluid infusion through the catheter should be discontinued, and a physician contacted. The extravascular catheter will be removed.

Central venous catheter migration into the right ventricle may produce premature ventricular contractions. This migration will be apparent when a right ventricular waveform appears on the oscilloscope. If right ventricular migration occurs, the catheter should be withdrawn into the right atrium.

Right atrial thrombus formation has been reported in infants and young children with long-dwelling right atrial catheters. Septic or aseptic thrombi should be suspected in any child with an indwelling line who develops fever or evidence of vena caval obstruction, and it can usually be confirmed using echocardiography. The thrombus will often require surgical evacuation, although occasional success in clot dissolution has been reported using urokinase.[8,22]

Arterial Pressure Monitoring

Arterial pressure monitoring should be instituted for any unstable, critically ill child. This monitoring permits constant visualization of the child's arterial pressure, and provides immediate information regarding the child's response to volume and vasoactive drug therapies. Intra-arterial monitoring also facilitates arterial blood sampling for blood gas and other laboratory analysis. Use of the Seldinger technique allows percutaneous insertion of catheters in even small arteries.

Intra-arterial monitoring is certainly helpful in determining the child's absolute arterial blood pressure. In fact, if the child's monitoring system is appropriately zeroed and calibrated, this form of monitoring will be more accurate than auscultated or oscillometric blood pressure measurements. The mean arterial pressure calculated (by a cardiac monitor) from the actual area under an arterial waveform will also be more accurate than arithmetic estimations of the mean arterial pressure from the systolic and diastolic pressures (see Chapter 6 for further information).

The appearance of the arterial waveform in the child is identical to that observed in the adult (refer to Chapter 6). Of course, the normal arterial pressure in the child will be much lower than that observed in the normal adult (see Table 11-1 for review of normal blood pressures in children).

Some congenital heart defects may produce characteristic changes in the arterial waveform. The child with patent ductus arteriosus or aortic insufficiency may demonstrate aortic runoff pulses, with a low diastolic and mean pressure, and a widened pulse pressure. Significant aortic valvular stenosis characteristically produces a biphasic pulse (with an anacrotic notch noted during the systolic upstroke of the waveform). Coarctation of the aorta will result in hypertensive pulses (and associated arterial waveform) in the upper extremities (or any arterial circulation arising from the aorta proximal to the narrowed segment), and hypotensive and dampened pulses in the lower extremities. Just as in the adult, the child with tamponade may demonstrate pulsus paradoxus (if the child's respiratory rate is sufficiently slow), and the child with myocarditis and very low cardiac output may demonstrate pulsus alternans.

Indications

Indications for placement of an arterial line in the child are virtually identical to those for the adult and include the need for continuous observation of arterial blood pressure, or frequent arterial blood sampling. As a rule, if the child requires arterial blood gas analysis several times daily, insertion of an intra-arterial catheter is recommended (over repeated arterial puncture) to minimize pain to the child and trauma to arteries.

The most common arteries used for intra-arterial monitoring in children include: radial artery, dorsalis pedis artery, posterior tibial artery, femoral artery, and umbilical artery. Technique for insertion of an umbilical artery catheter is summarized below. The technique for insertion of the catheter into a peripheral artery with the Seldinger technique is identical to that described for adults; for this reason, the technique for catheterization of all peripheral arteries will be presented only briefly below (see Chapter 6 for further details).

Umbilical Artery Catheterization

Umbilical artery catheterization may be performed during stabilization of the critically ill neonate, and it can be accomplished by an experienced clinician within moments. However, since the procedure can be associated with significant complications, including hemorrhage, thromboembolic phenomena, and infection, it is not recommended for routine intra-arterial or vascular access in the neonate.

Long catheters must be used for umbilical artery insertion, because the catheter must pass through the umbilical artery (approximately 7 cm in length in the full-term neonate) into the internal iliac artery, and then retrograde into the common iliac artery and into the aorta. Since the catheter lies in the descending aorta, it is useful as a standard arterial line, but it may also enable administration of intravenous fluids and drugs if another intravenous line is not available.

Insertion

An umbilical artery catheterization tray should be obtained (see the box on p. 268). The catheter used should be smooth and radio-opaque, with a single hole at the tip. A 5-French catheter is used if the infant weighs more than 1200 g, and a 3.5-French catheter is used if the infant weighs less than 1200 g.

Before insertion, the proper depth of catheter insertion should be estimated from published charts, or from measurement of the distance from the distal ends of the clavicles to the umbilicus (the length of the umbilical stump must be added), and the length indicated on the catheter (using sterile umbilical artery tape).

The infant should be placed in the supine position and restrained, and cardiac monitoring should be performed throughout the procedure. The umbilical cord and surrounding area is cleansed with a povidone-iodine solution, and the umbilical area is draped with sterile towels in such a manner that the infant's face remains visible, and chest wall movement can still be observed. The entire procedure is performed using strict sterile technique.

A sterile segment of umbilical tape is placed around the umbilicus and knotted loosely—this will reduce bleeding from the cord during cord trimming and catheterization. The tape should not be tied too tightly, or it will be impossible to thread the catheter through the umbilical vessels. The distal end of the cord is held upright, and a scalpel is used to cut the cord horizontally, to produce a perfect horizontal view of the vessels. Two curved hemostats are used to grasp the umbilical cord on each side, holding it taut and immobile, while the two umbilical arteries are identified (they are the two smaller, thick-walled vessels). The outer wall of the cord is grasped with forceps, near one of the arteries, and the artery is probed gently with curved forceps. The forceps are inserted two or three more times, to a depth of approximately 1 cm, and the tips of the forceps are spread, to dilate the artery. While the curved forceps are holding the artery open, the catheter is inserted gently into the arterial lumen. Once the catheter is inserted for approximately 2 to 3 cm, the forceps may be removed. It may be necessary to loosen the umbilical tape that is wrapped around the base of the umbilical cord stump, for the catheter to be threaded beyond the depth of the stump.

The catheter should be advanced gently to the appropriate depth (as indicated by the umbilical tape). The catheter should not be forced if resistance is felt. Once the catheter is in place, it will be possible to readily aspirate blood from the catheter. When the catheter is joined to the arterial monitoring system, a characteristic arterial waveform should be displayed.

Some umbilical artery catheters (UACs) are equipped with standard intravenous tubing connections, so they may be directly connected to a fluid-filled monitoring system. However, many umbilical catheters require insertion of a blunt-tipped needle into the distal end of the catheter to provide the proper connection to a tubing system. If a blunt-tipped needle is required, an 18-gauge needle is used with a 5-French catheter, and a 20-gauge needle is used with a 3.5-French catheter.

Following catheter insertion, the umbilical tape is removed from the base of the umbilicus, and a purse-string suture is placed around the cord, to prevent bleeding from the umbilical vein or the noncatheterized umbilical artery. The catheter should be secured in place using a bridge taping system (refer to the previous discussion under Umbilical Venous Catheterization). It is important to keep the umbilicus and catheter entry site free of dressings or ointment. The nurse should be able to inspect the site at all times, to detect any bleeding or inflammation.

Radiographic confirmation of proper catheter placement will be necessary. The tip of the catheter should be either near the diaphragm (usually at the level of the sixth thoracic vertebra) or within the lumbar aorta at the third or fourth lumbar vertebrae. *The umbilical artery catheter tip should not remain between the tenth thoracic and the second lumbar vertebrae, since the catheter can then obstruct renal and mesenteric arterial blood flow.*

Maintenance

The UAC must be flushed continuously or intermittently with a saline or heparinized saline solution. Continuous infusion of solution heparinized with 0.5 to 1 unit of heparin/ml may increase longevity of the catheter and improve catheter patency. Occasionally, the critically ill neonate develops hypernatremia. If this occurs, the umbilical catheter may be flushed with heparinized 0.45% normal saline, instead of heparinized 0.9% normal saline.

If the catheter is flushed continuously, a volume-controlled infusion pump should be used to ensure delivery of a known quantity of fluid at a constant rate. Use of pressure bags and rapid flush flow-limiting devices *is not* recommended since it is impossible to determine the exact amount of fluid delivered in a day. In addition, the use of the rapid-flush device may produce arterial spasm, and may result in retrograde flow into the aortic arch vessels (see the following discussion in the Maintenance section of Peripheral Artery Catherization). If intermittent irrigation of the catheter is necessary, a syringe should be used to gently flush the catheter over several minutes.

Medications may be administered through an umbilical artery line, if no other route of administration is available. However, complications of such medication administration will depend on the pH and osmolality of the medication, and on the adequacy of the infant's cardiac output—if cardiac output is critically low, there will be inadequate blood flow in the aorta to effectively dilute the administered medication, and the drug may flow undiluted into the lower extremity arterial circulation. The nurse should refer to unit and hospital policy before administering any medication or blood product through an umbilical artery catheter.

Any connections in the umbilical arterial monitoring system should have luerlocks, to reduce the risk of inadvertent tubing separation. The entire arterial line should be visible at all times, and the infant should not be covered with blankets, since this may prevent recognition of bleeding. The arterial pressure monitor with digital display and oscilloscope should be equipped with an audible low-pressure alarm. This alarm should be set to sound whenever the neonate's systolic or diastolic arterial pressure falls by 10%; this will ensure that tubing separation is detected immediately. Such alarms should only be equipped with temporary alarm silence features, and it should be impossible to permanently disable such an alarm.

The most common complication of umbilical artery catheterization is obstruction of renal, mesenteric, and femoral artery blood flow (as a result of the catheter or thromboembolic events). Whenever a UAC is in place, the neonate's urine output and perfusion of the lower extremities should be evaluated constantly. Lower extremity pulses (including femoral, dorsalis pedis, and posterior tibial arteries) should be palpated hourly, and the quality of the pulses, temperature of the feet and legs, color, and briskness of capillary refill should be documented at least hourly.

Blanching, mottling, cyanosis, pallor, decreased pulses, or cooling of the legs should be reported to a physician immediately. Such developments usually indicate arterial obstruction, and removal of the catheter is usually necessary. These observations may also be made if a thrombus forms in the descending aorta as a result of umbilical artery catheterization—surgical removal of the thrombus may be necessary.

Blood should be drawn from the UAC as from any arterial catheter in the infant or child—very little blood should be wasted, and it should not be necessary to flush any additional fluid following blood drawing (see the following section, Blood Sampling from Indwelling Lines). If irrigation of the catheter is necessary because of suspected catheter obstruction, gentle irrigation and aspiration should be performed.

The catheter should always be taped securely in place, so that accidental dislodgement is impossible. The nurse should measure the distance from the umbilicus to the first tubing connection, and record this distance on the nursing care plan, so that catheter migration will be easily detected.

The neonate should not receive enteral feedings while the UAC is in place. The catheter may result in compromise to mesenteric blood flow, and feeding may then increase the risk of development of necrotizing enterocolitis. Feeding may be resumed several hours after the catheter has been removed (if bowel sounds and respiratory status are satisfactory).

Before the UAC is removed, the purse-string suture is cut at the level of the umbilical cord stump, rather than at the level of the catheter. Sterile umbilical tape is wrapped around the umbilicus, and tied loosely. As the catheter is withdrawn slowly, the umbilical tape may be tightened to reduce bleeding. In many hospitals, the umbilical artery catheter is withdrawn in stages, over a period of several hours. During the withdrawal period, the nurse observes the patient closely for evidence of bleeding from the umbilicus.

Additional maintenance of the UAC will be similar to that required for maintenance of any arterial catheter (refer to the following section, Peripheral Artery Catheterization).

Complications

The most common complications associated with umbilical artery catheterization include: hemorrhage, peritoneal perforation, compromise of lower extremity perfusion, thromboembolic complications (including occlusion of renal, mesenteric, or spinal cord arteries), and infection. Paraplegia and leg necrosis have been reported following use of the UAC, and intimal damage to the aorta may also occur. These complications can be prevented or detected with careful observation of the catheter entrance site, arterial waveform, and tubing connections and constant assessment of urine output and lower extremity perfusion.

Peripheral Artery Catheterization

Insertion of a pediatric peripheral artery catheter is accomplished with techniques identical to those used for adult peripheral artery catheterization (refer to Chapter 6 for details of peripheral artery catheter insertion). In all but the smallest neonates, the radial artery is the preferred site for arterial cannulation, and the dorsalis pedis and posterior tibial arteries are also used commonly. Femoral artery catheterization is usually performed only under emergent conditions, because the entrance site is likely to become contaminated, and limb ischemia may also result. Temporal artery catheterization has been largely abandoned, since cerebral embolization has been reported following use of this site.[28]

Insertion

Before insertion of a radial artery catheter, the Allen test should be performed to assess adequacy of collateral circulation to the hand. The radial artery is occluded as the patient's hand is curled into a fist. The radial artery should remain occluded as the patient's hand is opened to the relaxed position; if the hand remains blanched for longer than 3 seconds, collateral circulation is inadequate, and that radial artery should not be catheterized. If the hand reperfuses quickly despite occlusion of the radial artery, the collateral circulation is adequate, and the radial artery can be catheterized.

The entrance site over the artery is scrubbed with a povidone-iodine solution, and draped. A small amount of 1% xylocaine should be instilled subcutaneously at the anticipated catheterization site. Using sterile technique, the clinician palpates the artery. A small nick in the skin may be made using a 20-gauge needle.

A 22-gauge catheter is suitable for peripheral artery catheterization for all but the smallest neonates. In the newborn ICU, a 24-gauge catheter may be used as an arterial catheter. If a catheter with stylette is used, the styletted catheter may be inserted directly into the artery, at a 30-degree angle from the plane of the arm. Once the artery is entered, the catheter is threaded over the stylette into the artery, and the stylette is removed.

The Seldinger technique may also be used to achieve percutaneous arterial catheterization. A needle is used to pierce the artery, then a guidewire is threaded through the needle, well into the artery, and the needle is withdrawn. The catheter is then threaded over the guidewire into the artery. Once the catheter is properly positioned, it should be sutured into place.

If percutaneous entry into the artery fails, an arterial cut-down may be performed. The technique for arterial catheterization through direct cut-down is identical to that performed in the adult patient, so the reader is referred to Chapter 4 for further information.

Once the catheter is in the artery, it is irrigated gently with a syringe containing normal saline until the catheter is joined to the arterial monitoring system and transducer. Placement of a short T-connector between the catheter and the monitoring tubing (Fig. 11-9) may reduce movement of the catheter, and facilitate blood sampling (refer to the following section, Blood Sampling from Monitoring Lines). Use of this T-connector usually will not reduce the quality of the arterial waveform signal (Fig. 11-10), but the nurse should ensure that no dampening of the displayed arterial waveform occurs.

Maintenance

Catheter patency is improved if peripheral pediatric arterial catheters are flushed continuously, rather than intermittently.[32] Use of heparinized flush solution rather than nonheparinized solution will also prolong catheter patency; most commonly, 1 unit of heparin/ml concentration is used, although concentrations ranging from 0.25 to 5 units/ml have been reported.[4]

The arterial line should be flushed at a rate of 1 to 3 ml/hour, to prevent clot formation. Pediatric catheters should *not* be flushed using pressure bags and continuous flush devices—such devices will deliver an unknown quantity of fluid at a rapid rate when the flush valve is opened. Catheter irrigation should be accomplished using a volume-controlled infusion pump and noncompliant tubing. The

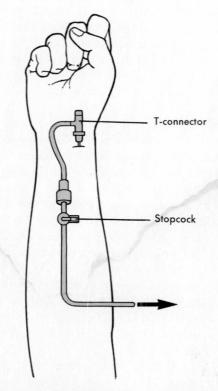

T-connector

Stopcock

Fig. 11-9. Arterial line infusion device with T-connector.

infusion fluid should be delivered through the valved continuous flush device (refer again to Fig. 11-7); the flush device will prevent dampening of the waveform signal by the continuous infusion.

If intermittent flushing of the pediatric arterial catheter and tubing is necessary (as a result of observed waveform dampening or blood back-up into the intravenous tubing), it should only be accomplished using gentle irrigation from a syringe. Rapid, forceful irrigation with a syringe or a flush device may result in retrograde flow of irrigant (and possibly air or thrombus) into the arch of the aorta and cerebral circulation. Such retrograde flow has been documented during irrigation of radial artery catheters in neonates, children, and adults.[3] All fluids used to flush the arterial line must be totalled and added to the child's hourly fluid intake.

Throughout the time the arterial catheter is in place, assessment of distal extremity perfusion and appearance of the catheter entry site must be performed and documented. Signs of distal limb ischemia include cooling, mottling, blanching, or cyanosis of the limb, or reduced arterial flow assessed by Doppler measurements. Such signs should be reported to a physician immediately, and removal of the catheter is usually necessary. If arterial spasm is suspected to be causing distal limb ischemia, a warm compress may be applied to the *contralateral* extremity, to induce reflex vasodilation (heat should *never* be applied to the ischemic extremity).

Bleeding at the catheterization site may occur during catheter insertion, or while the catheter is in place. The quantity of blood loss should be estimated on a

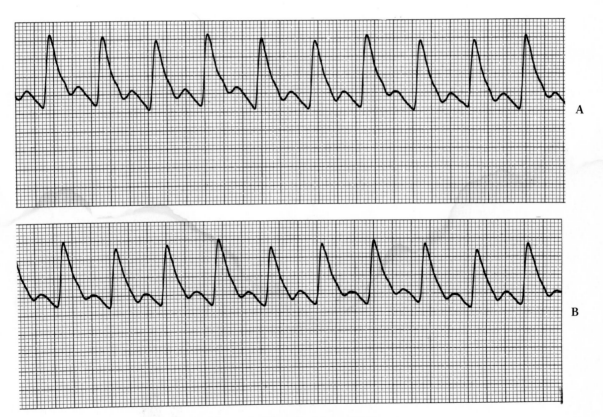

Fig. 11-10. Arterial waveform with (A) and without (B) T-connector.

regular basis, and blood replacement therapy discussed if blood loss is significant (see Table 11-3 for calculation of circulating blood volume).

While the catheter is in place, blood loss may occur if tubing connections separate. Luer-lock connections should always be used in monitoring systems, to prevent inadvertent tubing disconnection. Significant blood loss can occur as a result of only brief seconds of tubing separation—a 25-ml blood loss in a 3-kilogram infant is equivalent to a 12% hemorrhage. The monitor used to display digital arterial pressure and waveform should have a high- and low-pressure alarm. These alarms should be set to alert the clinician if the systolic or diastolic blood pressure falls by 10%—thus, an alarm will sound as soon as pressure loss occurs from a loose connection, before significant blood loss has occurred. The low-pressure alarm on the monitor should be active at all times—if the alarm is silenced during blood sampling or tubing changes, a temporary alarm silence option should be used; such temporary options will automatically reactivate the alarm within 90 seconds, and are much safer than options that may permanently disable the alarm. The catheterization site and all tubing connections should be visible at all times (never covered by blankets), so that tubing separation and blood loss will be readily visible.

The catheter insertion site should be dressed with sterile gauze and occlusive tape, or use of transparent, vapor-permeable occlusive film. Routine use of povidone-iodine ointment is not recommended, since it has not been shown to alter the incidence of catheter-related infection.[10,29] Throughout the catheterization period, the entrance site should be observed closely for evidence of inflammation, including: local tenderness, drainage, erythema, or warmth. The development of fever, leukocytosis, lymphangitis, and thrombocytopenia would strengthen the suspicion of infection or sepsis. The use of a transparent dressing will enable continuous observation of the catheter entrance site without the need for dressing changes.

Arterial line tubing and fluid are routinely changed every 48 hours. Although recent studies have documented that such frequent changing of tubing may not be necessary,[10] current Centers for Disease Control guidelines and published standards recommend the 48-hour tubing and fluid change[21] to reduce the incidence of system contamination and septicemia. Anytime the tubing or line is handled, aseptic technique must be employed.

Blood samping from arterial lines is reviewed in the following section, Blood Sampling from Indwelling Lines.

Complications

Distal extremity ischemia, infection, and bleeding are the most common complications reported after peripheral artery catheterization in infants and children. Presence of hypotension, need for administration of vasoactive agents, small patient size (less than 5 years) and prolonged (more than 4 to 6 days) catheterization time are consistent variables associated with increased risk of distal arterial occlusion and embolic complications.[30,33] Major ischemic/embolic complications are reported in approximately 1% to 3% of children requiring peripheral artery catheterization;[10,33] these include the loss of distal pulses, cooling and blanching of the extremity, and decreased capillary refill. Such complications should be detected quickly, and the catheter should be removed immediately. Embolic complications may require heparin therapy or surgical treatment. Minor reduction in distal limb blood flow may occur in as many as 57% of catheterized children.[24]

Catheter-related infection is most likely to develop in the pediatric patient if breaks in aseptic technique occur during catheter insertion or maintenance, if the catheter remains in place longer than 4 to 6 days, or if the patient has multiple invasive monitoring lines.[10,33] Infection should be suspected if local tenderness, drainage, or erythema are noted at the insertion site. In addition, infection should be suspected if the child develops fever, leukocytosis, thrombocytopenia, or lymphangitis. The septic neonate may demonstrate temperature instability.

Bleeding related to arterial catheterization in the child is most commonly caused by loose catheter connections. The catheterized extremity and the entire length of monitoring tubing should be visible at all times, and all connections should be luer-locked. At least hourly, every portion of the monitoring system should be closely inspected and palpated, so that kinks or loose connections will be detected immediately. If blood loss occurs as the result of catheterization or tubing separation, the quantity of blood loss should be estimated and considered as a percentage of the child's circulating blood volume—significant blood loss (more than 5% of circulating blood volume) must be reported to a physician immediately, and blood component therapy may be required.

Blood Sampling from Indwelling Lines

When blood is withdrawn from the pediatric patient for laboratory analysis, attempts must be made to minimize blood loss and fluid administration. Laboratory analysis must be performed rapidly, using "micro" techniques, so that blood sample volume is minimal (for example, arterial blood gas analysis should require no more than 0.3 to 0.5 ml of blood). Everyone who cares for the child should be aware of the minimal volume of blood required for each laboratory test and for typical combinations of tests (for example, the volume required for a CBC, electrolytes, and arterial blood gas is probably less than the sum of volumes required for each test). Minimal sample volumes should be posted in a prominent area in the unit; in some hospitals the director of laboratory services is asked to sign a copy of the notice, so that there will be no dispute about the sample volumes required. The total blood withdrawn for laboratory analysis should be totalled daily for any infant less than 6 months of age, and blood replacement should be contemplated if this volume approximates 5% to 7% of the child's circulating blood volume, or if the hematocrit is critically low.

Of course, all blood sampling must be performed using strict aseptic technique. Good handwashing is performed before and after each patient contact, and current CDC guidelines recommend use of gloves when handling blood products. Stopcock ports should be wiped with a povidone-iodine wipe whenever caps or syringes are added or removed; this will reduce the risk of contamination of the monitoring line.

During blood sampling, an adequate volume of discarded blood must be used to clear the sample tubing and stopcock of irrigant fluid, yet the child's actual blood loss for each sample should be limited to the sample volume itself (not the sample volume plus the discard volume). In many hospitals, the discarded blood is withdrawn from the sampling tubing into a syringe, then is reinfused into the patient after the blood sample is withdrawn. This practice is undesirable, because the discarded blood may begin to clot in the syringe, and may be mixed with bits of fibrin; reinfusion of this partially-clotted blood may result in thromboembolic phenomena.

The child should not receive an undetermined or large volume of irrigant fluid to clear the sample tubing of patient blood following the sampling procedure. Any net fluid administered following blood sampling must be added to the child's total hourly fluid intake. Excessive irrigant fluid administration may necessitate reduction of other sources of fluid intake, and may result in reduction of the volume of nutritional fluid administered to the child.

Use of the two-stopcock method for blood sampling first described by Cannon in 1985[5] allows blood sampling without significant patient blood loss, and without net fluid administration. This procedure has also been modified to allow blood sampling through the injection port of a T-connector. Both techniques are described below.

Blood sampling from a proximal and distal stopcock

The tubing and monitoring system should be constructed with two stopcocks; a proximal stopcock is positioned near the entrance of the catheter, and a distal stopcock is positioned adjacent to the transducer. The two stopcocks are separated by at least 6 inches of noncompliant tubing, or as much as 24 inches of tubing (Fig. 11-11, *A*). The greater the space between stopcocks, the larger the effective discard volume displaced during blood sampling.

1. Syringes are attached to both stopcocks, with the stopcocks turned off to the syringes (see Fig. 11-11). The syringe attached to the distal stopcock should contain exactly 2 ml of irrigation (flush) liquid (the fluid should be identical to that in the monitoring tubing).
2. The *distal* stopcock is turned off to the transducer, and irrigant fluid from the monitoring tubing is withdrawn into the distal syringe. This fluid aspiration will result in movement of patient blood into the monitoring tubing—this blood will act as the discard blood volume. It is extremely important that fluid be aspirated to draw blood toward but not *into* the distal stopcock—the distal stopcock and syringe should contain only irrigant fluid (Fig. 11-11, *B*).
3. The *proximal* stopcock is now turned off to the transducer. This will allow aspiration of blood from the patient into the proximal syringe. However, before sampling is performed, a small amount of blood (0.1 ml) should be withdrawn and discarded, and a second syringe is attached to the proximal stopcock for actual sampling of blood.
4. The blood sample is withdrawn into the proximal syringe (Fig. 11-11, *C*).
5. The proximal stopcock is turned off to the sampling port, and fluid from the distal syringe is used to flush patient blood back into the patient, and irrigation fluid back into the tubing. Gentle irrigation should be provided, and 2 ml of irrigant fluid should remain in the distal syringe at the end of the procedure (Fig. 11-11, *D*).
6. The proximal stopcock is turned off to the patient, and a small amount of the irrigant fluid in the distal syringe is used to flush out the sampling port of the proximal stopcock (Fig. 11-11, *E*).
7. When the sampling is complete, a sterile cap is placed on the sampling port of

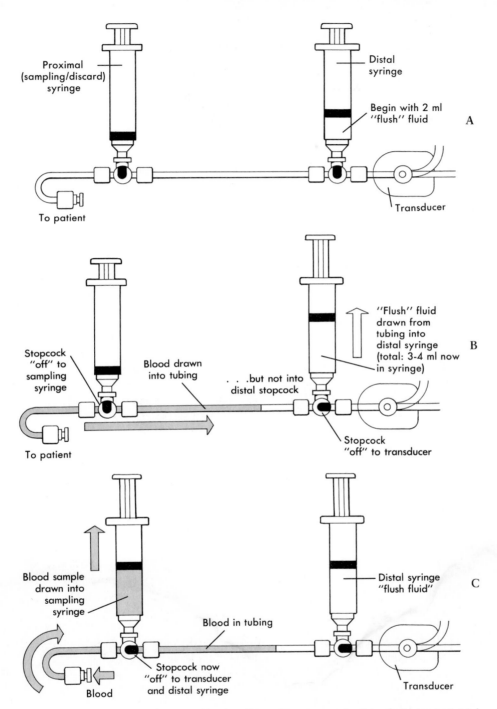

Fig. 11-11. Blood sampling from monitoring line using two-stopcock technique. **A,** Initial setup. Begin with 2 ml of irrigation (flush) fluid in distal syringe. **B,** Turn distal stopcock off to transducer, and aspirate until patient blood is drawn into monitoring tubing into distal syringe. **C,** Turn proximal stopcock off to transducer and distal syringe, and draw blood sample into syringe (after discarding initial 0.1 ml). *Continued.*

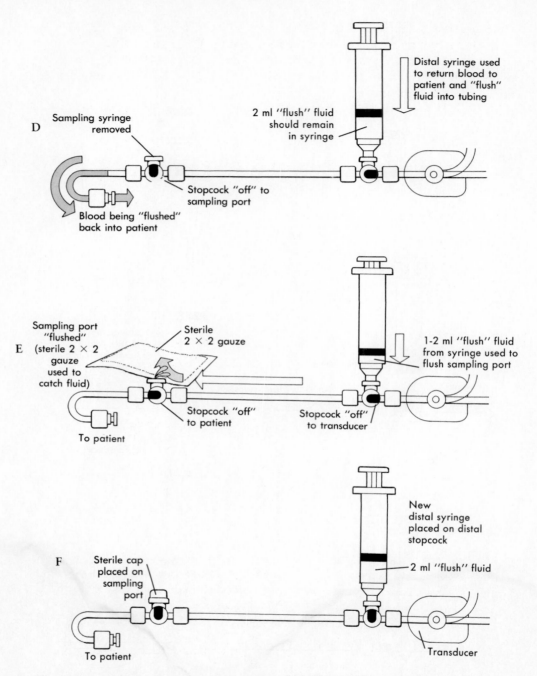

Fig. 11-11, cont'd. D, Turn proximal stopcock off to sampling port. Flush irrigation fluid from distal syringe into tubing and patient, until blood is cleared from monitoring tubing. 2 ml of fluid should remain in distal syringe. **E,** Turn proximal stopcock off to patient and use remaining fluid from distal syringe to irrigate sampling port. **F,** Turn proximal stopcock off to sampling port. Turn distal stopcock off to syringe. Waveform should be visible on monitor. Place sterile occlusive cap on sampling port of proximal stopcock and syringe containing 2 ml of irrigant on distal stopcock.

the proximal stopcock. A fresh syringe (containing exactly 2 ml of irrigant fluid) may be placed on the distal stopcock (Fig. 11-11, *F*).

The above sampling procedure results in patient blood loss equal to the sample volume plus 0.1 ml. No net fluid is administered to flush the monitoring line, if care is taken to begin and end the procedure (before flushing of the sampling port) with exactly the same volume of irrigation fluid.

Recently, a blood-drawing tubing system containing two sampling ports has become commercially available (LabSite, TM Migada Laboratories, marketed by Abbott Laboratories). The sampling ports replace stopcocks, and cumbersome manipulation of the stopcocks is avoided. Another modification of the two-stopcock blood drawing procedure uses a T-connector, described below.

Blood sampling using a T-connector

Sampling of blood from the injection port of the T-connector can be accomplished in two ways. In the first method, the T-connector is used just like the proximal stopcock of the two-stopcock technique described above. Blood is drawn past the T-connector, and toward but not into the distal stopcock—this blood will act as the discard volume. A small volume of blood is then drawn from the injector port of the T-connector and discarded; this blood clears irrigant fluid from the port of the T-connector. The blood sample is then drawn from the injection port of the T-connector, and the line is then flushed with irrigant fluid from the distal syringe (refer to procedure above for further details about the technique).

Blood sampling may also be accomplished through the injection port of the T-connector without use of a distal stopcock. This procedure is described in detail below.

1. Begin with the T-connector joined directly to the vascular catheter hub (Fig. 11-12, *A*). Wipe the T-connector injection port with a povidone-iodine wipe before insertion of any needles, to reduce the risk of contamination of the line.
2. Use the graduated clamp located on the T-connector tubing to clamp the tubing near the injection port. This will temporarily discontinue irrigation of the line. The volume-controlled infusion pump should continue fluid administration into the monitoring line; this will result in build-up of pressure into the monitoring line which will aid in flushing the line after sampling is completed.
3. Once the tubing is clamped, and the injection port is wiped with povidone-iodine solution, a 22-gauge needle is inserted (using aseptic technique) into the injection port. Four to six drops of patient blood should be allowed to flow out of the needle onto a sterile 2 × 2 or 4 × 4 piece of gauze (Fig. 11-12, *B*). This blood will act as the discard blood, and will passively clear the hub of the irrigation port of irrigation fluid.
4. Taking care to keep the needle in the same position in the injection port, attach a syringe to the needle, and allow the syringe to fill passively (Fig. 11-12, *C*). It may be necessary to aspirate gently to begin the flow of blood into the syringe, but forceful aspiration of arterial catheters should be avoided, since it is likely to produce arterial spasm. Use of a 3-ml syringe is preferable to use of smaller syringes, since the smaller syringes may result in more forceful aspiration (note that the sample volume should still be the smallest possible volume, regardless of the size of the sampling syringe).

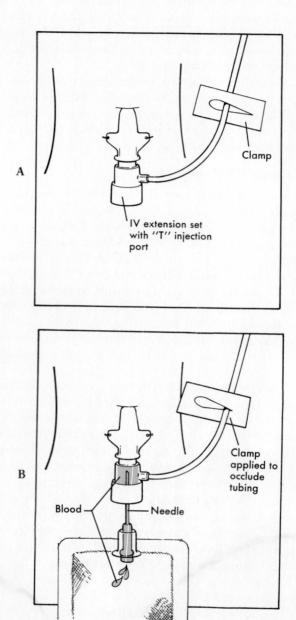

Fig. 11-12. Blood sampling from monitoring line using T-connector. **A,** Initial setup. **B,** Clamp tubing just distal to T-connector and insert needle into T-connector, allowing several drops of blood to drip onto sterile gauze pad.

Continued.

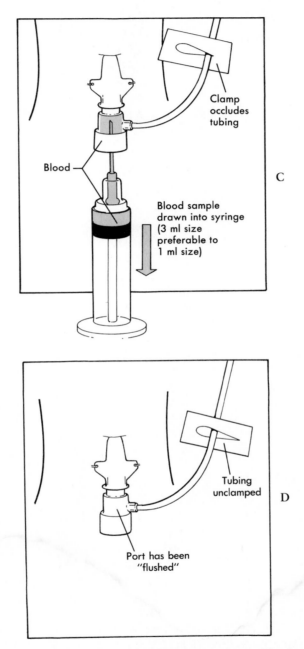

Fig. 11-12, cont'd. C, Attach syringe to needle, and gently aspirate blood sample. **D,** Withdraw syringe and needle from T-connector and unclamp tubing. Blood should be flushed from tubing.

5. Once the sample is drawn, the syringe and needle are removed from the injection port. The tubing is unclamped, and the pressure that has developed in the tubing system during the sampling procedure should be sufficient to flush patient blood from the T-connector and tubing (Fig. 11-12, D).

   Use of the T-connector for sampling in the above manner results in a loss of patient blood equal to the sample volume plus approximately 0.3 to 0.4 ml. There is no net fluid administration required to irrigate the tubing. However, blood will eventually accumulate in the sampling port—this blood will increase the risk of bacterial growth in the system, and may result in reduction of the quality of waveform transmission. It is important to change the T-connector whenever blood accumulation is observed.

Flow-Directed Balloon-Tipped Pulmonary Artery Catheterization

The assessment and manipulation of cardiac output is discussed very thoroughly in Chapter 7. This section is designed to summarize essential aspects of the use of flow-directed balloon-tipped pulmonary artery catheters and thermodilution cardiac output measurements in children, with particular reference to techniques and typical errors in measurements and derived calculations.

Indications

The flow-directed, balloon-tipped pulmonary artery catheter is used to measure pulmonary artery and pulmonary artery wedge pressures. If the catheter is wedged in an appropriate segment of the lung, and if no pulmonary venous obstruction is present, pulmonary artery wedge pressure will approximate left atrial pressure. In the absence of mitral valve disease, left atrial pressure will equal left ventricular end-diastolic pressure (LVEDP). Measurement of pulmonary artery pressure (PAP) is useful in the treatment of the child with pulmonary hypertension, and estimation of LVEDP will be helpful in the management of the child with suspected left ventricular dysfunction. Under these conditions, right ventricular end-diastolic pressure (and right atrial and central venous pressures) cannot be expected to resemble LVEDP.

In general, when the use of the pulmonary artery catheter is indicated, a pulmonary artery catheter which contains a thermistor bead is used, so that thermodilution cardiac ouput calculations may also be made from the same catheter. In older children, a fiberoptic pulmonary artery catheter may be inserted, to allow continuous display of the mixed venous (pulmonary artery) oxygen saturation ($S\bar{v}O_2$); $S\bar{v}O_2$ will generally trend directly with the child's cardiac output.

Indications for the use of the thermodilution balloon-tipped pulmonary artery catheter in children are as follows:
1. Shock unresponsive to volume therapy and short-term inotropic support
2. Septic shock with low cardiac output (since myocardial dysfunction can play such an important role in patient deterioration)
3. Anytime precise tracking of hemodynamic parameters is required (for example, during treatment with a drug that may produce myocardial depression, or use of new antiarrhythmic or vasoactive drugs, or during treatment of a child with severe cardiovascular instability)
4. Postoperative monitoring in the unstable patient

5. Anytime precise tracking of oxygen transport (Arterial oxygen content × Cardiac output) is required (for example, in manipulation of PEEP in the treatment of severe respiratory failure)
6. The catheter may also be used in the treatment of the child with severe pulmonary hypertension. However, some physicians consider the risks of using the catheter in these patients greater than the potential benefits.

Contraindications to pulmonary artery catheterization

In general, this catheter should be inserted only when the information it will yield is expected to influence therapy. Additional contraindications for use in children include:

1. Presence of large intracardiac shunts—the pulmonary artery catheter may inadvertently pass into the left side of the heart, and the balloon could wedge in the mitral or aortic valve, resulting in severe drop in cardiac output and cerebral perfusion.
2. Presence of serious dysrhythmias—malignant arrhythmias may develop during catheter passage through the right ventricle
3. Presence of severe coagulopathies—bleeding at the insertion site may be impossible to control
4. Presence of a very low cardiac output—the balloon may fail to float out of the right ventricle if cardiac output is extremely low
5. Anytime the potential risks of the procedure outweigh the potential benefits

Insertion

The pulmonary artery catheter is inserted into a large vein, most commonly the right internal jugular vein, the left subclavian vein, or the right femoral vein. The right internal jugular venous approach may be favored because it does not introduce the risk of pneumothorax; however, if bleeding occurs at this site, it is very difficult to control. This approach should not be used if increased intracranial pressure is present, because the catheter may obstruct cerebral venous return.

The left subclavian venous approach is preferred over the right subclavian venous approach, because the curve of the vein toward the superior vena cava facilitates catheter entry into the right atrium and right ventricle. The right subclavian venous approach may be used, however, if the left subclavian vein has already been used for venous access. The femoral venous approach is most often used in infants, since the catheter may not be long enough to float into the pulmonary artery if this approach is used in older patients.

If the child weighs less than 15 to 18 kg, a 5-French catheter is used, and if the child weighs more than 15 to 18 kg, a 7-French catheter is used. A 5-French catheter will be inserted through a 6.0-French introducer, and a 7-French catheter will be inserted through an 8.5 French introducer sheath.

The 5-French catheter contains smaller lumens, which may readily become occluded by fibrin material, so this catheter will require scrupulous attention to lumen irrigation. In addition, the thermal injection lumen of the 5-French catheter is very small, and provides a great deal of resistance to rapid injection of the thermal indicator, so excellent injection technique will be required for cardiac output determinations. Finally, insertion and proper placement of small catheters may take a long time (much longer than insertion of 7-French catheters in adult patients).

Strict sterile technique must be maintained during catheter insertion. Absolute aseptic technique is then maintained during manipulation of the catheter monitoring system. The procedure should be explained simply (as age-appropriate) to the child and informed consent obtained from the parents. If possible, the child should be premedicated with an analgesic before the procedure, and appropriate restraints should be applied. The placement technique is summarized in the following discussion.

1. Set up the pulmonary artery pressure monitoring system, and flush the transducer and all tubing. Zero and mechanically calibrate the transducer (refer again to the box on p. 263), and zero and electronically calibrate the monitor digital display and waveform. The waveform scale should be set at 0 to 30 or 0 to 60 during catheter insertion and preparations made to obtain a paper printout of the chamber waveforms and pulmonary artery wedge waveform. The printout should also be calibrated.

2. The catheter entrance site is scrubbed with a povidone-iodine solution and draped. A 1% xylocaine solution is injected into the subcutaneous tissue surrounding the insertion site. If the neck veins are used, the child will be placed in a Trendelenburg position, to reduce the possibility of air entry into the right atrium.

3. A needle is used to enter the desired central vein (refer to the previous section, Central Venous Pressure Monitoring, for further information about catheterization of specific veins), and the Seldinger technique is used to thread a guidewire into the large vein.

4. Once the guidewire is in place, a catheter introducer sheath is threaded over the guidewire and into the large vein, and the sheath is sutured in place. This sheath will facilitate entry of the pulmonary artery catheter into the large vein, and will also serve as an additional fluid administration port. Most introducer kits include a sterile, transparent sleeve that can be attached to the sheath; when the catheter is threaded through the sleeve into the sheath, it can be advanced and withdrawn without compromising its sterility (please refer to Chapter 5 for an illustration of the PA catheter, introducer sheath, and sterile sleeve).

5. Once the catheter introducer sheath and sleeve are in place, the pulmonary artery catheter is prepared for insertion. Each lumen of the pulmonary artery catheter is flushed with normal saline, and the proximal end of the pulmonary artery lumen is connected to the pulmonary artery pressure monitoring system, so that a digital display and waveform can be seen on the monitor.

6. The transducer of the system is placed at the level of the right atrium, and the tip of the catheter is held within the sterile field at the same height as the transducer and the patient's right atrium. The pressure reading from the transducer should be zero at this time. The tip of the catheter is then elevated 27 cm above the zero-reference point, and the pressure reading should be 20 mm Hg. If accurate readings are not obtained, the transducer and monitoring system should be checked.

7. The catheter balloon is inflated in a sterile container of normal saline or wa-

ter—if bubbles are visible, or the balloon fails to inflate, a new catheter should be obtained (and steps 5 and 6 are repeated). Carbon dioxide is the preferred gas for balloon inflation, because it is easily dispersed in the blood should balloon rupture occur. However, because this gas is not readily available in the clinical setting, air may be used to inflate the balloon. The maximum balloon inflation volume is printed on the catheter, and should be written on the nursing Kardex.

8. If the catheter will be used for thermodilution cardiac output measurements, the thermistor connector cable from the cardiac output computer (or from the monitor, if cardiac output calculations will be performed by the bedside monitor) should be connected to the thermistor hub of the catheter. The cardiac output computer or monitor should be turned on. If the thermistor is faulty, this will be indicated by the computer or monitor, and a new catheter should be obtained (and steps 5 and 6 repeated).

9. While monitoring the pressure waveform obtained through the pulmonary artery port, one threads the catheter into the introducer sheath. Once a venous waveform is displayed, the balloon may be inflated to half its normal inflation volume. The catheter is then advanced until it reaches the right atrium. Some physicians prefer to leave the balloon deflated until the catheter is clearly in the right atrium. Once the catheter is in the right atrium and a typical right atrial waveform is achieved (Fig. 11-13, A), the balloon is completely inflated with the recommended volume.

10. The catheter is then advanced as the balloon floats into the right ventricle and pulmonary artery, as illustrated by the appearance of appropriate waveforms (Fig. 11-13, B and C). During passage of the catheter through the right ventricle, everyone at the bedside should monitor the patient's electrocardiogram for evidence of premature ventricular contractions. If these develop, treatment with 1 mg/kg of xylocaine may be necessary.

11. Once a characteristic pulmonary artery wedge waveform is visualized (Fig. 11-13, D), advancement of the catheter should stop. The balloon is deflated, and a pulmonary artery waveform should appear. The balloon is again inflated, and the wedge waveform should again become apparent. If the wedge waveform occurs only intermittently during balloon inflation, it may be necessary to advance the catheter 1 to 2 cm further.

12. Once the catheter is thought to be in place, the length of catheter insertion is noted on the nursing Kardex and in the patient chart, and the catheter is taped securely to the transparent sleeve, where the catheter enters the sleeve. Note that it is not possible to suture the catheter to the sleeve, so caution must be taken to avoid any tension on the catheter or tubing.

13. Radiographic confirmation of proper catheter placement will be necessary.

14. The right atrial port should be joined to a fluid infusion and monitoring system. It is possible to join the right atrial and the pulmonary artery port to the same monitoring line, so both pressures can be monitored using a single transducer (with the turning of a stopcock). Use of a piece of noncompliant tubing with male-to-male connections will be helpful.

15. If thermodilution cardiac output calculations will be performed, the proximal right atrial port should be joined to the injection syringe and injection system.

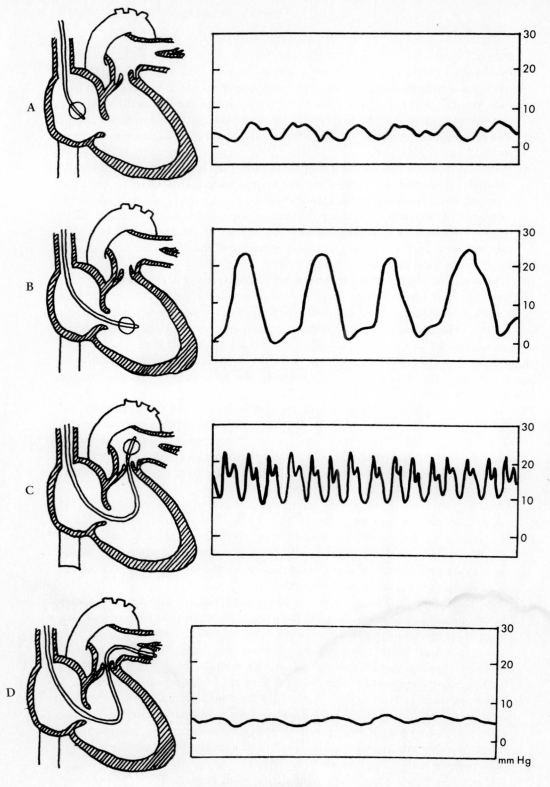

Fig 11-13. For legend see opposite page.

If a second right atrial port is present, it should be joined to a fluid infusion system.

16. If a fiberoptic pulmonary artery catheter has been inserted, the fiberoptic port must be joined to the optical module (which contains the light-emitting diodes) and the microprocessor (which continuously displays the mixed venous saturation in a fashion similar to that displayed by the pulse oximeter). If the patient's length and weight are entered into the microprocessor, the patient's expected cardiac output is displayed. The mixed venous oxygen saturation is normally approximately 75%, and a fall in this saturation usually indicates a fall in oxygen transport (as a result of a fall in arterial oxygen content, cardiac output, or both).

17. Pulmonary artery and pulmonary artery wedge waveforms should be recorded on graphic paper, and patient end-expiration should be marked. Both pressure measurements should be taken from the graph paper at end-expiration.

Maintenance

Care must be taken to ensure that the transducer and monitoring system are appropriately leveled and calibrated, and are free of air or kinks. Small, disposable transducers may be taped at the phlebostatic axis. The transducer and monitor should be zeroed to air at least once every shift, and whenever there is a change in patient or transducer position. The transducer should be mechanically calibrated (see box on p. 263) once every day. Irrigation fluid and intravenous tubing should be changed using aseptic technique every 48 to 72 hours.[34]

The pulmonary artery waveform should be displayed at all times, so that spontaneous wedging of the balloon or catheter movement into the right ventricle will be immediately detected. If such wedging or movement occurs, a physician should be contacted immediately, and the catheter should be repositioned. High- and low-pressure alarms should be set carefully so that spontaneous wedging or tubing disconnection (and resultant fall in pulmonary artery pressure) or change in patient condition will immediately trigger an audible alarm.

The pulmonary artery lumen should be flushed continuously with 1 to 3 ml/hr of heparinized normal saline (1 unit of heparin/ml is standard), and all fluids administered through the catheter should be added to the child's hourly fluid intake totals. Since the pulmonary artery lumen is very small, it can easily become occluded by fibrin, clots, or crystals from intravenous solutions. For this reason, this lumen should be used for pressure measurements only, and should *not* be used for infusion of antibiotics or drugs. It may be used as a lumen of last resort for vasoactive drug infusion.

Mixed venous blood samples from the pulmonary artery may be drawn through the pulmonary artery port, but such sampling may lead to the develop-

---

Fig. 11-13. Characteristic waveforms during insertion of PA catheter. **A,** RA position and waveform (normal mean pressure is 0 to 5 mm Hg). **B,** Right ventricular position and waveform insertion (normal pressure is approximately 30/5 mm Hg). **C,** Pulmonary artery position and waveform (normal pressure is approximately 30/15 mm Hg). **D,** Pulmonary artery wedge position and waveform (normal mean pressure 4 to 8 mm Hg).

ment of clot occlusion of the lumen. If blood sampling is performed, the catheter should be irrigated several times after the sampling is performed.

Pulmonary artery (PA) and wedge (PAW) pressure measurements

Pulmonary artery pressure measurements should only be performed if the transducer is appropriately zeroed, leveled, and mechanically calibrated. The measurement should *not* be taken from the digital display on the bedside monitor, since the display represents the average pressure over a several-second sampling period. Instead, the pulmonary artery and pulmonary artery wedge pressures should be derived from a graphic printout of the waveforms. Inspiration and expiration should be marked on the waveform, and the pressures at end-expiration should be calculated. A graphic printout of the pulmonary artery waveform should be added to the patient chart every 8 hours to document appropriate catheter placement and catheter patency.

When wedge pressure measurements are performed, the balloon should be inflated with the minimal volume necessary to wedge the catheter. The catheter should be left in the wedge position only long enough to obtain a graphic printout of the wedge waveform. The balloon should never be inflated with a larger volume than that recommended by the catheter manufacturer.

If pulmonary vascular resistance is normal, pulmonary artery end-diastolic pressure will equal pulmonary artery (mean) wedge pressure. If pulmonary artery end-diastolic pressure is significantly higher than pulmonary artery wedge pressure at end-expiration, pulmonary vascular resistance must be elevated (Fig. 11-14).

If pulmonary artery wedge pressure is to accurately reflect left atrial pressure (and LVEDP), there must be patent, fluid-filled, vasculature between the tip of the catheter and the left atrium. Therefore, accurate wedge pressure measurements require that the catheter be wedged in a zone III pulmonary artery (posterior, inferior portion of the lung, below the level of the left atrium). In this area of the lung,

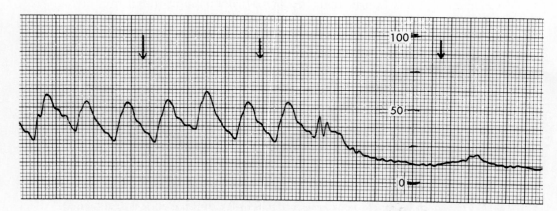

Fig. 11-14. Relationship between pulmonary artery end-diastolic pressure and pulmonary artery wedge pressure when PVR is elevated. Pulmonary artery end-diastolic pressure is 27 mm Hg and pulmonary artery wedge pressure is 12.5 mm Hg. All pressures are recorded only at end-expiration (*arrows*).

pulmonary artery and venous pressures are nearly always greater than alveolar pressure, so the vessels will remain patent even during positive pressure ventilation. Thus, pulmonary artery wedge pressure will accurately reflect pulmonary venous, left atrial, and left ventricular end-diastolic pressure. Placement of the catheter in a zone III artery will result in minimal wedge pressure variation during positive pressure inspiration and expiration (Fig. 11-15, A).[35]

If the pulmonary artery catheter is wedged in a zone I or zone II artery (at the apex or center of the lung, above the level of the left atrium), the pulmonary capillaries and small arteries and veins may be compressed during positive-pressure inspiration. In these portions of the lung, the wedge pressure will not accurately reflect left atrial pressure (and LVEDP), and significant variation in the wedge pressure will be observed during the respiratory cycle (Fig. 11-15, B).[25,35]

Normal pulmonary artery pressure (PAP) in children is 30/8 mm Hg. Pulmonary artery pressure is elevated with some forms of congenital heart disease resulting in increased pulmonary blood flow. PAP is also elevated in children with pulmonary hypoplasia, primary pulmonary hypertension, pulmonary hypertension

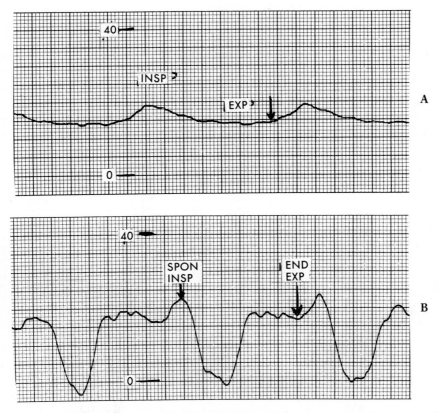

Fig. 11-15. Variations in accuracy of pulmonary artery wedge pressure measurements with changes in catheter tip location. **A,** Zone III wedge pressure. Note minimal difference during respiratory cycle. End-expiratory pressure is 14 mm Hg. **B,** Zone II wedge pressure. Note wide inspiratory and expiratory excursion. End-expiratory wedge pressure is 17 mm Hg, but the wedge pressure varies from −3 to 20 mm Hg during the respiratory cycle.

secondary to cardiac or pulmonary disease, or pulmonary venous obstruction. In addition, PAP may be increased by alveolar hypoxia, acidosis, hypothermia, and agitation in neonates, infants, and children with reactive pulmonary vascular beds. PAP may also be elevated if the pulmonary artery wedge pressure is significantly elevated.

Normal pulmonary artery wedge (PAW) pressure in the child is 4 to 8 mm Hg. PAW will be elevated in children with obstruction to pulmonary venous return (such as total anomalous pulmonary venous return with obstruction, or pulmonary venous constriction), mitral stenosis or insufficiency, or left ventricular failure.

Errors in pulmonary artery pressure measurement may occur as the result of problems in the monitoring system and transducer (refer, again, to the box on p. 264). Causes of errors in pulmonary artery wedge pressure measurements are listed in the box below, and include improper leveling or calibration of transducer, respiratory artifact, catheter obstruction, or catheter migration.[25]

Complications

Complications of pulmonary artery catheterization in children consist of those related to catheter insertion, and those related to the continued presence of the catheter in the pulmonary artery. Complications of placement include bleeding at the site, pneumothorax (particularly if the subclavian approach is used), and arrhythmias (as the catheter passes through the right ventricle).

Complete obstruction of the right ventricular outflow tract during balloon passage through the pulmonary valve has been reported in a child with severe pulmonary valvular stenosis; the catheter was withdrawn without incident. Knotting of the catheter in the right ventricle may occur if frequent, prolonged attempts are required to float the balloon into the pulmonary artery. If knotting occurs, attempts to withdraw the catheter gently should be made, but surgical removal of the catheter may be necessary.

Once the catheter is in place, complications include pulmonary infarctions, pulmonary artery rupture, thromboembolic events, and infection. Pulmonary infarctions are thought to result from occlusion of blood flow to a lung segment as the result of prolonged balloon inflation or migration and spontaneous wedging of the catheter itself. This complication will result in hypoxemia, the development of an infiltrate on chest radiograph, and possible hemoptysis. It should be prevented if

---

Typical errors in pediatric pulmonary wedge pressure measurements

Faulty monitoring system (noncalibrated transducer, air)
Transducer inappropriately leveled
Respiratory artifact (obtain wedge pressuremeasurement from graphic printout at end-expiration)
Catheter tip in zone I or zone II artery
Failure to wedge or overwedging
Obstructed catheter

the pulmonary artery waveform is displayed and observed continuously, and balloon inflation time is reduced to a minimum.

Pulmonary artery rupture has been reported in adults, rather than in pediatric patients. This complication is more likely to occur in older patients with pulmonary hypertension (and friable pulmonary artery tissue), and those with coagulopathies.

Thromboembolic phenomena and septic complications are more likely to develop if the patient is septic when the catheter is inserted, if the catheter is manipulated (repositioned) many times, if the catheter remains in place longer than 72 hours, if the catheter is inserted without complete sterile technique, or if breaks in aseptic technique occur during catheter care. Sepsis should be suspected if the child develops fever, leukopenia, leukocytosis, thrombocytopenia or other signs of disseminated intravascular coagulation (DIC). Use of teflon-coated pulmonary artery catheters has reduced the development of thrombocytopenia related to platelet-coating of the catheter, so that a significant fall in the child's platelet count (a decrease of more than 25,000) may indicate development of sepsis.

The catheter should be removed after 72 hours to minimize risk of contamination. If PA or PAW measurements or CO calculations are still necessary beyond 72 hours, a new catheter may be inserted at the same or another site.

Cardiac output determinations

Although there are several methods of determining cardiac output in the critically ill child, use of the thermodilution method with injection into a pulmonary artery catheter is the most common. This is the only method of cardiac output determination which will be reviewed here; for further information on indicator-dilution cardiac output calculations, and the Fick equation, the reader is referred to a thorough presentation in Chapter 7.

When a thermodilution cardiac output calculation is made, a small, known quantity of thermal indicator (iced or room temperature dextrose and water) is injected into the right atrium. This fluid will, in effect, function as a thermal indicator. As the injected fluid passes through the right ventricle, it mixes with the (body temperature) blood ejected by the right ventricle, and cools the blood. A thermistor located in the pulmonary artery portion of the catheter measures the temperature change in the pulmonary artery from body temperature to cooler temperature, and then back to body temperature. The computer plots the change in blood temperature over time, and integrates the data to calculate the area beneath the time-temperature change curve.

The area under the time-temperature curve will be inversely proportional to the flow rate of blood, or the cardiac output. Thus if the child's cardiac output is high, flow through the right ventricle and pulmonary artery is rapid, and only a small, brief temperature change will be produced by the cool injectate; so high cardiac output is associated with a small area under the time-temperature curve. Anything that artificially reduces the magnitude of the temperature change in the pulmonary artery will result in falsely high cardiac output calculations.

If, on the other hand, the child's cardiac output is low, flow through the right ventricle and pulmonary artery will be slow, and the temperature change produced by the cool injectate will be significant and it will persist for a long period of time;

thus low cardiac output is associated with a large area under the time-temperature curve. Anything that artificially increases the magnitude of the temperature change in the pulmonary artery will result in falsely low cardiac output calculations.

The major differences between thermodilution cardiac output measurements in the child and similar measurements in adults relate to the volume of the injectate, and to small pediatric cardiac outputs. The child will not be able to tolerate multiple, large-volume injections; as a result, smaller injectate volumes are used. Since small injectate volumes produce a small temperature change, use of iced injectate is recommended to increase the temperature change in the child's pulmonary artery. This increase in signal size will reduce the significance of minor errors in injection.

The small cardiac output of the child may mean that *small errors in injection technique will result in relatively significant errors in cardiac output calculations.* As a result, it is imperative that the technique for cardiac output calculation be standardized, so that error may be eliminated or standardized.

When cardiac output calculations are to be performed, the appropriate *equipment* must be assembled. The pulmonary artery catheter is in place, and monitoring systems are joined to the right atrial and pulmonary artery ports of the catheter. Multiple stopcocks will be used to join the cardiac output injection syringe and temperature probe to the proximal injectate port or hub of the catheter (Fig. 11-16).

The following equipment must be assembled to enable cardiac output calculations by thermodilution:

1. Closed injection system with cooling coils—this system is preferred over use of syringes to more carefully standardize injectate temperature and to reduce the risk of infection.
2. Sterile injectate solution (5% dextrose or normal saline). Prime the closed injection system tubing and cooling coil with this injectate solution as soon as possible.
3. Cooling container—fill this container with iced water and submerge the (primed) cooling coil in the iced water as soon as possible—this will ensure that cooled injectate will be prepared when you are ready to perform cardiac output determinations (cooling will take approximately 20 to 30 minutes).
4. Cardiac output computer or monitor cartridge, with temperature probe, thermistor/catheter connector, and recorder.
5. Two luer-lock stopcocks
6. One large (35 ml) luer-lock syringe

Once the equipment is assembled, and the injectate fluid is cooling in the cooling container, the insulated injection syringe is joined by stopcock to the proximal injection (right atrial) port of the pulmonary artery catheter. The computer temperature probe is clipped to the housing between the injection syringe and the stopcock. This will allow measurement of injectate temperature with every injection.

A 35-ml waste syringe should be joined by stopcock to the injection system. This will allow collection of the initial test injections into a syringe, and will reduce fluid administration to the child during the procedure (refer again to Fig. 11-16).

When all equipment is prepared, the cardiac output computer is plugged in and turned on. The computer should be joined by cable to a strip chart recorder. The recorder should also be turned on, and the recorder paper speed set at 5 mm/sec.

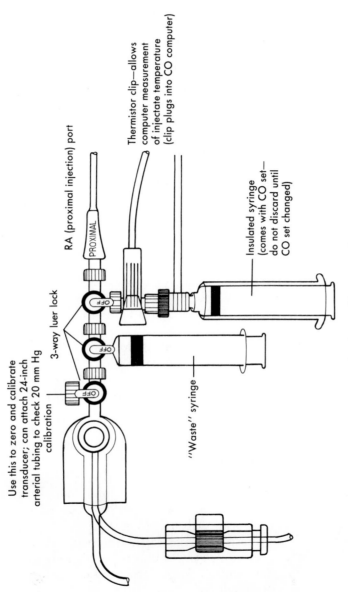

Use this to zero and calibrate transducer; can attach 24-inch arterial tubing to check 20 mm Hg calibration

3-way luer lock

RA (proximal injection) port

PROXIMAL

Thermistor clip—allows computer measurement of injectate temperature (clip plugs into CO computer)

Insulated syringe (comes with CO set— do not discard until CO set changed)

"Waste" syringe

Fig. 11-16. Set up for thermodilution cardiac output injections.

It is important that the technique of cardiac output injections be standardized—everyone in the unit should perform the injections in the same manner, so that most potential error is eliminated, and remaining error is standardized. This will increase the value of the cardiac output measurements for evaluating patient condition over several hours or days.

To perform the thermodilution cardiac output measurement:

1. Check the patient's pulmonary artery waveform to ensure that the catheter remains in the pulmonary artery.

2. Set the appropriate computer calibration (or computation) constant. This number varies with the size of the catheter and the volume and temperature of the injectate. It is essential that this constant be set accurately, and *appropriate constant setting should be verified before any cardiac output determination.* This constant allows for the loss of some of the thermal indicator as it passes through the catheter external to the body (which is at room temperature) and within the body (at body temperature). Iced injections of 3 ml are usually used for pediatric cardiac output determinations. In the adolescent, 5 ml iced injections may be used (with appropriate change in calibration constant.)

3. When the monitor or computer is adequately warmed up, push the "Injectate Temperature" button, so that the injectate temperature will be displayed.

4. Turn the injection syringe off to the patient, and open to the waste syringe (turn the stopcock on the waste syringe off to the transducer and open to the injection syringe—see Fig. 11-16). Aspirate the exact appropriate injectate volume into the insulated syringe, then quickly inject it past the temperature probe, into the waste syringe.

5. Once the injectate temperature is less than 10 degrees centigrade, cardiac output determination may be performed. Note that the closed injection system and coils will contain only approximately 20 to 25 ml of cold fluid; if this fluid is wasted in documenting the injectate temperature, room temperature fluid will be drawn rapidly through the coils and into the syringe during cardiac output injections. Try to ensure that the injectate fluid is cooled sufficiently before CO determinations are required.

6. Turn the waste syringe stopcock off to the waste syringe. Turn the injection syringe stopcock off to the transducer and monitoring system and open to the proximal right atrial injection port.

7. Switch the computer or monitor control to cardiac output. If possible, temporarily interrupt any large-volume fluid infusions into the right atrium (via the introducer sheath or another right atrial port).

8. When the computer or monitor flashes "Ready," carefully aspirate exactly 3 ml (or 5 ml in the adolescent) into the injection syringe.

9. Depress the start button on the computer, monitor, or remote foot pedal, and quickly inject the 3 ml into the proximal right atrial injection port (within 3 to 4 seconds) during patient end-expiration.

10. Within seconds, the patient's cardiac output will be displayed, and graphic representation of the pulmonary artery time-temperature change curve will be made by the strip chart recorder.

11. Repeat steps 7, 8, and 9 two more times, for a total of three injections. Each injection should be performed during patient end-expiration. Inspect the injection curves, to ensure that all injections were uniform in speed, and that simi-

lar time-temperature curves resulted (Fig. 11-17, *A*). If there is significant variation in injection curves, perform a fourth injection.

12. To determine the child's cardiac output, look at the results of the three injections. Discard the first injection (since a large portion of the cold injectate filled the lumen of the catheter, this first injection will produce a falsely high cardiac output calculation), and average the second and third injection results as long as they do not vary by more than 10%.

13. To determine the child's cardiac index, divide the resulting cardiac output by the child's body surface area. Normal cardiac index in the child is approximately 3.5 to 4.5 L/min/m^2 body surface area. Note that the computer calibration constant may be adjusted so that a cardiac index (rather than a cardiac output) result is displayed after injections, but such changes in standard constants may be confusing—therefore, it is probably easier to ensure that everyone check the posted manufacturer's recommended calibration constants and determine the child's cardiac index later.

Because the child's cardiac output is small, small sources of error may produce significant errors in cardiac output calculations. Typical sources of error are summarized in the box below. In general, anything that artificially reduces the magnitude of the temperature change in the pulmonary artery will result in erroneously high cardiac output results. Warming of the injectate (by, for example, a hand wrapped around the injection syringe), excess tubing dead space between the injection syringe and the injection port, loss of some injectate (caused by tubing, syringe, or stopcock separation during the injection), or an inaccurately high calibration constant are examples of such error. If the child is receiving a large volume of room temperature fluid into the catheter introducer sheath (or another right atrial port), this fluid can reduce the change in the pulmonary artery temperature caused by the iced injectate, and will result in falsely high cardiac output calculations—if possible, the fluid infusion should be briefly interrupted during injections.

Anything that artificially increases the magnitude of the temperature change in the pulmonary artery will result in erroneously low cardiac output calculations. If, for example, the computer calibration constant is set for a 3 ml injection, and a 3.5

Typical errors in pediatric thermodilution cardiac output calculations

Inaccurate computer calibration constant
Inappropriate injectate volume/temperature
   Falsely high cardiac output calculations will result from:
      Inaccurately small injectate volume
      Tubing dead space between injectate syringe and right atrial port
      Warming of injectate temperature before injection
      Large volume right atrial or catheter introducer sheath infusions (at room
         temperature)
   Falsely low cardiac output calculations will result from:
      Inaccurately large injectate volume
      Iced injectate with calibration constant set for room temperature injectate
Poor injection technique
Computer or catheter malfunction

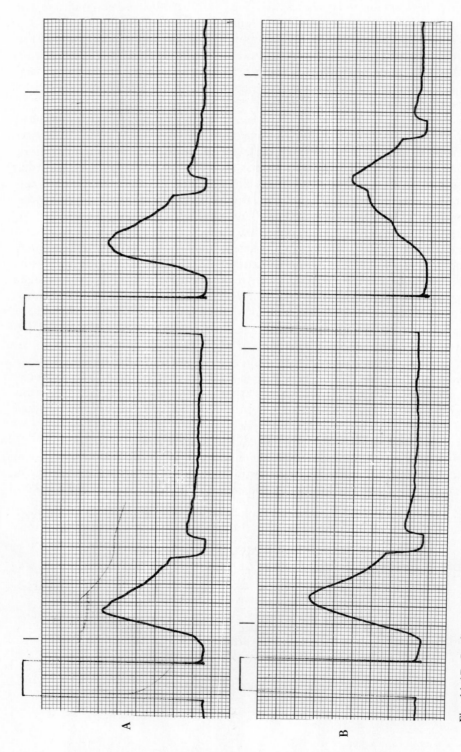

Fig. 11-17. Cardiac output injection curves. **A**, Identical curves consistent with good injection technique. **B**, Inconsistent injection technique (second injection is uneven and too slow).

Continued.

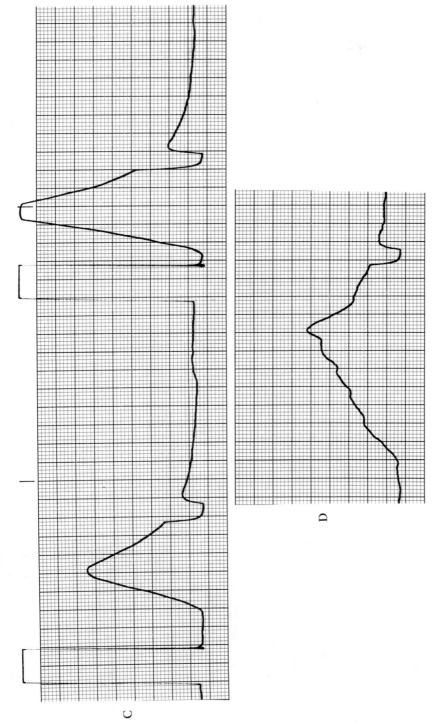

Fig. 11-17, cont'd. C, Inconsistent injection volume (second injection used 5 ml instead of 3 ml, and produced a falsely low cardiac output calculation). **D,** Excessively slow and uneven injection.

ml or 5 ml injection is performed, an inaccurately low cardiac output calculation will result. If iced injectate is used, and the calibration constant is appropriate for room temperature injections, the cardiac output calculation will be falsely low.

If the injection curves are inspected, they should be identical in height and configuration (see Fig. 11-17, *A*). Changes in curve configuration from injection to injection or from clinician to clinician indicates lack of standardization or error in injection technique (Fig. 11-17, *B*).

Slow or uneven injection technique will also produce error in cardiac output determinations. The computer or monitor will record the temperature change only after the start button or foot pedal is depressed; therefore, false calculations can result if the injection begins before the computer begins recording (Fig. 11-17, *C*). Slow injection will usually result in inaccurate cardiac output determinations—injections should take no longer than 4 seconds, and the curve should be no wider than 4 to 5 seconds.

Continuous monitoring of mixed venous oxygen tensions

Mixed venous oxygen saturation ($S\bar{v}o_2$) is the percentage of hemoglobin that is saturated with oxygen in a well-mixed systemic venous blood sample. The most accurate mixed venous oxygen saturation is obtained in the pulmonary artery, since superior and inferior vena caval blood is well-mixed in the pulmonary artery.

Fiberoptic catheters are now available in sizes as small as 4-French. When a fiberoptic catheter is placed in the child's pulmonary artery, and the catheter is joined to a microprocessor, a continuous display of the child's $S\bar{v}o_2$ can be obtained in a manner similar to that employed during pulse oximetry. Normal $S\bar{v}o_2$ is approximately 75%.

The $S\bar{v}o_2$ is influenced by arterial oxygen saturation, cardiac output, and tissue oxygen consumption; generally there is a direct relationship between changes in $S\bar{v}o_2$ and CO. However, $S\bar{v}o_2$ will also fall if the patient develops significant hypoxemia, such as may be observed in the child with severe respiratory disease or cyanotic heart disease. The $S\bar{v}o_2$ will rise when cardiac output rises, but it may also increase in the presence of sepsis (and resultant decreased tissue oxygen use) despite a fall in cardiac output.

Although continuous display of the $S\bar{v}o_2$ may provide immediate indication of changes in the child's cardiac output, verification of the change by use of thermodilution injections will often still be necessary. The $S\bar{v}o_2$ monitor may be a useful monitor during titration of PEEP therapy—when arterial oxygen content is improved significantly without a compromise in cardiac output, the $S\bar{v}o_2$ will rise. If, however, PEEP therapy compromises cardiac output proportionately more than it improves arterial oxygen content, oxygen delivery and the $S\bar{v}o_2$ will fall.

Transthoracic Right or Left Atrial or Pulmonary Artery Catheterization

During cardiovascular surgery, individual catheters may be inserted through the chest wall and placed directly into the right atrium, left atrium, or pulmonary artery. Generally, a 2- to 3-French catheter is used and the principles of monitoring using these catheters are the same as those discussed for any invasive intravascular catheter.

The right atrial catheter is used in a fashion identical to a CVP line, and will accurately reflect right ventricular end-diastolic pressure. This catheter may be used for RA pressure measurements, infusion of fluids, or administration of medications. Care should be taken to prevent air or clot entry into the catheter. *If the child has unrepaired cyanotic congenital heart disease, any air entering the right atrial catheter may be shunted to the left side of the heart and into the systemic circulation, ultimately producing a cerebral air embolus (stroke).*

The left atrial catheter is used to monitor left ventricular end-diastolic pressure when the surgeon wishes to avoid the need to place a pulmonary artery catheter. When the left atrial catheter is joined to the monitoring and flush system, and throughout the use of this catheter, scrupulous care must be taken to prevent air entry into this line—*air entry into the left atrial catheter can result in cerebral air embolus.* This catheter should *not* be entered once it is joined to the monitoring system, and only irrigation fluid should be flushed through the catheter. If dampening of the LA waveform occurs, a physician should be consulted and the line should be aspirated, and then irrigated gently *only* with physician approval, if no particulate matter is observed in the catheter or tubing.

A pulmonary artery catheter may be placed directly into the pulmonary artery to allow postoperative monitoring of pulmonary artery pressure. Use of this catheter will not allow pulmonary artery wedge pressure measurements. However, if the child's pulmonary vascular resistance is known to be normal, pulmonary artery end-diastolic pressure will be equal to mean pulmonary artery wedge pressure (note that normal pulmonary vascular resistance will *not* be present in most children with congenital heart disease and pulmonary hypertension).

Small (2.5-French) pulmonary artery catheters are available with thermistor beads. During cardiovascular surgery, while the chest is open, the tip of the catheter will be passed through a small incision in the child's chest, and placed directly in the pulmonary artery. The proximal end of the catheter is joined to a cardiac output computer and a monitoring/fluid infusion system. Thermodilution cardiac output calculations may be performed using this catheter if a right atrial line is in place to allow right atrial fluid injections. However, it will be necessary to check with the catheter manufacturer to determine the computer calibration constant, and the precise recommended volume and temperature of right atrial injections. Such information is also available in the literature.[1]

Transthoracic catheters are generally left in place for several days. After this time, a small tract has formed through the chest wall. Then if bleeding occurs following catheter removal, the blood should be evacuated through the tract, instead of accumulating in the mediastinum. The catheters are removed only with physician order, and the patient should be monitored closely for evidence of bleeding or tamponade following catheter removal.

Summary

Accurate hemodynamic monitoring of pediatric patients requires careful attention to construction of a reliable monitoring system, and standardization of measurement techniques. Measurements and derived calculations of hemodynamic variables should always be evaluated in light of the patient's condition and general appearance. The best monitoring system is the presence of a skilled clinician at the bedside.

REFERENCES

1. Baskoff JD and Maruschak R: Correction factor for thermodilution determination of cardiac output in children, Crit Care Med 9:870, 1981.
2. Boxer RA, Gottesfeld I, Singh S, LaCorte MA, Parnell VA, and Walker P: Noninvasive pulse oximetry in children with cyanotic congenital heart disease, Crit Care Med 15:1062, 1987.
3. Butt WW, Gow R, Whyte H, Smallhorn J, and Koren G: Complications resulting from use of arterial catheters: retrograde flow and rapid elevation in blood pressure, Pediatrics 76:250, 1985.
4. Butt WW, Shann F, McDonnell G, and Hudson I: Effect of heparin concentration and infusion rate on the patency of arterial catheters, Crit Care Med 15:230, 1987. Note: this article refers to pediatric catheters.
5. Cannon K, Mitchell KA, and Fabian TC: Prospective randomized evaluation of two methods of drawing coagulation studies from heparinized arterial lines, Heart Lung 14:392, 1985.
6. Carroll GC: Blood pressure monitoring, Crit Care Clin 4:411, 1988.
7. Chameides L, editor: Textbook of pediatric advanced life support, Dallas, 1988, American Heart Association and the American Academy of Pediatrics.
8. Delaplane D, et al: Urokinase therapy for a catheter-related right atrial thrombus, Journal of Pediatrics 100:149, 1985.
9. Diprose GK, Evans DH, Archer LN, and Levene MI: Dinamap fails to detect hypotension in very low birthweight infants, Arch Dis Child 61:771, 1986.
10. Ducharme FM, Gauthier M, Lacroix J, and Lafleur L: Incidence of infection related to arterial catheterization in children: a prospective study, Crit Care Med 16:272, 1988.
11. Eisenberg PR, Jaffe AS, and Schuster DP: Clinical evaluation compared to pulmonary artery catheterization in the hemodynamic assessment of critically ill patients, Crit Care Med 12:549, 1984.
12. Fanconi S, Doherty P, Edmonds JF, Barker GA, and Bohn D: Pulse oximetry in pediatric intensive care: comparison with measured saturations and transcutaneous oxygen tension, J Pediatr 107:362, 1985.
13. Green GE, Hassell KT, and Mahutte CK: Comparison of arterial blood gas with continuous intra-arterial and transcutaneous PO2 sensors in adult critically ill patients, Crit Care Med 15:491, 1987.
14. Hansen TN and Tooley WM: Skin surface carbon dioxide tension in sick infants, Pediatrics 64:942, 1979.
15. Hazinski MF: Children are different. In Hazinski MF, editor: Nursing care of the critically ill child, St Louis, 1984, The CV Mosby Co.
16. Hazinski MF: Nursing care of the critically ill child: the 7-point check, Pediatr Nurs 11:453, 1985.
17. Hazinski MF: Discrepancies between intra-arterial and oscillometric blood pressure measurements in critically ill infants and children, Unpublished manuscript, 1989.
18. Horgan MJ, Bartoletti A, Polansky S, Peters JC, Manning TJ, and Lamont BM: Effect of heparin infusates in umbilical arterial catheters on frequency of thrombotic complications, J Pediatr 111:774, 1987.
19. Huch R, Huch A, and Lubbers DE: Transcutaneous measurement of blood PO2 (tcPO2): method and application in perinatal medicine, J Perinat Med 1:183, 1973.
20. Katz RW, Pollack MM, and Weibley RE: Pulmonary artery catheterization in pediatric intensive care, Adv Pediatr 30:169, 1983.
21. Maki DG, Botticelli JT, LeRoy ML, and Thielke TS: Prospective study of replacing administration sets for intravenous therapy at 48- vs 72-hour intervals, JAMA 258:1777, 1987.
22. Mandoza GJB, et al: Intracardiac thrombi complicating central total parenteral nutrition: resolution without surgery or thrombolysis, J Pediatr 108:610, 1985.
23. Milliken J, Tait GA, Ford-Jones EL, Mindorff CM, Gold R, and Mullins G: Nosocomial infections in a pediatric intensive care unit, Crit Care Med 16:233, 1988.
24. Miyasaka K, et al: Complications of radial artery lines in the pediatric patient, Can Anaesth Soc J 23:9, 1979.
25. Morris AH, Chapman RH, and Gardner RM: Frequency of wedge pressure errors in the ICU, Crit Care Med 13:705, 1985.
26. Nicolson SC, Sweeney MF, Moore RA, and Jobes DR: Comparison of internal and external jugular cannulation of the central circulation in the pediatric patient, Crit Care Med 13:747, 1985.
27. Park MK, and Menard SM: Accuracy of blood pressure measurement by the Dinamap monitor in infants and children, Pediatrics 79:907, 1987.
28. Prian GW, et al: Apparent cerebral embolization after temporal artery catheterization, J Pediatr 93:115, 1978.

29. Ricard P, Martin R, and Marcoux A: Protection of indwelling vascular catheters: incidence of bacterial contamination and catheter-related sepsis, Crit Car Med 13:541, 1985.

30. Riggs CD, and Lister G: Adverse occurrences in the pediatric intensive care unit, Pediatr Clin North Am 34:93, 1987.

31. Rudolph AM: Cardiac catheterization and angiocardiography. In Rudolph AM: Congenital diseases of the heart, Chicago, 1974, Year Book Medical Publishers, Inc.

32. Sellden H, Nilsson K, Larsson LE, and Ekstrom-Jodal, B: Radial arterial catheters in children and neonates: a prospective study, Crit Care Med 15:1106, 1987.

33. Smith-Wright DL, Green TP, Lock JE, Egar MI, and Fuhrman BP: Complications of vascular catheterization in critically ill children, Crit Care Med 12:1015, 1984.

34. Snydman DR, Donnelly-Reidy M, Perry LK, and Martin WJ: Intravenous tubing containing burettes can be safely changed at 72-hour intervals, Infect Control 8:113, 1987.

35. Sprung CL, Rackow EC, and Civetta JM: Direct measurements and derived calculations using the pulmonary artery catheter. In Sprung, CL, editor: The pulmonary artery catheter: methodology and clinical applications, Baltimore, 1983, University Park Press.

36. Walsh MC, Noble LM, Carlo WA, and Martin RJ: Relationship of pulse oximetry to arterial oxygen tension in infants, Crit Care Med 15:1102, 1987.

37. Wareham JA, Haugh LD, Yaeger SB, and Horbar JD: Prediction of arterial blood pressure in the premature neonate using the oscillometric method, Am J Dis Child 141:1108, 1987.

38. West P, George CF, and Kryger MH: Dynamic in vivo response characteristics of three oximeters: Hewlett-Packard 47201A, Biox III, and Nellcor N-100, Sleep 10:263, 1987.

Chapter 12

Hemodynamic Monitoring of the Patient with Acute Myocardial Infarction

PATHOPHYSIOLOGY

The actual event that precipitates the dramatic, sudden onset of an acute myocardial infarction is poorly understood. In more than 95% of patients who die of myocardial infarction, there is associated severe occlusive atherosclerosis in the coronary arteries that supply the area of infarction. In recent studies investigators have performed coronary arteriography within a few hours of onset of angina in patients suspected of having a myocardial infarction. Most of these studies have shown complete occlusion of those coronary arteries supplying the infarcted area. In many instances the clot appeared fresh, as evidenced by staining with the angiographic dye. These findings have set the stage for the use of thrombolytic therapy, which will be discussed later in this chapter. The evidence of fresh thrombus in the majority of patients with acute myocardial infarction suggests that a platelet thrombus, caused either by disruption of the endothelium over an atherosclerotic plaque or perhaps by focal spasm, is an important etiologic factor in the onset of myocardial infarction. Recent clinical investigation indicates that aggressive treatment with thrombolytic agents such as streptokinase or tissue plasminogen activator (TPA) to dissolve the occluding clot may result in improved myocardial function and survival. The role of immediate or later angioplasty of the underlying stenotic lesion is under study. In general, it appears that the provision of thrombolytic therapy as soon as possible after the onset of chest pain and angioplasty 2 to 3 days later may result in optimal infarct reduction and survival. In addition, a few groups have taken a highly aggressive attitude toward acute infarction and used emergency coronary arteriography and coronary bypass surgery in the treatment of patients. It has been difficult to document the efficacy and extent of infarct reduction accomplished with these treatment approaches. It is certainly likely that the longer the patient has angina and myocardial ischemia before these interventions can be accomplished, the less myocardium can be salvaged.

A rare event that may precipitate infarction is hemorrhage beneath an atherosclerotic plaque, resulting in sudden occlusion of the coronary artery. Spasm of a severely atherosclerotic vessel can also cause irreversible ischemia. If this event occurs, there is a vicious cycle of ischemia → decreased myocardial function → further ischemia → decreased myocardial function → decreased coronary perfusion and infarction.

Within 30 seconds of the onset of ischemia, metabolic changes occur in the myocardial cells that affect their function. Effective ventricular contraction ceases almost immediately, and there are changes in membrane electropotential. These changes are associated with ECG changes, including marked S-T elevation and peaking of the T waves, probably resulting from the loss of sodium pump activity and a change in transmembrane potassium gradient. Cessation of oxidative phosphorylation results in a rapid fall in myocardial temperature. Anaerobic glycolysis is initiated for cellular high-energy phosphate production in lieu of the aerobic Krebs cycle. This anaerobic process results in lactate production from glucose.

In experimental animals these ischemic changes are reversible up to 15 or 20 minutes after the onset of coronary occlusion. When the occlusion is released, function is restored within a few minutes, and after several hours cellular structure is essentially normal. The time period of reversible ischemia can be markedly prolonged, however, by lowering the temperature of the myocardium during the ischemic result. This procedure is commonly performed during cardiac surgery, particularly for congenital heart disease, when regional and total body hypothermia are used on infants too young to be placed on cardiopulmonary bypass. In cardiac transplantation the intact denervated heart can be preserved with iced saline for several hours during the interval before coronary blood flow is reinstituted in the recipient's body.

Attempts at reversing myocardial ischemia, decreasing infarct size, or stabilizing the electrophysiologic system require an understanding of the acute metabolic effects of ischemia. The point where these anaerobic processes become associated with irreversibility is more difficult to analyze. Irreversibility relates to a number of pathologic processes, including rupture of lysozymes, structural defects in sarcolemma, marked rises in intracellular acidity that may result in protein denaturation, and other irreversible changes in the structure of the cell. Although initially these abnormalities may be reversible, after approximately 20 minutes they become irreversible. One can attempt to prevent irreversible damage by delivering oxygen, stabilizing cell membranes, and administering hydrogen receptors to combat lactic acidosis. It is important to note, however, that irreversible infarction occurs in the center of the infarcted zone; there is an increasing number of normal or near-normal cells toward the periphery, and it is this borderline or "twilight" zone that is the most susceptible to pharmacologic and physiologic intervention to maintain myocardial function and prevent necrosis.

The clinical picture of the patient with acute myocardial infarction may not necessarily indicate the status of the patient's myocardial function unless the ischemic area is extensive. Decreased coronary blood flow, resulting in ischemia and segmental akinesia, leads to myocardial dysfunction manifested by a decreased rate

Table 12-1. Hemodynamic findings after a myocardial infarction

Clinical status	Patients (%)	Blood pressure	Cardiac output	Heart rate	Peripheral vascular resistance	CVP	PAW or PA diastolic Pressure (mm Hg)
Uncomplicated	30	N*	N	↑ or ↓	N	N	3 to 12
Mild LV failure	45	N	N	↑ or ↓	N	N	12 to 15
Severe LV failure	15	N or ↓	↓	↑	↑	N or ↑	15 to 20
Cardiogenic shock	10	↓	↓	↑	↑	↑ or ↓	15 to 30

*N, Normal range; ↑, increased; ↓, decreased.

of LV pressure development (dp/dt), decreased LV ejection rate, and decreased stroke volume. These abnormalities are accompanied by a compensatory increase in LV diastolic filling pressure and end-diastolic volume. The extent of the infarction can be closely related to the degree of LV dysfunction. This correlation is particularly accurate in the patient with a single infarction and no evidence of previous ventricular damage. The full spectrum of LV dysfunction seen in patients with myocardial infarction ranges from cardiogenic shock or pump failure (which occurs when over 40% of the left ventricle is infarcted) to essentially normal or near-normal pressures and cardiac output.

Our understanding of LV function and dysfunction following an acute myocardial infarction has been broadened by the development of the Swan-Ganz catheter for monitoring PAW pressures. Table 12-1 outlines the variety of hemodynamic abnormalities that can be seen following an acute myocardial infarction. In the clinically uncomplicated patient with a small infarction, hemodynamic measurements are usually normal, although approximately 25% of these uncomplicated patients have a slight increase in their PAW pressure or LVEDP. In the majority of patients who develop a transient mild LV failure (usually during the first 4 days after the infarction), hemodynamic measurements reveal an abnormal PAW pressure, reflecting an abnormal LVEDP. These patients experience further deterioration with any challenge, such as an increase in afterload as a result of a rise in blood pressure. Of the remaining 25% with acute infarction, about 15% develop severe LV failure, of which about one half will show marked improvement after a week's convalescence. These patients exhibit serious elevations in LVEDP and have abnormally low stroke volume and cardiac output.

The hemodynamic patterns of the patient who has developed cardiogenic shock (resulting from severe congestive heart failure) may show an increase in CVP and PAW pressure, associated with a fall in arterial blood pressure and cardiac output. A small percentage of patients, however, have a low cardiac output with normal, or even decreased, CVP and PAW pressures. These patients require challenging with fluid to separate hypovolemic shock from the true low-output cardiogenic shock. (This procedure is discussed in the section on cardiogenic shock.) In most circumstances the range of hemodynamic patterns can be correlated to the extent of the infarction.

PHYSIOLOGIC CONCEPTS OF TREATMENT
Maintenance of Optimal Cardiac Function
Maintaining electrophysiologic stability

More than 90% of patients who have an acute myocardial infarction develop arrhythmias some time during the first 72 hours of the infarction. As many as 50% of patients with an infarction develop a lethal ventricular arrhythmia at the onset of the infarction, and this arrhythmia precipitates sudden death before hospital admission. The seriousness of any arrhythmia will be dependent not only on the type of arrhythmia but on the degree of myocardial dysfunction.

A number of clinical factors are associated with an increased potential for developing an arrhythmia:

1. Myocardial ischemia
2. Systemic hypoxemia
3. Cardiomegaly
4. Conduction abnormalities
5. LV failure
6. Acidosis
7. Increased sympathetic tone
8. Hypokalemia

Myocardial ischemia increases vulnerability to ventricular fibrillation by altering conduction velocity, automaticity, and membrane potentials. Systemic hypoxemia associated with LV failure may aggravate myocardial ischemia, further enhancing susceptibility to arrhythmias. Other factors associated with arrhythmias (and probably reflecting the severity of the cardiac disease) include an enlarged heart, preexisting impairment in conduction, and pacemaker abnormalities. The degree of either systemic or local acidosis caused by peripheral or cardiac anaerobic metabolism is thought to cause changes in transmembrane potassium potential and cellular function, which may alter the potential for cardiac arrhythmias. Anxiety, fear, and pain cause increases in catecholamine secretion. Experimental studies have shown that sympathetic activity markedly affects susceptibility to ventricular fibrillation. Metabolic abnormalities, particularly hypokalemia, may also cause arrhythmias.

Atrial arrhythmias occur less frequently than ventricular arrhythmias in the patient with an acute myocardial infarction. Their development is important, however, since the loss of atrial systole can result in a 20% or more decrease in cardiac output. In the undigitalized patient, atrial fibrillation and the associated rapid ventricular rate, decreased diastolic filling period, and increased myocardial oxygen demand may precipitate a fatal outcome. The occurrence of atrial arrhythmias reflects a serious prognosis and may be caused by extensive infarction involving the atrium, atrial distention resulting from ventricular failure, or pericarditis.

Ventricular arrhythmias may be caused by alterations in automaticity, abnormalities in conduction that allow a reentry mechanism to develop or a combination of the two. Normal cardiac conduction tissue (not myocardial contractile cells) is characterized by a phase IV depolarization, which at a given threshold triggers depolarization of the cell. Abnormalities may occur either in the *rate* (slope) of phase IV depolarization or in the *threshold* for depolarization (Fig. 12-1). It is thought

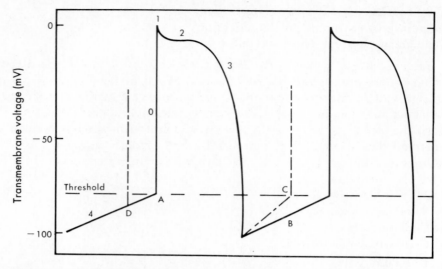

Fig. 12-1. Transmembrane electropotential of cardiac conduction tissue. Normally, there is a gradual rise in voltage from the low point of—90mV. At a given threshold the cell depolarizes; then myocardial contractile cells depolarize and contract. During repolarization, a peak negative transmembrane voltage is again attained, and the sequence recurs. *A,* Normal threshold for depolarization; *B,* normal slope of depolarization; *C,* increased slope of depolarization reaching threshold for firing prematurely (as might occur with ischemia); *D,* decreased threshold also causing premature firing.

that ischemia, as well as local metabolic factors, can affect this rate and threshold of depolarization.

Altered conduction of the cardiac impulse, rather than increased automaticity, probably accounts for the majority of arrhythmias related to ischemic heart disease. Concepts about the development of these arrhythmias are based on the premise that there is a unidirectional conduction block in the ischemic tissue surrounding the infarction area. Thus a given propagating cardiac impulse may be blocked or slowed through a zone of ischemic injury, but the impulse spreads normally through the terminal branches of nonischemic tissue. Because of slowed conduction through the ischemic muscle, the normal conduction tissue has had time to repolarize, so that when the propagating impulse finally leaves the ischemia area, it can repolarize the normal conductive tissue, giving rise to a premature ventricular beat. A reentry tachycardia can develop from this mechanism, precipitating ventricular tachycardia or ventricular fibrillation.

Maintaining optimal electrophysiologic function is aimed at eliminating or decreasing factors known to be associated with increased susceptibility to ventricular fibrillation. Administering oxygen and treating LV failure may be important in eliminating or decreasing the frequency of premature contractions. This treatment alone, however, is usually inadequate, particularly during the first 72 hours after the onset of an acute myocardial infarction. Prophylactic administration of antiarrhythmic drugs can decrease or prevent primary ventricular fibrillation in patients in the coronary care unit.

The development of a second- or third-degree block complicates acute myocardial infarction in about 10% of patients. When the heart block is associated with an anterior wall infarction, the prognosis is poor because of the implication of extensive septal damage. In the majority of patients with a heart block caused by an inferior myocardial infarction, the arrhythmia has been resolved by 1 to 2 weeks after the infarction. When the heart block is complete, or 2:1, insertion of a temporary pacemaker may be required to maintain an adequate heart rate and cardiac output. Insertion of a temporary pacemaker is a relatively simple procedure in a coronary care unit equipped for invasive monitoring. External pacing can be used to maintain the patient's heart rate until the intracardiac pacing wire can be placed.

Maintaining adequate coronary perfusion

Sufficient coronary circulation is important not only for electrophysiologic stability but also for maintenance of myocardial contraction. Approximately 70% of the coronary blood flow occurs during the diastolic phase of the cardiac cycle. Normally, there is a certain degree of autoregulation of coronary flow, so that an increase in aortic diastolic pressure without an increase in myocardial demand will result in an increase in resistance to the coronary circulation. This autoregulation is operative until a mean diastolic pressure of 80 mm Hg is reached. Below this level there is complete vasodilation of the coronary bed, and flow through the coronary circulation is more linearly related to the perfusion pressure at the coronary ostia. Although coronary blood flow may be normal in patients with occlusive coronary disease, there are inadequacies or inequities in the distribution of the blood flow, determined by the severity and distribution of the occlusive disease. It has been demonstrated that an atherosclerotic plaque has little impact on blood flow through the artery until the vessel becomes approximately 75% occluded. After this point, however, there is rapidly increasing resistance to flow, and greater pressure falls across the partially occluded area. In addition, the length of the occluded area has marked hemodynamic impact on blood flow.

Since 70% of the coronary flow to the left ventricle occurs during diastole, the heart rate, which determines the length of diastole, is an important factor in myocardial oxygen delivery. With an increasing heart rate, there is less time for distole and therefore less time for coronary perfusion. This problem is aggravated by the increased myocardial oxygen required for the increased work of a rapidly beating heart.

Studies in animal coronary circulation indicate that the coronary circulatory bed can regulate itself (autoregulation) and vasodilate in response to decreased flow or increased metabolic demands. However, in the diseased human coronary arterial system, evidence suggests that inappropriate increase in vasomotor tone or

Table 12-2. Factors affecting myocardial oxygen demands

Factor	Clinical measurement
Heart rate	Heart rate
Afterload	Arterial systolic pressure or SVR
Preload	LVEDP, PAW pressure, or PA diastolic pressure
Inotropic state or ejection time	Requires LV volume and pressure measurements

even occlusive spasm may occur in the setting of an anginal attack or acute infarction. Therefore the use of vasodilators such as nitroglycerin sublingually or as a paste may improve coronary perfusion when not accompanied by excessive diastolic hypotension. Nitrates thus may act to improve myocardial ischemia by decreasing afterload via peripheral arterial vasodilation, by decreasing preload via peripheral venodilation, and by direct coronary artery dilatation.

Decreasing myocardial oxygen demands

The four major factors determining myocardial oxygen demands are heart rate, afterload (arterial systolic pressure or SVR), preload (LVEDP), and ejection time or contractility (Table 12-2). Continous bedside monitoring of these factors provides a basis for maintaining optimal cardiac function while decreasing myocardial oxygen demands in the critically ill patient.

The patient with minimal LV dysfunction can tolerate a wide range of heart rates without a serious effect on the cardiac output. Many patients with inferior infarction have a heart rate as low as 55 beats/min in the early phase of acute infarction. Normally, this low rate is adequately compensated for by an increase in stroke volume as a result of a prolonged diastolic filling period. In the patient with a compromised left ventricle, however, the heart rate is an important determinant of cardiac output. An increase in heart rate to maintain output and coronary perfusion must be balanced against its adverse effect on increasing myocardial oxygen demands and decreasing diastolic filling time.

Afterload, or arterial systolic pressure, is particularly important in determining myocardial oxygen demands because of the frequent association of systemic hypertension with coronary artery disease. Even in the patient with long-standing systemic hypertension, both diastolic and systolic pressure usually can be reduced without seriously impeding adequate renal or coronary blood flow. A systolic pressure decrease of 30 to 40 mm Hg may have a dramatic effect on cardiac function directly (by allowing an increase in stroke volume) and indirectly (by decreasing myocardial oxygen demands) and therefore on cardiac ischemia.

Preload, or LVEDP, is the third determinant affecting myocardial oxygen demands. LVEDP can be monitored with a PA catheter; either the PA diastolic pressure or the PAW pressure is used as a reflection of the diastolic filling pressure of the left ventricle. Again, changes in pressure must be related to the effect on cardiac output. If the ventricle is compromised, a filling pressure between 16 and 20 mm Hg is thought to be optimal for maintaining stroke volume. An LV diastolic filling pressure above 20 mm Hg probably has deleterious effects because of increased pulmonary congestion and myocardial oxygen demands occurring with minimal further increase in stroke volume.

The fourth factor affecting myocardial oxygen demands is the contractile state of the ventricle, that is, the degree of myocardial fiber shortening at any given preload and afterload. This factor is not directly monitored at the bedside, since it requires simultaneous ventricular pressure and volume measurements. However, an evaluation of the contractile state of the ventricle can be obtained through the use of ventricular function curves. Fig. 12-2 illustrates various states of contractility as indicated by the amount of ventricular work performed at specific fiber lengths (preload).

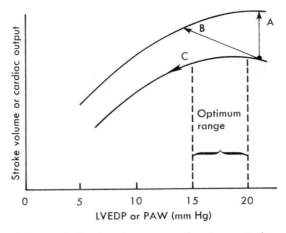

Fig. 12-2. Schematic left ventricular function curves showing an index of LV performance such as stroke volume or cardiac output on the vertical axis and pulmonary artery wedge (PAW) pressure as a reflection of LV filling pressure on the horizontal axis. As the PAW (or LVED) pressure rises, myocardial fiber shortening increases (Frank-Starling law), resulting in increased CO. Increases in PAW pressure over 20 mm Hg usually produce little or no improvement in the CO, as reflected by flattening of the curve. *A,* Arrow reflects a shift to a higher ventricular function curve and stroke volume without a change in preload (this occurs with positive inotropic therapy). *B,* Arrow reflects a shift to a higher ventricular function curve and stroke volume at a lower preload level (this occurs with vasodilator therapy). *C,* Arrow reflects a shift to a lower preload and stroke volume while remaining on the same ventricular function curve (this occurs with diuretic therapy).

Myocardial oxygen demands can be markedly affected by pharmacologic intervention, such as the use of vasodilators to decrease peripheral resistance, or by mechanical assistance to improve LV function by diastolic counterpulsation.

Reduction of Infarct Size

Studies by Jennings and others have demonstrated the development of irreversible structural changes in cell mitochondria after 20 minutes of ischemia; however, it is known that the process of myocardial infarction is a dynamic process that may progress over at least 24 hours. According to Cox and coworkers, the size of an ischemic zone may continue to increase for up to 18 hours; the region of central necrosis extends out from the central area. These data, plus the lack of a clear demarcation between infarcted and normal tissue, have promoted the concept of an ischemic or twilight zone of myocardium surrounding the central necrotic area of infarction. Presumably, the quantity of oxygen delivered to this area and the oxygen demands of an ischemic area (based on myocardial work requirements) determine the outcome of the twilight area. With this phenomenon in mind, Maroko and Braunwald have systemically studied a number of interventions that might reduce myocardial injury and perhaps infarction. These studies have been limited by the lack of suitable methods for accurately determining the extent of infarction in patients. Serial enzyme curves, precordial S-T mapping, and radioisotope techniques have been important but are not yet quantitative for determining infarct size. Nevertheless, there is a great deal of physiologic experimental data in-

Table 12-3. Methods of reducing myocardial ischemia

Desired effect	Method
↓ Myocardial oxygen demand	Treatment of tachycardia or arrhythmia
	Treatment of hypertension
	Beta-adrenergic blockade
	Treatment of LV failure
	Mechanical assist
↑ Myocardial oxygen delivery	Maintenance of normal Po_2
	Maintenance of arterial diastolic pressure around 80 mm Hg
	Maintenance of normal hemoglobin
	Intra-aortic balloon counterpulsation
	Thrombolytic therapy
	Coronary bypass surgery
	Acute angioplasty
↓ Cell injury	Administration of calcium antagonists
	Administration of hydrogen receptors
	Administration of oxygen free radicals

dicating that pharmacologic and physiologic interventions probably can reduce infarct size.

Recent clinical studies have shown that early administration of IV beta-blockers reduces ventricular arrhythmias and may reduce infarction size. The routine use of nitroprusside for afterload reduction remains controversial, however, with some studies showing either no or deleterious effects and other studies demonstrating some beneficial effect. These differing results, coupled with the lack of precise measurements of actual infarction size, characterize the problem of routinely attempting to reduce infarction size in the patient with uncomplicated myocardial infarction. Table 12-3 describes factors or interventions that may decrease myocardial ischemia during active infarction.

Acute Thrombolytic Therapy

Early studies documenting complete occlusion of the corresponding coronary artery in patients presenting with an acute myocardial infarction led to the concept of thrombolytic therapy, initially administered by the intracoronary route. Subsequently it has been shown in large clinical trials that intravenous administration of streptokinase results in decreased mortality, particularly if it is provided in the first 4 to 6 hours after onset of symptoms. Other large clinical trials have demonstrated reduced infarct size and improved left ventricular function with early thrombolytic therapy. Early IV thrombolytic therapy with streptokinase or TPA results in lysis of the clot in 70% to 85% of patients, manifested clinically by rapid resolution of chest pain and reduction of the ST elevation on ECG. Left ventricular function may recover more slowly from the ischemic insult. Thrombolytic therapy is contraindicated when decreased clotting ability might be dangerous to the patient. These new developments have revolutionized our approach to the heart attack patient.

The majority of patients in whom coronary flow is reestablished by thrombolytic therapy demonstrate severe occlusive atherosclerotic lesions underlying the area of the thrombus. Thus these patients are at high risk for reocclusion and require continued anticoagulation therapy and calcium blocker administration to prevent coronary spasm. Angioplasty at the time of acute thrombolytic therapy has been successful but carries some risk because of the anticoagulated state. Recent clinical studies have demonstrated that it is better to wait 24 to 72 hours after thrombolytic therapy to perform the angioplasty procedure. Complications of acute thrombolytic therapy include hemorrhage, hemorrhagic stroke, and gastrointestinal bleeding. Furthermore, re-occlusion may occur, necessitating restudy or acute angioplasty. Postprocedure heparin infusion and calcium blockers are routinely used to decrease the frequency of this problem.

Treatment of Associated Symptoms

The complexities and attention required of biomedical monitoring may divert attention away from other symptoms associated with the myocardial infarction. Pain and anxiety not only cause psychologic discomfort but can produce hemodynamic abnormalities that can jeopardize the patient's cardiovascular status.

Pain causes an increased sympathetic discharge, resulting in tachycardia and increased blood pressure. Because these factors increase myocardial oxygen requirements, immediate treatment is important. Severe pain may also precipitate a vasovagal reaction, resulting in marked sinus bradycardia and hypotension caused by excessive parasympathetic activity. In this case atropine, as well as a narcotic for pain relief, may be useful.

Simlilar hemodynamic responses occur with the situational anxiety of hospitalization; sedation is both effective and necessary in the majority of patients.

Treatment of Complications

Treatment of complications of an acute infarction is directed at returning cardiovascular function toward normal, either by pharmacologic or by physiologic means. In general, the patient with an acute myocardial infarction is considered to be a high risk for cardiac surgery, and aggressive medical treatment is used before surgical intervention. This section deals with the complications most commonly seen after an acute myocardial infarction and the physiologic concepts of treatment.

Hypoxemia

Approximately 60% to 70% of patients suffering a myocardial infarction develop LV dysfunction and elevation of LVEDP. This elevation, in turn, increases pulmonary venous pressure, resulting in transudation of fluid from the pulmonary capillaries into the alveoli. The presence of fluid in the alveoli interferes with the transfer of oxygen at the alveolocapillary level and results in systemic hypoxemia. This hypoxemia may not be evident clinically but is documented by arterial blood gases. Because hypoxemia may contribute to cardiac arrhythmias and further myocardial ischemia, oxygen is administered to return the Po_2 to normal levels. Sufficient oxygen delivery can usually be achieved with a nasal cannula at low flow rates of 2 to 6 L/min. Repeated arterial blood gas measurements are necessary to document adequate oxygen administration. Abnormally high Po_2 levels may cause rises in systemic pressure and actually increase myocardial work.

Arrhythmias

Treatment for arrhythmic complications is discussed in the section on maintaining electrophysiologic stability.

Thromboembolism

Pulmonary embolism and infarction continue to contribute to the mortality of patients in the coronary care unit. These conditions are fostered by advanced age, inactivity, decreased cardiac output, and invasive cardiac catheters. Many clinicians routinely prescribe anticoagulation for the high-risk patient who has a history of thromboembolic disease, obesity, or congestive heart failure. Minidose heparin (5000 units subcutaneously every 12 hours) may be useful prophylactically in these situations with few, if any, complications. Recurrent small pulmonary emboli should be suspected in the patient with repeated, unexplained episodes of tachypnea, tachycardia, dyspnea, cyanosis, or hypotension.

The rise in PA pressure with the occurrence of a pulmonary embolus causes a delay in the closure of the pulmonic valve, and there is fixed or wide splitting of the second sound. There may be an RV gallop. In severe cases there may be accompanying transient tricuspid insufficiency because of pulmonary hypertension. Recurrent small pulmonary emboli may precipitate pulmonary edema or recurring bouts of chest pain without roentgenographic evidence of an infarction. The occurrence of hemoptysis or a pleural friction rub, however, should be considered evidence of a pulmonary infarction. Hemodynamic monitoring can help establish the diagnosis of pulmonary embolus by demonstrating a high PA pressure in the presence of a low or normal PAW pressure.

Systemic emboli may occur from a thrombus on the endocardium in the area of infarction. Studies using echocardiography in acute myocardial infarction patients have demonstrated mural thrombus in a high percentage of patients with anterior myocardial infarction. Although the incidence of mural thrombi is high, the incidence of arterial emboli of clinical consequence is low, and it has not been established whether aggressive anticoagulation therapy in this patient group is useful in preventing morbidity and mortality. Anticoagulation and warfarin sodium (Coumadin) may be useful in speeding dissolution of the clot and reducing the risk of a systemic embolus, particularly in the patient with a protruding or mobile left ventricular thrombus or with an anterior myocardial infarction and congestive heart failure. Thrombolytic therapy with TPA or streptokinase may provide an additional approach to the patient with this complication.

Pericarditis

A pericardial friction rub can be heard in at least 10% to 20% of patients with a myocardial infarction, particularly those with an anterior myocardial infarction. The rub is usually transient, occurring on the second through the fifth day after the infarction. If the pain is severe, it may require analgesics or anti-inflammatory drugs.

Ventricular aneurysm

A ventricular aneurysm occurs in a later phase of a myocardial infarction at any time from a few days to several weeks after the infarction. The diagnosis is difficult to establish by physical examination, although in midsystole and late systole there may be outward bulging when the precordium is palpated. It can be suspected in the patient with refractory heart failure, in the patient with an abnormally large cardiac silhouette or unusual shadow on a roentgenogram, and in the patient with paradoxical movement of the cardiac silhouette during fluoroscopy. A small group of patients have drug-resistant ventricular tachycardia associated with the aneurysm.

Surgical removal of the aneurysm is usually not performed during the first 6 to 12 weeks to allow time for cardiac function to stabilize. Earlier surgical intervention may be necessary, however, in the patient who is hemodynamically deteriorating.

Mitral insufficiency

More than 50% of patients with a myocardial infarction develop a transient systolic murmur at the apex, consistent with papillary muscle dysfunction. This complication usually occurs within the first few days after an acute myocardial infarction. There are varying degrees of mitral insufficiency, depending on the extent of the infarction and ischemia of the papillary muscles. Vasodilator therapy during hemodynamic monitoring is an ideal treatment for these patients, because it not only decreases LVEDP but also decreases afterload. This reduction in afterload tends to promote forward cardiac output and minimize mitral regurgitation. An increase in forward flow decreases LV volume, which may improve function of the subvalvular apparatus of the mitral valve. When the condition is severe, continuing vasodilator therapy, either orally or intravenously, may allow an optimal waiting period before mitral valve replacement.

Occasionally, an infarcted papillary muscle can rupture, resulting in flagrant mitral regurgitation. This complication is clinically characterized by the sudden onset of a loud holosystolic murmur and pulmonary edema that is resistant to drug treatment. Hemodynamic evidence of the development of mitral regurgitation consists of an abnormal elevation of the v wave of the PAW pressure tracing (see Fig. 5-30). The patient may be managed temporarily by afterload reduction with vasodilators, but the majority of patients require immediate mitral valve replacement after cardiac catheterization and coronary arteriogaphy.

RV infarction

Infarction of the right ventricle is important to recognize because of a relatively good prognosis if managed properly. This diagnosis is suspected when there is evidence of RV failure during an acute inferior infarction. Clinical findings usually include extensive inferior myocardial infarction and distended neck veins but absence of LV failure with clear lungs and no S_3 gallop. Hypotension and heart block may be present. The cause is proximal occlusion of a dominant right coronary artery, resulting in extensive damage to the walls of both left and right ventricles and the intraventricular septum.

The marked venous distention can easily lure the physician into treatment with diuretics if infarction is not considered in the differential diagnosis. Diuresis decreases intravascular volume and LV filling pressures, resulting in further hypotension and lowered cardiac output. The diagnosis of right ventricular infarct must be considered when there is apparent right ventricular failure in the setting of an acute inferior myocardial infarction. The ECG can be useful to establish the diagnosis by demonstrating ST elevation in right-sided chest leads such as V_{2-4}. Hemodynamic monitoring is very useful in establishing the diagnosis of RV infarction by demonstrating a high CVP and RA pressure in the presence of a lower or normal PAW pressure. Therapy is directed at volume loading to maintain high intravascular volume and adequate cardiac output. Close monitoring and maintenance of PAd or PAW mean pressures in the range of 10 to 15 mm Hg are required during fluid therapy in an effort to maintain adequate LV filling pressures without precipitating pulmonary edema. As the patient improves, IV fluid therapy can be decreased and hemodynamic monitoring discontinued.

Cardiac rupture

Cardiac rupture almost inevitably leads to sudden death and accounts for approximately 10% of hospital patient deaths caused by infarction. Physical examination and cardiovascular monitoring are not helpful in the prediction or care of this problem.

Ventricular septal defect

Rupture of the ventricular septum is a well-known complication and occurs with both anterior and inferior myocardial infarctions, usually within 2 to 10 days after the infarction. This complication is characterized by the sudden onset of a palpable thrill and a loud pansystolic murmur at the lower left sternal border. Hemodynamic evidence of a VSD consists of a step-up in the oxygen saturation of an RV or PA blood sample compared with that of an SVC or RA blood sample. Depending on the size of the VSD, left-to-right shunting can cause cardiac failure and pulmonary overcirculation. Because early surgical intervention results in high patient mortality, treatment with afterload reduction decreases the left-to-right shunting and allows time for initial healing of the infarcted area. In the patient who develops shock with drug-resistant heart failure, however, early surgical repair of the VSD may be required.

Congestive heart failure

Congestive heart failure developing during acute myocardial infarction is closely related to the extent of the infarction and generally implies a more serious prognosis. As indicated in Table 12-1, approximately 25% of patients with myocardial infarction develop LV failure or cardiogenic shock. Primary treatment for congestive heart failure is directed toward correction of systemic metabolic factors, such as acidosis, hypoxemia, and arrhythmias, that may compromise cardiac output. Maintaining electrophysiologic stability and adequate coronary perfusion and reducing myocardial oxygen demands, as discussed previously, are also important.

The medical therapy for LV failure associated with an acute infarction is based on three hemodynamic objectives. The *first objective* is to maintain adequate arterial pressure to perfuse vital organs, particularly the heart. In some cases, this objective may also be accomplished by increasing cardiac output with afterload reduction. However, in more severe cases of LV failure, the patient may require peripheral vasoconstrictors to prevent the vicious downward cycle that can occur once hypotension leads to myocardial ischemia and further LV dysfunction.

The *second objective* is to maintain adequate cardiac output and tissue perfusion to provide life-sustaining organ functions. This objective may be achieved by simply reducing afterload or, in more severe cases, by also administering positive inotropic agents to improve LV ejection.

Because elevation of LVEDP is the hallmark of LV failure, the *third objective* is to reduce the LVEDP (PAW) if it is greater than 20 to 25 mm Hg. This treatment will not only relieve symptoms of dyspnea and improve arterial oxygenation but will decrease preload, reducing myocardial oxygen demands. Although diuretic therapy is the initial step to achieve this objective, afterload reduction using a vasodilator has become increasingly recognized as valuable therapy and will be discussed in detail shortly.

Hemodynamic Guidelines to Therapy

This section will discuss hemodynamic variables and the appliction of pharmacologic agents to optimize cardiac function during congestive heart failure occurring during an acute myocardial infarction.

Preload

The ventricular function curve is a useful tool when assessing the functional status of the left ventricle. Fig. 12-2 shows the relationship between cardiac output or stroke volume on the vertical axis and the PAW pressure (preload) on the horizontal axis. Swan and others have demonstrated that, in patients with acute myocardial infarction, LV fiber shortening and stroke volume continued to improve as LV volume increased (as reflected by LVEDP and PAW pressure rising to the 15 to 20 mm Hg range). Beyond that range, however, the ventricular function curve tends to become flat, with little or no further increase in stroke volume. In addition, PAW pressure exceeding 20 mm Hg causes transudation of fluid from the pulmonary capillary intravascular space into lung interstitial and alveolar spaces, resulting in progessively severe pulmonary edema.

In a patient who manifests moderate or severe congestive heart failure, monitoring the PAd or PAW pressure through a balloon-tipped catheter helps assess the degree of LV abnormality and indicates appropriate treatment. For example, if the PAW pressure (LVEDP) is higher than 20 mm Hg, the patient can be treated with IV diuretics such as furosemide. This agent causes an immediate venodilation with a reduction in central venous return and preload that is manifested hemodynamically as a fall in LVEDP and PAW pressure and clinically as a reduction of pulmonary venous congestion. The later diuretic effect of the drug decreases intravascular volume and further reduces venous congestion and pulmonary edema. Assessing optimal preload prevents excessive reduction of PAW pressure to that point on the ventricular function curve where stroke volume or cardiac output fails.

PAW pressure assessment can also aid a patient with mild congestive heart failure who was treated simply with diuretics. This patient may respond with excessive diuresis and develop unrecognized intravascular volume depletion with a reduction in stroke volume and cardiac output that mimics cardiogenic shock or low output syndrome. Confirmation of low ventricular filling pressures by PAW pressure measurement suggests the correct therapy of volume replacement; up to 1000 ml of 5% dextrose in normal saline administered at a rate of 100 ml every 5 to 10 minutes helps replace intravascular volume. The use of salt-poor albumin to increase the intravascular oncotic pressure also helps temporarily maintain a greater intravascular volume and preload without precipitating pulmonary edema.

Afterload reduction

In the patient with more severe LV failure and flatter ventricular function curves, reduction of a high PAW pressure (preload) alone may decrease cardiac output, even though it improves respiratory status (see Fig. 12-2). In the past a positive inotropic and vasoconstrictive agent, such as norepinephrine, was administered to increase the blood pressure and improve LV contractility in an attempt to increase cardiac output. However, this increased SVR and contractility, leading to additional stroke work and myocardial oxygen demands, frequently resulted in further LV failure rather than improvement. A therapeutic approach using peripheral vasodilating drugs has found increasing use in the treatment of congestive heart failure during acute myocardial infarction. The administration of these IV agents requires both PA or PAW and systemic arterial pressure monitoring because of their rapid onset of action, potential hypotensive effects, and occasional excessive reduction in preload.

Because of a balanced vasodilation of both arterioles and venules, sodium nitroprusside is usually the initial drug of choice in treating the patient with LV pump failure and high PAW pressures. As the agent is administered, increasing degrees of peripheral vasodilation occur. Central venous return falls because of venous dilatation and venous pooling, resulting in a decrease in preload and a reduction in pulmonary venous congestion. For this reason, this agent is used primarily when the PAW pressure is over 20 mm Hg. The SVR also decreases because of arterial dilatation, reducing impedance to ejection of blood from the left ventricle. This effect results in improved LV ejection fraction or stroke volume at the same or reduced preload (LVEDP) (see Fig. 12-2). These afterload reducing agents can cause severe hypotension and are generally not used if the initial arterial blood pressure is lower than 90/60 mm Hg. Because of their peripheral vasodilation effects, however, the increase in stroke volume and cardiac output usually compensates for the decrease in SVR, and little change in blood pressure may occur. The relationship between blood pressure, cardiac output, and SVR is indicated by the following formula:

$$BP = CO \times SVR$$

Thus, even though the blood pressure may remain the same, the reduction of SVR has unloaded the heart and allowed the left ventricle to increase cardiac output without an increase in work. Pharmacologic afterload-reducing agents administered intravenously during careful hemodynamic monitoring may markedly improve cardiac output and decrease pulmonary congestion. As progressive peripheral vasodilation occurs, careful attention must be paid to preload. If PAW pressure (LVEDP) falls below the 15 to 20 mm Hg optimal range, additional fluid, preferably with the addition of salt-poor albumin, is needed to maintain optimal LV function.

Afterload reduction and positive inotropic agents

In the patient with extreme LV failure or cardiogenic shock, afterload reduction alone may be insufficient, and the addition of a positive inotropic agent may be needed to improve cardiac output and still maintain arterial pressures high enough for adequate myocardial and tissue perfusion. The patient with low output and hypotension may even require initial treatment with an agent such as dopamine or dobutamine to maintain adequate arterial perfusion pressures while initiating hemodynamic monitoring and afterload reduction. The use of dobutamine or dopamine provides a positive inotropic effect that increases contractility and shifts the LV function curve to a higher curve (see Fig. 12-2); that is, it allows increased stroke volume at the same preload or LVEDP. With improved stroke volume, blood pressure rises and improves tissue perfusion ($BP = CO \times SVR$). However, this improved myocardial contractility increases myocardial oxygen demands, and care must be taken to add just enough inotropic agent to achieve the desired therapeutic goals.

The goal of hemodynamic monitoring and IV pharmacologic therapy is to continually assess and optimize LV function and perfusion of the heart and other body tissues during the acute infarction and initial healing process. Prevention of further myocardial ischemia and infarction is an important consideration when using positive inotropic and vasodilating agents. Because the patient with LV dysfunction tends to improve over a period of 3 to 7 days, these combined IV pharmacologic agents can be administered temporarily and adjusted appropriately during hemodynamic monitoring.

Recently, there has been a tendency to prefer IV nitroglycerine (TNG) over nitroprusside as the initial afterload reduction agent in the setting of an acute myocardial infarction. Clinical studies with IV TNG have demonstrated less ST segment elevation on the electrocardiogram. Many groups have found that IV TNG also results in reduction in chest pain during the acute event, suggesting reduction in the degree of myocardial ischemia. As with nitroprusside, the dose and systemic blood pressure must be monitored carefully to avoid an excessive fall in blood pressure. As the patient improves, the goal is to taper and stop the positive inotropic agents and assess the need for continued afterload reduction. As afterload reduction therapy is tapered, a rise in PAW pressure and a fall in cardiac output indicating continued LV dysfunction may indicate the need for long-term afterload-reducing therapy. Although there are a number of oral therapeutic agents that result in peripheral vasodilation and afterload reduction, either hydralazine, with a primarily arteriolar vasodilation effect, or prazosine, with a more balanced arteriolar and venular vasodilation effect, is recommended as the IV drugs are tapered and stopped. Studies suggest that patients with residual LV failure can be maintained on oral afterload-reduction agents for long periods with continued reduction of congestive heart failure symptoms and minimal adverse side effects. Long-acting nitrates such as isosorbide dinitrate have also been shown to be effective. More recently, angiotensin-converting enzyme (ACE) inhibitors such as captopril have become increasingly important in the treatment of *chronic* congestive heart failure by reducing afterload. The choice of agents and the transition from short- to long-term therapy for congestive heart failure will depend on the patient's course and the prior status of the left ventricle.

CARDIOGENIC SHOCK

Cardiogenic shock will develop in 8% to 10% of patients entering the coronary care unit with an acute myocardial infarction. The primary physiologic hallmark of cardiogenic shock is inadequate perfusion and oxygen delivery to body tissues. Other accompanying changes include varying decreases in arterial pressure, cardiac output, and LV function. Clinical manifestations of cardiogenic shock may include hypotension, a cardiac index of less than 2.1 L/min/m^2, a urinary output of less than 20 ml/hr, tachycardia with a poor pulse contour, mental confusion, and decreased peripheral perfusion.

Pathologic studies have demonstrated that patients who die during cardiogenic shock have at least 40% of their myocardium infarcted. Therefore cardiogenic shock reflects extensive myocardial necrosis, usually associated with severe triple-vessel occlusive coronary artery disease. Attempts to identify the high-risk patient who will develop cardiogenic shock have not been entirely successful. Ratshin, Rackley, and Russell have found an LVEDP or PA end-diastolic pressure over 28 mm Hg with a cardic index of less than 2.3 L/min/m^2 to be associated with 100% mortality. Early identification of the high-risk patient for cardiogenic shock may provide a basis for earlier pharmacologic or surgical intervention to decrease the infarction size and prevent the development of shock.

As progressive cardiogenic shock and hypotension occur, there is decreased coronary perfusion, leading to development of other areas of focal necrosis and marked subendocardial ischemia throughout both ventricles. This progressive ischemia and infarction lead to further deterioration of LV function and death. A patient may have such extensive initial infarction because of occlusion of a major coronary artery (such as the proximal left anterior descending or main left coronary artery) that the patient dies rapidly from cardiogenic shock. On the other hand, in some patients, progression of cellular necrosis into areas of ischemia leading to this cycle may be amenable to pharmacologic or surgical intervention.

Physiologic Concepts of Medical Treatment

Cardiogenic shock, as well as other forms of shock, causes multiple systemic abnormalities that must be identified and corrected to provide optimal chance for recovery. Most of these abnormalities are the result of decreased perfusion. Correction of factors that contribute to decreased tissue perfusion, as discussed earlier in this chapter, is important. Cardiac arrhythmias, hypoxemia, and pain require attention and treatment. In cardiogenic shock lactic acidosis occurs because of inadequate oxygen delivery to the tissues, leading to anaerobic metabolism and lactate production. The acidosis can only be partially compensated for by hyperventilation and other buffer mechanisms. Use of sodium bicarbonate temporarily reverses the acidosis, promotes an optimal transmembrane potassium gradient, and improves the myocardial response to inotropic drugs.

Hemodynamic Guidelines to Therapy

Bedside hemodynamic monitoring during the administration of pharmacologic agents is essential to provide optimal hemodynamic function for the acutely infarcted heart when congestive heart failure or cardiogenic shock ensues. The initial goal of treatment is to provide adequate tissue perfusion to maintain the patient's life. Longer-term goals consist of providing temporary assistance to the left ventricle until spontaneous improvement in LV function occurs or stabilizing the critically ill patient for surgical therapy. Because of the marked response variability to these potent therapeutic agents, it is mandatory that hemodynamic monitoring be initiated before using many of them.

Evaluation of the hemodynamic data also helps determine whether any factors other than pump failure are contributing to the cardiogenic shock. The development of a ruptured papillary muscle causing severe mitral insufficiency or a ruptured ventricular septum can be diagnosed at the time of initiation of bedside hemodynamic monitoring, as discussed elsewhere in this chapter. Because both of these problems are amenable to aggressive afterload reduction and subsequent surgical therapy, the diagnosis can be critical.

Once hemodynamic monitoring has established baseline data, decisions about pharmacologic therapy are directed toward optimizing LV function at the lowest level of myocardial oxygen demands. These principles are similar to the treatment of LV failure, except that hypotension may be a more predominant part of this profile. Studies have shown that a coronary perfusion pressure below 80 mm Hg is directly related to coronary flow; collapse of the coronary artery occurs at approximately 40 mm Hg (Fig. 12-3). Thus every effort should be made to maintain coronary artery perfusion pressure at 60 to 80 mm Hg, even though this pressure may be at the expense of increasing myocardial oxygen demands. Table 10-4 lists a number of vasoactive agents and indicates the relationship between their effect on improving contractility and their effect on constricting peripheral arterioles to increase SVR. Because peripheral vasoconstriction and a high SVR are usually associated with cardiogenic shock, agents that improve LV contractility and ejection fraction with minimal peripheral effects, such as dopamine or dobutamine, are usually the initial drugs of choice. These agents shift the patient's left ventricle to a higher function curve at the same level of preload (PAW) pressure (see Fig. 12-2). Thus adequate coronary perfusion pressure and cardiac output can be maintained temporarily while assessing other potentially correctible problems.

The use of a positive inotropic agent should not be a substitute for providing optimal LVEDP (preload) in the 15 to 20 mm Hg range. The patient in cardiogenic shock occasionally may have a low or normal PAW pressure in association with hypotension and a markedly reduced cardiac output. In this case treatment would be aimed at increasing PAW pressure to the optimal range of 15 to 20 mm Hg by administration of IV fluid. As the diastolic volume and pressure in the left ventricle increase during IV fluid administration, stroke volume will also increase, as indicated in Fig. 12-2. If there is any possibility of a low PAW pressure, fluid loading as previously described should be initiated until the PAW pressure reaches 25 mm Hg.

Once the patient's blood pressure is stabilized and optimal or high preload is determined, a trial of afterload reduction can be initiated to increase stroke volume at the same or lower preload. Use of nitroprusside in this situation requires ex-

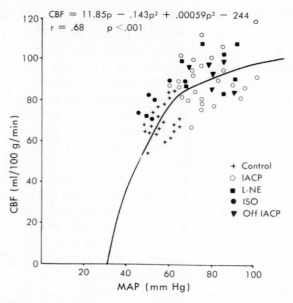

Fig. 12-3. Pressure-flow relationship in severely diseased coronary vascular bed. The graph demonstrates that L-norepinephrine, *L-NE,* and intra-aortic counterpulsation, *IACP,* increase mean aortic pressure, *MAP,* and coronary blood flow, *CBF.* As MAP falls, CBF decreases; with a MAP of 30 or 40 mm Hg, the projected fall of CBF is to zero. (From Mueller H et al: Trans NY Acad Sci, Series II 34(4):309-333, 1972.)

treme caution because of the accompanying hypotension in the patient with cardiogenic shock. As the afterload agent is increased, the stroke volume may improve sufficiently to prevent any fall in blood pressure and may allow a gradual tapering of the dopamine over several days.

Mortality remains high in the cardiogenic shock patient because of inadequate spontaneous improvement in the infarcted left ventricle to maintain sufficient cardiac output and blood pressure. Some of these patients are excellent candidates for intra-aortic balloon pumping to further improve the relationship between LV work and output (see Chapter 9), especially if a definitive surgical procedure such as LV aneurysmectomy is planned.

Physiologic Concepts of Surgical Intervention

Because the mortality of patients with cardiogenic shock approaches 100%, dramatic methods to lower mortality have been undertaken. Pathologic studies indicate an area of ischemia surrounding the central necrosis, and theoretically this ischemic area could be converted to functioning myocardium if oxygen delivery could be improved. This conversion would result in improved LV function and patient prognosis. The concept of surgically bypassing areas of occlusion and thereby increasing myocardial perfusion provides a basis for surgery for these patients. Before surgical intervention, selective coronary arteriography and IV angiography must be performed to ascertain the extent of coronary occlusion and LV dysfunction. These procedures frequently are performed with circulatory assist because of their inherent danger and the difficulty in maintaining optimal hemodynamic monitoring and treatment. The exact indications for coronary bypass surgery vary, but they are based on the premise that increased coronary perfusion via the bypass will convert areas of dysfunction caused by ischemia to functioning myocardium. Except for the period of cardiopulmonary bypass, circulatory assist is continued during surgery to maintain optimal tissue perfusion. If there is difficulty in taking the patient off cardiopulmonary bypass, circulatory assist can be reinstituted. This approach allows early operative procedures with minimal risk. Mortality in this group of surgically treated patients is approximately 50%, in contrast to the 80% to 100% mortality of medically treated patients.

Other surgical approaches have been tried to lower the mortality of patients with cardiogenic shock. Infarctectomy has the theoretic possibility of decreasing LV and intramyocardial tension. It has not been successful in lowering mortality, however, because the additional trauma to the surrounding zones of ischemia and the impact of cardiopulmonary bypass outweigh the mechanical advantage accomplished by the procedure. In contrast, when a mechanical or anatomic complication is causing the cardiogenic shock, such as rupture of papillary muscle or a VSD, surgical intervention and correction can be lifesaving. As cardiac transplantation has become more commonly available, with survival rates of 80% at 1 year and 60% to 70% at 5 years, this alternative has become more feasible for treatment of acute myocardial infarction.

PATIENT EXAMPLES

The following cases are presented to give an overall picture of the types of complications of LV failure that may develop during acute infarction. Please consult the bibliography for further guidance to medical therapy of these patients.

Case 1

A 72-year-old woman was admitted to the coronary care unit with severe chest pain, and an anterior myocardial infarction was indicated on the ECG. Her initial vital signs were within normal limits. However, because of bibasilar lung rales, she was given 40 mg of fu-

Case 1

Hemodynamic parameter	Admission	24 hr	48 hr	49 hr	50 hr
Rx	IV furosemide	PO furosemide	IV normal saline	IV normal saline	—
BP (mm Hg)	110/88	102/72	96/75	105/85	110/84
HR (beats/min)	85	90	94	88	86
RA (mm Hg)	—	—	0	2	4
PA (mm Hg)	—	—	20/7	22/10	30/15
PAW (mm Hg)	—	—	7	10	15
CO (L/min)	—	—	2.5	2.9	3.4
SVR (units)	—	—	32	30	26
Urinary output (ml/hr)	30	60	10	15	20
LV function curve point (Fig. 12-4)	—	—	1	2	3

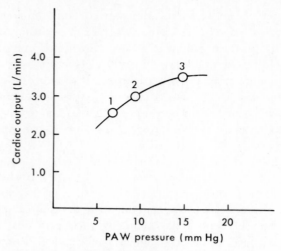

Fig. 12-4. LV function curve for case I (see text).

rosemide IV. After 24 hours, her blood pressure was 102/72 mm Hg; she appeared in distress, so she was given a second dose of furosemide. After 48 hours, she had symptoms of low CO as manifested by decreasing urinary output, orthostatic hypotension, and confusion. Her neck veins were flat, indicating a low CVP. Hemodynamic monitoring was initiated and revealed a low CO of 2.5 L/min, PAW of 7 mm Hg, and RA pressure of 0 mm Hg. A diagnosis of hypovolemia-induced hypotension was made, and administration of 100 ml of IV normal saline every 10 minutes was initiated. One hour later, blood pressure and urinary output had improved. Fluid replacement was continued until the PAW reached 16 mm Hg and then was maintained with 2 units of salt-poor albumin per 8-hour shift for the next 24 hours.

The high SVR of 32 units also indicated compensatory peripheral vasoconstriction in response to the low intravascular volume and falling stroke volume. This also was improved with fluid therapy. Hemodynamic monitoring can quickly and accurately establish the diagnosis and allow more rapid replacement of fluid without jeopardizing the patient.

Case 2

A 62-year-old man was admitted with a history of an inferior myocardial infarction with uneventful recovery 2 years ago. He was now suffering from 3 hours of severe crushing chest pain. He had been taking no drugs but had hypertension in the past. Initial evaluation

Case 2

Hemodynamic parameter	Admission	6 hr	24 hr
Rx	Morphine	IV nitroprusside	—
BP (mm Hg)	150/105	100/60	105/80
HR (beats/min)	105	110	90
RA (mm Hg)	—	5	2
PAW (mm Hg)	—	35	20
CO (L/min)	—	2.8	3.9
SVR (units)	—	28	23
LV function curve point (Fig. 12-5)	—	1	2

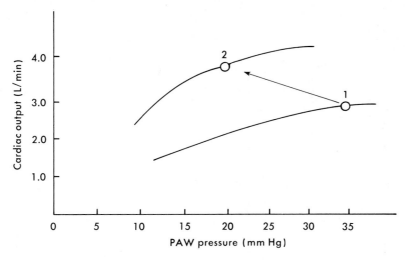

Fig. 12-5. LV function curve for case 2 (see text).

revealed dyspnea, blood pressure of 150/105 mm Hg, heart rate of 105 beats/min, and bilateral lung rales. Administration of 5 mg morphine sulfate IV resulted in some symptomatic improvement. However, 6 hours later rales had risen to the midchest level and hemodynamic instrumentation was accomplished. Data revealed a low CO of 2.8 L/min with a PAW of 35 mm Hg and blood pressure of 100/60 mm Hg.

Based on these hemodynamic data, initial therapy was directed at decreasing afterload with peripheral vasodilators to increase stroke volume while decreasing myocardial work and oxygen demands. This approach would also decrease preload, relieving the marked pulmonary venous congestion. Intravenous nitroglycerin was started at 0.5 µg/kg/min and increased to 2 µg/kg/min over 1 hour. Because of its rapid onset of action and potential hypotensive effect, intra-arterial blood pressure was monitored carefully. The reduction in arteriolar resistance by nitroprusside caused the SVR to fall dramatically, allowing stroke volume to increase without requiring the addition of a positive inotropic agent. Blood pressure remained relatively stable because the increase in CO compensated for the fall in SVR (BP = CO × SVR). Furthermore, the reduction in preload with the PAW decreasing from 35 to 20 mm Hg dramatically reduced the pulmonary venous congestion by decreasing central venous return. This reduction is preload also contributed to decreasing myocardial work and reducing LV radius.

The patient's initial tachycardia, resulting from the fall in CO and chest pain, gradually returned toward normal as these other abnormalities were improved. The initial tachycardia and hypertension both had increased myocardial oxygen demands, which most likely contributed to progressive ischemic dysfunctions of the left ventricle, aggravating the situation.

Over the next 4 days the patient continued to improve. The nitroglycerin was tapered and stopped without occurrence of hypotension or pulmonary venous congestion.

Case 3

A 39-year-old man was admitted with 30 minutes of severe chest pain, palpitations, and pallor. Electrocardiograms revealed an extensive anterior myocardial infarction with marked ST elevation across the precordium. In the emergency room he received 100 mg of lidocaine IV for PVCs and was started on dopamine 2 µg/kg/min because of a blood pressure of 90/60 mm Hg and cool extremities. In the coronary care unit he complained of dyspnea and appeared confused. Increasing the level of dopamine improved his blood pressure but had little effect on tissue perfusion or his confusion. Hemodynamic monitoring was ini-

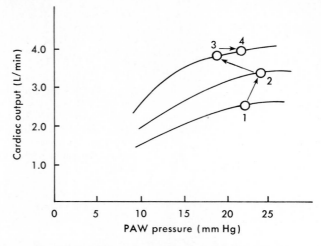

Fig. 12-6. LV function curve for case 3 (see text).

Case 3

Hemodynamic parameter	ER	CCU		6 hr	48 hr	74 hr
Rx	Dopamine	Dopamine increased		Dopamine and nitroprusside	Nitroprusside	Hydralazine
BP (mm Hg)	90/60	88/60	108/70	100/80	102/80	105/80
HR (beats/ min)	125	98	106	92	90	90
RA (mm Hg)	—	10	9	5	6	7
PAW (mm Hg)	—	22	24	18	20	18
CO (L/min)	—	2.5	3.2	3.9	3.8	3.7
SVR (units)	—	24	30	22	22	22
LV function curve point (Fig. 12-6)	—	1	2	3	4	—

tiated and revealed hypotension, depressed CO and PAW of 22 mm Hg. Dopamine was discontinued and a trial of IV nitroprusside alone was started. This resulted in further hypotension. Dopamine was reinstituted at 4 µg/kg/min to raise the blood pressure to maintain adequate coronary perfusion and resulted in a rise in blood pressure to 100/80 mm Hg but little improvement in Co. Nitroprusside at 1 µg/kg/min was then begun and slowly increased. This resulted in a rise in CO to 3.9 L/min without producing a fall in the blood pressure. After several days, the dopamine was tapered without a significant fall in blood pressure. However, attempts to taper IV nitroprusside resulted in recurrence of PAW pressure rise to 30 mm Hg and symptomatic pulmonary edema. The patient was then started on oral afterload reduction with hydralazine, initially at a dosage of 25 mg 3 times a day, which was increased to 75 mg 4 times a day over 24 hours. This therapy allowed tapering of IV nitroprusside and subsequent cessation of hemodynamic monitoring.

REFERENCES

Armstrong PW: Contributions of hemodynamic monitoring to the treatment of chronic congestive heart failure, Can Med Assoc J 121:913-918, 1979.

Arven S, and Boscha K: Prophylactic anticoagulation for left ventricular thrombi after acute myocardial infarction: a prospective randomized trial, Am Heart J 113:688-693, 1987.

Ayres SM, and Mueller H: The overall approach to the patient with hypotension, Heart Lung 3:463-476, 1974.

Barden RM et al: Right ventricular infarction, Cardiovasc Nurs 19:7-10, 1983.

Bodai BI, and Holcroft JW: Use of the pulmonary arterial catheter in the critically ill patient, Heart Lung 11:406-415, 1982.

Bolooki H et al: Clinical, surgical, and pathologic correlation in patients with acute myocardial infarction and pump failure, Circulation 44:1034-1042, 1971.

Braunwald E: The myocardium: failure and infarction, New York, 1974, The Hospital Practice Publication, Inc.

Cairns JA: Hemodynamic monitoring in acute myocardial infarction, Can Med Assoc J 121:905-910, 1979.

Chatterjee K, and Parmley WW: The role of vasodilator therapy in heart failure, Prog Cardiovasc Dis 19:301-325, 1977.

Chatterjee K et al: Beneficial effects of vasodilator agents in severe mitral regurgitation due to dysfunction of subvalvar apparatus, Circulation 48:684-690, 1973.

Cohn JN et al: Right ventricular infarction: clinical and hemodynamic features, Am J Cardiol 33:209-214, 1974.

Corday E, and Swan HJC: Myocardial infarction, Baltimore, 1974, Williams & Wilkins.

Cox JL, Daniel TM, and Boineau JP: The electrophysiologic time-course of acute myocardial ischemia and the effects of early coronary perfusion, Circulation 48:971-983, 1973.

Crexells C et al: Optimal level of filling pressure in the left side of the heart in acute myocardial infarction, N Engl J Med 289:1263-1266, 1973.

Deepak V et al: A simplified concept of complete physiological monitoring of the critically ill patient, Heart Lung 10:75-82, 1981.

Dikshit K et al: Renal and extrarenal hemodynamic effects of furosemide in congestive failure after acute myocardial infarction, N Engl J Med 288:1087-1090, 1973.

Dugall JC, Pryor R, and Blount SG, Jr: Systolic murmur following myocardial infarction, Am Heart J 84:577-583, 1974.

Epstein SE et al: Reduction of ischemic injury by nitroglycerin in acute myocardial infarction, N Engl J Med 292:29-35, 1975.

Flaherty JT et al: Intravenous nitroglycerin in acute myocardial infarction, Circulation 51:132-139, 1975.

Forrester JS, Diamond GA, and Swan HJC: Correlative classification of clinical and hemodynamic function after acute myocardial infarction, Am J Cardiol 39:137-145, 1977.

Forrester JS et al: Medical therapy of acute myocardial infarction by application of hemodynamic subsets. Parts I and II, N Engl J Med 295:1356-1362, 1404-1414, 1976.

GISSI trial: long-term effects of intravenous thrombolysis in acute myocardial infarction—final report of the GISSI study, Lancet 2:871-874, 1987.

Gunnar RM, and Loeb HS: Use of drugs in cardiogenic shock due to acute myocardial infarction, Circulation 45:111-124, 1972.

Heikkila J, Kresoja M, and Luomanmaki K: Ruptured intraventricular septum complicating acute myocardial infarction, Chest 66:675-681, 1974.

Isner JM: Right ventricular myocardial infarction, JAMA 259:712-718, 1988.

Jennings RB: Early phase of myocardial ischemic injury and infarction, Am J Cardiol 24:753-765, 1969.

Kelly DT et al: Use of phentolamine in acute myocardial infarction associated with hypertension and left ventricular failure, Circulation 47:729-735, 1973.

Kennedy JW et al: Western Washington randomized trial of intracoronary streptokinase in acute myocardial infarction, N Engl J Med 312:1477-1482, 1983.

Kent KM, Smith ER, Redwood DR, and Epstein SE: Beneficial electrophysiologic effects of nitroglycerin during acute myocardial infarction, Am J Cardiol 33:513-516, 1974.

Khaja F et al: Intracoronary fibrinolytic therapy in acute myocardial infarction, N Engl J Med 308:1305-1318, 1983.

Lewis PS: Evaluation of the patient sustaining a right ventricular infarction and nursing implications, Crit Care Nurse, pp 50-54, Jan-Feb 1983.

Loeb HS, and Gunnar RM: Hemodynamic monitoring in a coronary care unit, Heart Lung 11:302-320, 1982.

Maroko PR, and Braunwald E: Modification of myocardial infarction size after coronary occlusion, Ann Intern Med 79:720-723, 1973.

Mathewson HS: Pharmacologic regulation of hemodynamic variables, J Cardiovasc Pulmonary Technology, pp 33-49, April-May 1982.

Miller RR et al: Combined dopamine and nitroprusside therapy in congestive heart failure, Circulation 55:881-884, 1977.

Mueller HS: Shock following acute myocardial infarction: assessment, pathophysiology, and therapy, J Cardiovasc Pulmonary Technology, pp 19-25, June-July 1980.

Mundth ED et al: Surgery for complications of acute myocardial infarction, Circulation 40:1279-1291, 1972.

Page DL et al: Myocardial changes associated with cardiogenic shock, N Engl J Med 285:133-137, 1971.

Parmley WW: The post-MI role of hemodynamic monitoring, Hosp Pract 17:169-175, 1982.

Rahimtoola S: Treatment of pump failure in acute myocardial infarction, JAMA 245:2093-2096, 1981.

Ratshin RA, Rackley CF, and Russell RO, Jr: Hemodynamic evaluation of left ventricular function in shock complicating myocardial infarction, Circulation 45:127-139, 1972.

Scheidt S, Alonso DR, Wilner G, and Killip T: New concepts of cardiogenic shock: preservation of ischemic myocardium, Bull NY Acad Med 50:247-254, 1974.

Shaver JA: Hemodynamic monitoring in the critically ill patient (corespondence), N Engl J Med 308:277-279, 1983.

Smith B, and Kennedy JW: Thrombolysis in the treatment of acute transmural myocardial infarction, Ann Int Med 106:414, 1987.

Sonnenblick EH, Frishman WH, and LeJemtel TH: Dobutamine: a new synthetic cardioactive sympathetic amine, Med Intelligence 300:17-22, 1979.

Spann JF: Changing concepts of pathophysiology, prognosis, and therapy in acute myocardial infarction, JAMA 74:877-886, 1983.

Symposium on vasodilator and inotropic therapy of heart failure, Am J Med 65:101-216, 1978.

Topol EJ: Tissue-type plasminogen activator in acute MI, Cardio 57-60, April 1988.

Topol EJ et al: A randomized, multicenter trial of intravenous tissue plasminogen activator and emergency coronary angioplasty in acute myocardial infarction: results from the TIMI study group, N Engl J Med 317:518-588, 1987.

Verstraete M: New thrombolytic drugs in acute MI: theoretical and practical consideration, Circulation 76(suppl II):II-31, 1987.

Weil MH, and Shubin H: Critical care medicine, New York, 1976, Harper & Row, Publishers, Inc.

Chapter 13

Hemodynamic Monitoring of the Patient with Pulmonary Disease

The close relationship between the heart and the lungs results in interactions that can alter the usual interpretation of hemodynamic data. Pulmonary disease imposes alterations in and limitations to hemodynamic evaluation of cardiac function. Thus it is essential not only to interpret hemodynamic data in relation to the overall clinical picture but also to have a basic understanding of the hemodynamic changes that can occur in patients with pulmonary disease.

HEMODYNAMIC ALTERATIONS IN PATIENTS WITH PULMONARY DISEASE

The relationships between right- and left-sided heart pressures and CO undergo variable changes in patients with primary pulmonary disease. Although it is possible for pulmonary disease to be present without any cardiac involvement, the interrelationship between the heart and the lungs more frequently leads to some degree of cardiac dysfunction. The cardiovascular effects of pulmonary disease are often categorized as (1) the "low cardiac output pattern" of dysfunction, with clinical features of the "pink-puffer" or "emphysematous type" associated with chronic obstructive lung disease, or (2) the "hypoxemic pattern" of dysfunction, with clinical features of the "blue-bloater" or "bronchial type" associated with obstructive lung disease.

Patients with pulmonary disease frequently have marked swings in intrathoracic pressure. The hemodynamic pressures measured in these patients parallel these intrathoracic pressure changes, with excessive drops in hemodynamic pressures during spontaneous inspiration.

The following hemodynamic alterations may be observed in patients with pulmonary disease.

RA Pressure

The RA pressure may be normal in patients with mild pulmonary disease (particularly in low output states) or moderately elevated in patients with more severe pulmonary disease. Elevated RA pressures resulting from pulmonary disease denote increased right heart dysfunction caused by increased PVR (afterload). Elevations in PVR can occur with primary pulmonary hypertension or as the result of vasoconstriction caused by hypoxemia and acidosis or by pulmonary obstructive processes such as severe obstructive lung disease and pulmonary embolus. With increases in resistance to flow through the right side of the heart, the *a* wave of the RA waveform becomes more dominant (Fig. 13-1).

Wide swings in the RA pressure can occur in conjunction with the respiratory cycle and large changes in intrathoracic pressure. For this reason it is important to obtain a mean RA pressure at end-expiration preferably over three to four respiratory cycles. This may require the use of a strip chart recorder to accurately assess end-expiration.

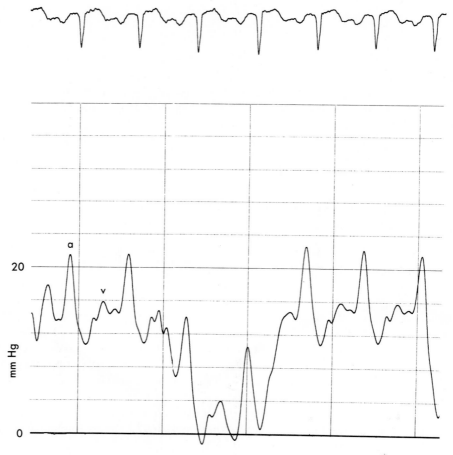

Fig. 13-1. RA pressure waveform with an elevated, dominant *a* wave secondary to pulmonary hypertension.

PA Pressure

The degree to which the PA pressure is changed as a result of pulmonary disease depends on the degree to which the PVR and/or the CO is altered. When evaluated in terms of the relationship between pressure, flow, and resistance (pressure = flow × resistance), it is apparent that the PA pressure could remain normal or be only mildly elevated in those patients with the "low cardiac output pattern" of pulmonary disease. This can be true in spite of mild elevations in PVR. However, with progressive pulmonary disease, PVR becomes markedly elevated even at rest. This results in elevated PA systolic, diastolic, and mean pressures. In the critical care setting, it is more common to find high PA pressures (pulmonary hypertension) resulting from pulmonary disease (Fig. 13-2).

PAW or LA Pressure

In patients without pulmonary disease or increases in PVR, the PA end-diastolic pressure equals the PAW or LA pressure (within a few mm Hg) and reflects the pressure in the LV at end-diastole. Because of the close approximation between the

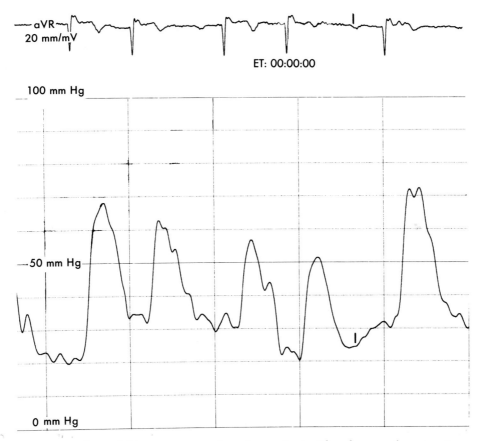

Fig. 13-2. Elevated PA pressure waveform in a patient with pulmonary hypertension.

PAEDP and the PAW or LA pressure, it is prudent to use the PAEDP as a reflection of LVEDP and thereby avoid the risks inherent in obtaining the PAW pressure (see Chapter 5). However, in the patient with pulmonary disease, or high PVR, this relationship is often altered. Although the PA pressure becomes elevated, reflecting the increased resistance to flow (PVR), the PAW or LA pressure may be normal; in the case of the "low cardiac output pattern" of pulmonary disease, the PAW or LA pressure may be low (Fig. 13-3). The PAW pressure does not reflect the increase in PVR for several reasons. First, when the balloon of the catheter is inflated to obtain a PAW pressure, forward blood flow ceases through the vessel in which it is located. The only pressure obtained is the retrograde reflection of pulmonary venous or LA pressure through the compliant pulmonary vasculature. Second, in patients with pulmonary disease, the marked reduction of lung compliance often prevents the transmission of increased pleural pressure to the pulmonary microvasculature.

However, errors in the measurement of PAW pressure in patients with pulmonary disease can be introduced and are important to bear in mind when evaluating hemodynamic data. Exaggerated increases in intrathoracic or alveolar pressures during expiration can be transmitted to the pulmonary microvasculature. This is more likely to occur in patients with chronic obstructive lung disease who have markedly increased airway resistance. Generally, this transmission of pressure occurs only when intrathoracic pressure changes are high (greater

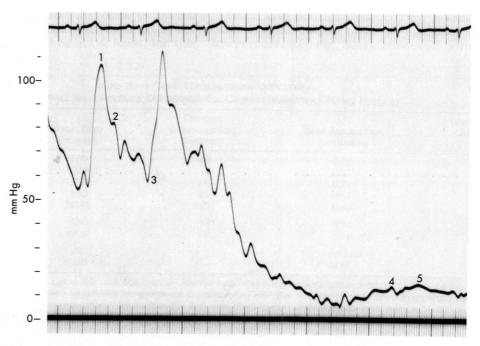

Fig. 13-3. Markedly elevated PA pressure (110/55 mm Hg) with a normal PAW pressure of approximately 11 mm Hg indicating increased PVR without cardiac dysfunction. (From Daily EK, and Schroeder JS: Hemodynamic waveforms: exercises in identification and analysis, St Louis, 1983, The CV Mosby Co.)

than 20 mm Hg) and in patients with compliant lungs, such as with emphysema. Additionally, increases in alveolar pressure could result in expanded zones I or II and invalidate the PAW pressure measurement (see the discussion below). However, in most patients with pulmonary disease, the PAW pressure approximates LVEDP.

Arterial Pressure

The alterations in arterial pressure that occur in conjunction with pulmonary disease are variable and depend primarily on alterations in CO. With low CO the arterial pressure may be normal or low, depending on the degree of reflex vasoconstriction. Paradoxical pulse may also be observed in the arterial pressure in patients with airway obstruction (Fig. 13-4).

Cardiac Output

Patients with relatively mild pulmonary disease generally have low normal CO values, whereas the CO tends to decrease to abnormally low levels in patients with severe obstructive pulmonary disease. An increase in right-sided afterload (PVR) is the major limiting factor of cardiac output in patients with pulmonary disease (Fig. 13-5). As a result of the low CO, the arteriovenous oxygen difference is abnormally wide. Further reductions in CO can occur if the patient develops LV dysfunction resulting from severe hypoxemia.

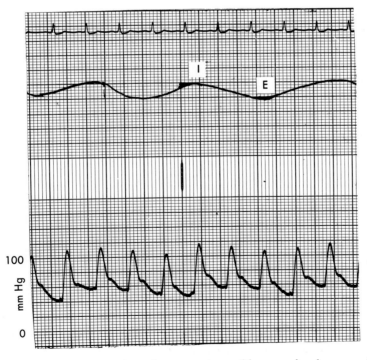

Fig. 13-4. Arterial pressure waveform demonstrating mild reversed pulsus paradoxus with an increase of approximately 14 mm Hg during mechanical inhalation. (Note pneumotachograph on upper portion of tracing indicating inhalation *(I)* and exhalation *(E)*.)

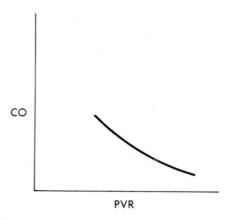

Fig. 13-5. Relationship between CO and PVR illustrating the effects of increased PVR on CO.

$S\bar{v}O_2$

Patients with pulmonary disease frequently have a lower than normal $S\bar{v}O_2$ as a result of increased oxygen extraction as a compensatory response to decreased oxygen delivery. If the CO is not adequately increased, or if it falls, $S\bar{v}O_2$ values decline.

HEMODYNAMIC MEASUREMENT AND INTERPRETATION IN PATIENTS WITH PULMONARY DISEASE

Alterations in hemodynamic pressures as a result of pulmonary disease require some precautions in interpretation of hemodynamic data. As previously discussed, errors in PAW measurement can occur with location of the tip of the catheter in either zone 1 or 2 of the lung. Although actual confirmation of catheter placement in zone 3 is done by a lateral chest x-ray examination, this is not always possible. However, there are some clinical clues that can aid in assessing catheter location. First, PAW pressure is always equal to or lower than PA diastolic pressure. If the PAW pressure exceeds the PAEDP, it is likely that it is artifactually increased, reflecting increased alveolar pressure as measured in zones 1 or 2. The absence of *a* and *v* waves in the PAW pressure contour and the appearance of a high, damped waveform with marked respiratory variation are other indications that the catheter may be located in zone 1 or 2, thus measuring alveolar pressure (Fig. 13-6).

Patients with chronic obstructive pulmonary disease frequently have increased chest diameters. This introduces the possibility of error in placement of the air-reference port of the transducer at the level of the RA. In the normal-sized chest, it is assumed that the heart lies in the midchest position, and therefore zeroing is performed with the air-reference port at this position. Increases in the diameter of the chest can alter this relationship and result in erroneous placement of the zero reference. Caution must be used in interpreting the absolute hemodynamic data in this situation, although trend monitoring can still be helpful.

Difficulty is commonly encountered in obtaining satisfactory PA and PAW

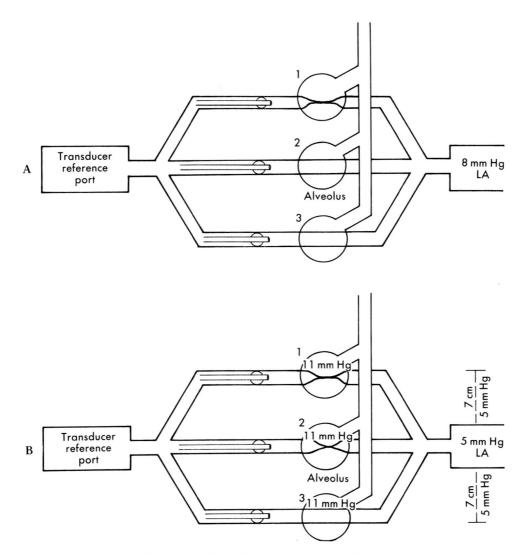

Fig. 13-6. Schematic illustration of the PA catheter in zones 1, 2, and 3 of the pulmonary circulation. **A,** Represents pressures in these areas with normal, spontaneous respiration. **B,** Represents these pressures with PEEP of 15 cm H_2O (11 mm Hg). Even in patients without increased airway pressure, the PAW pressure may not reflect LA pressure if the catheter tip is in zone 1, as in **A,** Increased airway pressure of 11 mm Hg results in collapse of the microvasculature when the catheter tip is located in either zones 1 or 2 *and* the LA pressure is low.

pressures in patients with pulmonary hypertension. Marked respiratory variation is usually noted in hemodynamic pressure measurements in patients with pulmonary disease. This mirrors the wide swings in intrathoracic pressure. Accurate hemodynamic pressure readings can be measured by obtaining an end-expiratory pressure reading and averaging the pressure reading over three to four respiratory cycles. This requires the use of either a paper write-out or a calibrated oscilloscope. Digital values displayed on the monitor represent the average of the current scope sweep and therefore cannot be correlated with the respiratory cycle.

HEMODYNAMIC MONITORING OF PATIENTS ON MECHANICAL VENTILATION

Mechanical ventilatory management in critically ill patients is used to: (1) improve oxygenation, (2) treat alveolar hypoventilation, and (3) reduce the work of breathing. Positive end-expiratory pressure (PEEP) is frequently applied to allow the reduction of the fractional concentration of oxygen in inspired gas (FiO_2) and to improve functional residual capacity and oxygen transport across the lungs. These interventions increase intrathoracic pressure and improve lung compliance and therefore affect hemodynamic pressure measurements. However, their beneficial aspects can be offset by a deleterious reduction in CO. The cardiovascular effects of mechanical ventilation correlate linearly with increases in intrapleural pressure. This, in turn, is influenced by the particular mode of ventilation and the level of positive pressure applied. Since PEEP produces the most deleterious effects on the cardiovascular system, much of the discussion will be directed toward its effects.

The normal respiratory variation is reversed in patients receiving mechanical ventilation. Cardiac and vascular pressures rise during mechanical inhalation and subsequently fall during mechanical exhalation.

RA Pressure

Measurement of the RA pressure relative to the atmosphere reveals an elevated RA pressure, reflecting the increase in intrathoracic pressure with mechanical ventilation. However, the actual RA transmural pressure (referenced to intrapleural pressure) often decreases as a result of the decrease in venous return that occurs when intrathoracic pressures are increased. The degree to which venous return is impeded, and hence the amount the RA transmural pressure falls, depends primarily on the amount of increase in mean intrapleural or airway pressure. Since PEEP applies pressure at end-expiration (when airway pressure normally is at its lowest point), it greatly increases the mean airway and intrapleural pressure.

PA Pressure

PA systolic, diastolic, and mean pressures are all usually elevated in patients receiving mechanical ventilation and PEEP. This is caused by the increase in PVR that occurs with increased airway pressure. Although venous return, pulmonic flow, and therefore CO fall as airway or intrapleural pressures are increased, the PVR increases dramatically (Fig. 13-7). This increase in RV afterload, coupled with the decrease in RV preload or filling, may be responsible for the major physiologic effect of increased airway or intrapleural pressure.

PAW and/or LA Pressure

PAW and/or LA pressures measured in reference to the atmosphere are usually elevated in patients with increased intrapleural pressure. However, the transmural left atrial filling pressures (measured directly or indirectly via the PAW pressure)

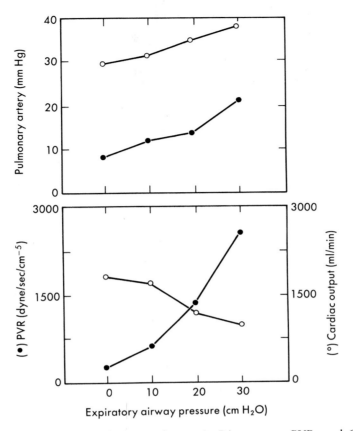

Fig. 13-7. Graphic illustration depicting changes in PA pressure, PVR, and CO with increased levels of PEEP. Note the marked increase in PVR with concomitant fall in CO as airway pressure is increased. The increase in PA pressure is much less dramatic because, although the PVR is high, the flow is low (P = F × R).

usually fall as airway or intrapleural pressures are increased and venous return and hence diastolic filling volumes decrease.

The degree to which the PAW pressure actually reflects the left-sided filling pressure (LA) depends on the alveolar or airway pressure, the compliance of the lung, the location of the catheter tip, and the pulmonary venous or LA pressure. Transmission of increased airway pressure can be markedly reduced when lungs become stiff and noncompliant. However, it is possible for the PAW pressure to reflect alveolar pressure rather than pulmonary venous or LA pressure. As described in the previous section, this can occur if (1) the catheter tip is located in either zone 1 or 2 of the lung (see Fig. 13-6), (2) alvelor pressures are increased to levels above the pulmonary intravascular pressure, and (3) the pulmonary venous or LA pressures are low. Fig. 13-6 illustrates the altered relationship between PAW and LA pressures and increased airway pressure with the catheter tip in two locations, above and below the LA. With the catheter tip in zone 1, the PAW reflects the increased alveolar pressure rather than the LA pressure. However, when the

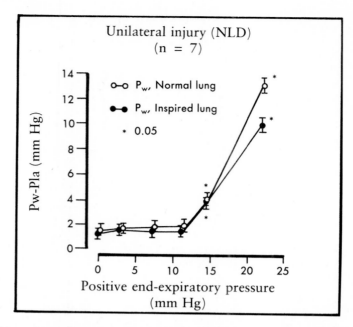

Fig. 13-8. Comparison of mean (± SEM) PAW - LA pressure differences obtained from injured and normal lungs at various PEEP levels in dogs with unilateral acid pneumnonitis positioned with the normal lung in the dependent position (NLD). Asterisk denotes significant increase in PAW-LA difference which occurs at PEEP levels above 15 mm Hg. (From Hasan FM, Weiss WB, Braman SS, and Hoppin FG: Influence of lung injury on pulmonary wedge-left atrial pressure correlation during positive end-expiratory pressure ventilation, Am Rev Respir Dis 131:246-250, 1985.)

catheter tip is positioned in zone 3 (below the level of the LA), the PAW pressure reflects LA pressure until the airway pressure exceeds 10 cm H_2O.

In patients with unilateral lung injury who receive PEEP therapy, the relationship between the PAW and LA pressures may also depend on location of the catheter in the injured or the normal lung. In these patients, the PAW pressure may correlate more closely with the LA pressure when the catheter is in the injured lung rather than in the normal lung. This may be because of alveolar flooding and localized atelectasis which protects intra-alveolar capillaries in the injured lung from the effects of increased airway pressure with PEEP. If the catheter tip is located in the normal lung, more accurate PAW pressure measurements can be obtained by placing the patient in a lateral position with the "normal" lung down (Fig. 13-8). However, with PEEP pressure above 15 mm Hg (11 cm H_2O), neither PAW or LA pressure accurately reflects LV preload or filling.

Although the PAW pressure usually reflects the LVEDP and volume, this relationship may also be altered in patients with increased PVR. It has been noted that elevations in PVR cause the intraventricular septum to deviate to the left, thereby decreasing LV end-diastolic volume in spite of increases in the LVEDP. This alteration in the pressure-volume relationship of the LV may overestimate the LVEDP (as reflected by the PAW pressures) in the presence of reduced LV end-diastolic volume (Fig. 13-9).

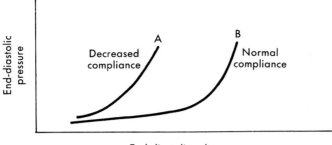

Fig. 13-9. Relationship between ventricular end-diastolic volume and end-diastolic pressure illustrating the effects of decreased compliance *(curve A)* on this relationship. With normal ventricular compliance, relatively large increases in end-diastolic volume are accompanied up to a point *(curve B)* by relatively small increases in end-diastolic pressure. In the noncompliant ventricle, small increases in end-diastolic volume are associated with marked increases in end-diastolic pressure.

Arterial Pressure

Peripheral arterial pressures remain unchanged or decrease with mechanical ventilation and PEEP. This is correlated to the decrease in CO that occurs with increasing levels of intrapleural pressure. The degree to which the arterial blood pressure falls depends on the amount of compensatory vasoconstriction that occurs with the decreased CO. The pulse pressure usually becomes narrower, reflecting decreased stroke volume. Exaggerated changes in the systolic arterial pressure in patients on mechanical ventilation are referred to as "reverse" or "positive pulsus paradoxus." A greater than 10 mm Hg *increase* during mechanical exhalation is felt to be an indication of hypovolemia, and can be reduced with volume administration (see the discussion see Fig. 13-4).

Cardiac Output

The greatest disadvantage of mechanical ventilation, particularly PEEP, is its deleterious effect on CO. The decrease in venous return and hence CO is directly correlated to increases in intrapleural or airway pressure (see Fig. 13-7) and is thought to be caused by the actual compressive effect of increased lung inflation that limits preload or cardiac filling. Increases in PVR, or right heart afterload, impose further limitation on ventricular output. Reductions in cardiac output are most significant in the presence of underlying hypovolemia.

Since tissue oxygenation depends not only on the oxygen saturation of blood but also on the rate of flow, the effects of mechanical ventilation on CO must be carefully assessed.

$$\text{Oxygen transport (OT)} = \text{CO} \times \text{Arterial oxygen content}$$

This formula for calculating oxygen transport shows the significance of both CO and the oxygen content in oxygen delivery or transport. If CO is severely depressed despite improvement in arterial oxygenation, it is highly possible to reduce rather than improve oxygen transport at the tissue level.

EXAMPLE: OT = CO × Arterial oxygen content (Hb × Oxygen saturation × 1.34 ml/g
Hb × 10)
884 ml/min = 5 L × 177 vol% (15 g × 0.88 × 1.34 ml/g Hb × 10)

Normally, oxygen transport is greater than 1000 ml O_2/min. Despite the fact that the CO is normal, oxygen delivery to the tissues is reduced because of hypoxemia (arterial saturation of 88%).

EXAMPLE: OT = CO × Arterial oxygen content
579 ml/min = 3 L × 19.3 vol% (150 gL × 0.96 × 1.34 ml/g Hb × 10)

This example illustrates the actual reduction in oxygen transport to the tissues that can occur with marked reductions in CO as a result of mechanical ventilation. In this case mechanical ventilation has improved oxygenation, as indicated by the increase in arterial saturation from 88% to 96%. However, coupled with a low CO, this is insufficient for adequate oxygen delivery. This points out the need to assess all the factors that contribute to oxygen supply rather than relying solely on the level of arterial oxygen saturation improvement.

Since hemodynamic measurements obtained with mechanical ventilation are altered by the increases in intrapleural pressure, various attempts have been made to more accurately measure transmural hemodynamic pressures during mechanical ventilation. These have included (1) the use of esophageal balloons and pericardial cannulas to record intrathoracic pressures, which are then subtracted from the measured hemodynamic pressures to obtain effective or transmural pressures, (2) the discontinuance of mechanical ventilation of PEEP during the hemodynamic measurement, and (3) measurement of pressures at end expiration as verified with transduced airway pressure. Discontinuing mechanical ventilation is generally not acceptable for several reasons. The sudden discontinuance of mechanical ventilation or PEEP can result in catastrophic hypoxemia and an immediate fall in functional residual capacity (FRC) and can also cause an initial sudden rise in venous return that does not reflect the true cardiovascular physiologic state of the patient. The use of esophageal balloons and intrapericardial cannulas to measure intrapleural pressures is fraught with a certain amount of vagaries and technical difficulties that precludes widespread clinical application.

One clinically valuable method of calculating transmural cardiac pressures is by estimation of intrapleural pressure and subtraction of it from the measured cardiac pressure.

Normal spontaneous respiration causes the intrapleural pressure to become negative (<760 mm Hg atmospheric pressure). Mean intrapleural pressure is normally about −5 cm H_2O or −3 mm Hg. The true transmural pressures therefore would really be the measured pressure minus this estimated intrapleural pressure.

EXAMPLE: PAWm − Pleural pressure = Transmural PAWm pressure
8 mm Hg − (−3 mm Hg) = 11 mm Hg

Because this difference is small and remains relatively constant during normal spontaneous breathing, it is not necessary to calculate the actual transmural hemodynamic pressures by subtracting −3 mm Hg from each pressure reading. However, if intrapleural pressures are increased to varying levels, the effect on measured hemodynamic pressures is more appreciable. The extent to which the intrapleural pressure is increased depends on the mode of ventilation. Control mode ventilation (CMV) increases mean airway and intrapleural pressure 5 to 10 cm H_2O or 3 to 7 mm Hg. The factors that influence the extent to which CMV increases intrapleural pressure are (1) the inspiratory/expiratory ratio, (2) the peak airway pressure, (3) the airway resistance, and (4) the lung compliance.

PEEP therapy increases the mean airway pressure during expiration. Because the critical care patient whose condition warrants the use of mechanical ventilation with PEEP usually has lungs that are stiff and noncompliant, it is felt that only about 30%, or one third or less, of the applied airway pressure is transmitted to the intrapleural space.

For further discussion of the methods of estimating intrapleural pressure for calculation of transmural pressure, the reader is referred to Phillips' article in the chapter references.

CLINICAL MANAGEMENT BASED ON HEMODYNAMIC PARAMETERS

The usefulness of monitoring hemodynamic parameters in patients receiving mechanical ventilation lies in its contribution to the formulation and titration of therapy. Since a definite balance must be struck between the beneficial effects of improved oxygenation and the deleterious effects of decreased CO, hemodynamic monitoring provides essential information to maintain this balance. The following are some of the more common therapeutic interventions employed to achieve this state of counterpoise.

Volume

With the drastic reductions in venous return and hence CO that can occur with increased intrathoracic pressure, it is frequently necessary to volume load the patient even before mechanical ventilation is initiated. Hemodynamic signs of hypovolemia, decreased ventricular filling, and hypoperfusion include:

1. Low transmural CVP or RAm pressure
2. Low transmural PAWm or LAm pressure
3. Low CO value

Clinical indications of decreased venous return and CO are flat neck veins, restlessness and confusion, reduced urine output, and cool, clammy skin. Volume infusion of a balanced electrolyte solution is often necessary to maintain transmural filling pressures of 15 to 18 mm Hg in an attempt to optimize CO according to the Starling law. This can be graphically plotted as a ventricular function curve when CO measurements are made in addition to monitoring the transmural PAW pressure.

Positive Inotropic Agents

A low CO in patients on mechanical ventilation can result from causes other than decreased venous return and ventricular filling. Severe hypoxemia can result in myocardial ischemia even in the presence of normal coronary arteries. This results in LV dysfunction and reduced contractility and ejection fraction. Hemodynamic evidence of this includes:

1. Low CO
2. Normal or high transmural PAWm or LAm pressure

Since the transmural PAWm pressure is normal or high, further increases in volume would be inappropriate and could result in pulmonary congestion and increased interference with oxygenation. Positive inotropic agents such as dopamine, dobutamine, and epinephrine may be necessary to improve ventricular contractility and hence stroke volume.

Vasodilators

As CO falls with the use of mechanical ventilation, sympathetic stimulation causes reflex vasoconstriction in an attempt to maintain an adequately perfusing blood pressure. This results in increased SVR. However, marked increases in SVR serve to further reduce CO by increasing afterload. Vasodilating agents or afterload-reducing agents are often necessary to interrupt this vicious circle. Hemodynamic data that suggest the need for a vasodilator such as nitroprusside or nitroglycerin include:

1. Low CO
2. Normal or high transmural PAWm or LAm pressure
3. High SVR

Precise hemodynamic monitoring allows support of the cardiovascular system during mechanical ventilation with or without PEEP, thereby minimizing the negative effects on the cardiovascular system. Several interventions can be used to improve cardiac performance during mechanical ventilation. Additionally, the use of intermittent mandatory ventilation (IMV) has been shown to be very useful in offsetting the negative effects of positive pressure ventilation. IMV lowers the overall *mean* intrathoracic pressure by allowing normal negative inspiratory pressures to occur several times each minute. This improves venous return and CO even at higher levels of PEEP.

Patient Example

A 69-year-old male with cancer of the pancreas and signs and symptoms of pyloric obstruction underwent a vagotomy and gastrojejunostomy. His postoperative course was stormy, and the patient manifested acute postoperative respiratory distress requiring FiO_2 greater than 60% and controlled ventilatory management. The patient's hemoglobin was also reduced to 12 g/dl (or 120 g/L). To maximize oxygen delivery and minimize dead space,

Table 13-1. Hemodynamic profile with *measured* hemodynamic pressures

Hemodynamic data	PEEP levels			
	0 cm H_2O	5 cm H_2O	10 cm H_2O	15 cm H_2O
Arterial saturation (%)	78	81	98	98
Arterial O_2 Content (vol%)	125	130	158	158
CO (L/min)	4.8	4.9	4.3	3.7
MAP (mm Hg)	78	77	74	71
RAm (mm Hg)	3	5	6	5
PAWm (mm Hg)	11	10	12	13
SvO_2 (%)	51	52	59	50

PEEP therapy was added. A pulmonary artery and arterial catheter had been inserted before the operation in this high-risk surgical patient. The measured hemodynamic data in Table 13-1 were obtained just before and following the institution of mechanical ventilation with gradual increments of PEEP therapy.

The hemodynamic data in Table 13-1 reveal a CO value within normal range until a PEEP level of 15 cm H_2O is reached. The MAP, PAWm, and RAm pressures all fall within the normal range and are obtained at end-expiration while the patient is on mechanical ventilation. The *transmural* RAm and PAWm pressures were calculated after estimating the patient's intrapleural pressure using the following formula:

$$\text{Intrapleural pressure} = \text{Normal pleural pressure} + \text{CMV pressure} + 1/3 \text{ PEEP}$$

Table 13-2 reveals the estimated intrapleural pressure for each level of PEEP and the esitmated transmural RA and PAW pressures when the intrapleural pressure is subtracted. It also reveals the oxygen transport at each level of PEEP obtained from the following formula:

$$\text{Oxygen transport} = \text{CO} \times \text{Arterial oxygen content (Hb} \times \text{Oxygen saturation} \times 1.34)$$

The data from Table 13-2 reveal an increase in arterial oxgenation from 78% to 81% at 5 cm H_2O PEEP. Since the CO remained approximately the same, this resulted in a desirable increase in oxygen delivery (from 600 to 637 ml/min), although it is still at a subnormal level. A look at the transmural RA and PAW mean pressures shows a decline in both filling pressures at 5 cm H_2O PEEP.

When PEEP is increased to 10 cm H_2O, there is a substantial increase in arterial oxygenation to 98%. Although the CO is reduced to 4.3 L/min, the proportionately larger increase in oxygen saturation results in improved oxygen transport to 679 ml/min. The transmural RA and PAW mean pressures remain low.

At 15 cm H_2O PEEP, the arterial oxygen saturation remains the same, but the CO is further reduced. The net result of this is a reduction in oxygen delivery despite improved arterial oxygenation. The transmural RA and PAW mean pressures remain low, reflecting reduced ventricular filling.

Thus in this patient it appears that a PEEP level of 10 cm H_2O is optimal in striking the balance between improved oxygenation and adequate cardiovascular function.

Subsequently, this patient's PEEP level was dropped to 10 cm H_2O and two units of

Table 13-2. Hemodynamic proile with *estimated* transmural hemodynamic pressures

Hemodynamic data	PEEP levels			
	0 cm H_2O	5 cm H_2O	10 cm H_2O	15 cm H_2O
Arterial saturation (%)	78	81	98	98
SvO_2(%)	51	52	59	50
Arterial O_2 Content (vol%)	125	130	158	158
CO (L/min)	4.8	4.9	4.3	3.7
MAP(mm Hg)	78	77	74	71
RAm (measured and transmural) (mm Hg)	3(6)	5(2)	6(2)	5(1)
PAWm (measured and transmural)(mm Hg)	11(14)	10(7)	12(8)	13(8)
Estimated intrapleural pressure (mm Hg)	−3	+3	+4	+5
Oxygen transport (ml/min)	600	637	679	585

Table 13-3. Hemodynamic profile with measured and estimated transmural hemodynamic pressures following transfusion

Hemodynamic data	PEEP level 10 cm H_2O
Arterial saturation (%)	99
Arterial O_2 content (vol%)	186
CO (L/min)	5.1
Svo_2 (%)	72
MAP (mm Hg)	80
RAm, measured (transmural) (mm Hg)	9(5)
PAWm, measured (transmural) (mm Hg)	20(16)
Estimated intrapleural pressure (mm Hg)	+4
Oxygen transport (ml/min)	947

whole blood were given to increase the patient's hemoglobin and filling pressures and thus improve tissue oxygenation. This resulted in a hemoglobin level of 14 g/dl and the hemodynamic data found in Table 13-3.

The administration of blood resulted in several improvements. First, it increased the filling pressures (RA and PAW), which resulted in improved CO according to the Starling law. Second, in increasing the hemoglobin to 14 g/dl, it increased oxygen transport to a normal level. Further increases in oxygen delivery to the tissues might be obtained by additional increases in CO, hemoglobin, or oxygen saturation of blood.

This case illustrates the benefits of careful measurement and interpretation of hemodynamic parameters in a patient receiving mechanical ventilation with PEEP and its use in guiding and titrating therapy. It allows the ability to select the appropriate intervention that will permit the best improvement in cardiovascular function and oxygenation.

REFERENCES

Agostoni E: Mechanics of the pleural space, Physiol Rev 52:57-128, 1972.

Bemis EC et al: Influence of right ventricular filling pressure on left ventricular pressure and dimension, Circ Res 34:498-504, 1974.

Benotti JR, and Dalen JE: Pulmonary embolism. In Horwitz LD, and Groves BM (editors): Signs and symptoms of cardiology, Philadelphia, 1985, JB Lippincott Co.

Benumof JL et al: Where pulmonary arterial catheters go: intrathoracic distribution, Anesthesiology 46:336-338, 1977.

Burrows B et al: The emphysematous and bronchial types of chronic airways obstruction: a clinicopathological study of patients in London and Chicago, Lancet 1:830-835, 1966.

Burrows B et al: Patterns of cardiovascular dysfunction in chronic obstructive lung disease, N Engl J Med 286:912-917, 1972.

Cengiz M, Crapo RO, and Gardner RM: The effect of ventilation on the accuracy of pulmonary artery and wedge pressure measurements, Crit Care Med 11:502-507, 1983.

Ditchey RV, Costello D, and Shebetai R: Effects of pressure and lung volume on left ventricular transmural pressure-volume relationships in humans, Am Heart J 106:46-51, 1983.

Esteban A, Gomez-Acebo E, and de la Cal MA: Pulsus paradoxus in acute myocardial infarction, Chest 81:47-50, 1982.

Filley GF et al: Chronic obstructive bronchopulmonary disease: oxygen transport in two clinical types, Am J Med 44:26-38, 1968.

Francis PB: Acute respiratory failure in obstructive lung disease, Med Clin North Am 67:657-668, 1983.

Gallagher TJ, Civetta JM, and Kirby RR: Terminology update: optimal PEEP, Crit Care Med 6:323-326, 1978.

Guyton, AC: Textbook of medical physiology, Philadelphia, 1981, WB Saunders Co.

Hasan FM, Weiss WB, Braman SS, and Hoppin FG: Influence of lung injury on pulmonary wedge-left atrial pressure correlation during positive end-expiratory pressure ventilation, Am Rev Respir Dis 131:246-250, 1985.

Hoffman J et al: Stroke volume in conscious dogs: effect of respiration, posture and vascular occlusion, J Appl Physiol 20:265-277, 1965.

Hudson LD: Ventilatory management of patients

with adult respiratory distress syndrome, Semin Respir Med 2(3):128-139, 1981.

Klose R, and Oswald PM: Effects of PEEP on pulmonary mechanics and oxygen transport in the late stages of acute pulmonary failure, Intensive Care Med 7:165-170, 1981.

Lozman J et al: Correlation of pulmonary wedge and left atrial pressures: a study in the patient receiving positive and expiratory pressure ventilation, Arch Surg 109:270-277, 1974.

Mathru M et al: Hemodynamic response to changes in ventilatory patterns in patients with normal and poor left ventricular reserve, Crit Care Med 10:423-426, 1982.

Matthay RA, and Berger HJ: Cardiovascular function in cor pulmonale, Clin Chest Med 4:269-295, 1983.

Moser KM, and Spragg RG: Use of the balloon-tipped pulmonary artery catheter in pulmonary disease, Ann Intern Med 98:53-58, 1983.

Nelson LD, Houtchens BA, and Westenskow DR: Oxygen consumption and optimal PEEP in acute respiratory failure, Crit Care Med 10:857-862, 1982.

Nelson LD, and Snyder, JV: Technical problems in data acquisition. In Snyder JV, and Pinsky MR: Oxygen transport in the critically ill, Chicago, 1987, Year Book Medical Publishers, Inc.

Philip C: Think transmural, Crit Care Nurse, 2(2):36-43, 1982.

Pierson DJ, and Hudson LD: Monitoring hemodynamics in the critically ill, Med Clin North Am 67:1343-1360, 1983.

Prewitt RM et al: Effect of positive-end expiratory pressure on left ventricular mechanics in patients with hypoxemic respiratory failure, Anesthesiology 55:409-415, 1981.

Primiano FP, Jr et al: Mean airway pressure: theoretical considerations, Crit Care Med 10:378-383, 1982.

Shapiro BA: Noncardiogenic edema, adult respiratory distress syndrome, and PEEP therapy. In Cane RD, and Shapiro BA (editors): Case studies in critical care medicine, Chicago, 1985, Year Book Medical Publishers, Inc.

Shapiro BA et al: Clinical application of respiratory care, ed 2, Chicago, 1979, Year Book Medical Publishers, Inc.

Simonneau G et al: A comparative study of the cardiorespiratory effects of continuous positive airway pressure breathing and continuous positive pressure ventilation in acute respiratory failure, Intensive Care Med 8:61-67, 1982.

Wiedmann HP, Matthay MA, and Matthay RA: Cardiovascular—pulmonary monitoring in the intensive care units, Chest 85:537-549 and 656-668, 1984

Chapter 14

Hemodynamic Monitoring of the Postoperative Cardiac Surgery Patient

PAT O. DAILY

The outcome for a patient undergoing cardiac surgery is determined by many factors. Three essential considerations are the patient's preoperative left ventricular function; the performance of the operation in an expedient, technically excellent manner and the provision of optimum conditions for postoperative recovery. Preoperative left ventricular dysfunction will predispose the patient to the likelihood of low cardiac output and left ventricular failure postoperatively. This should be anticipated, and the patient should be monitored vigilantly. Although an excellently performed operation may minimize postoperative problems, inadequate postoperative care may nullify that advantage and serve to increase morbidity and mortality.

The goals of optimum postoperative care are to (1) recognize, monitor, and assess all essential parameters, (2) anticipate potential hemodynamic or pulmonary instability for a given condition or situation, (3) detect deviations from acceptable ranges, and (4) intervene appropriately to reestablish optimum function.

Postoperative monitoring is the basis for appropriate postoperative management. Effective monitoring requires not only specific monitoring techniques, but also the knowledge of particular deviations that may occur. The techniques of hemodynamic monitoring that are employed after cardiac surgery are discussed in Chapters 5, 6, 7, and 8. This chapter emphasizes specific problems detected during monitoring of the patient following cardiac surgery.

Maintenance of a balance between myocardial oxygen supply and demand is imperative in the postoperative setting during which the myocardium is particularly vulnerable to ischemia. Fig. 14-1 schematically illustrates the determinants of myocardial oxygen consumption ($M\dot{V}O_2$), namely preload, afterload, and contrac-

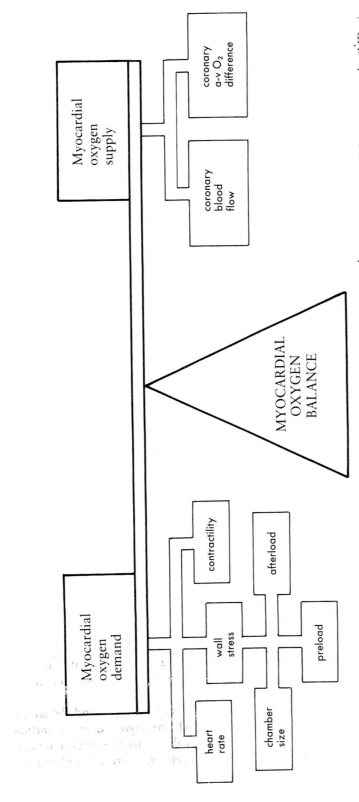

Fig. 14-1. Schematic illustration depicting the determinants of myocardial oxygen consumption ($\dot{M}Vo_2$) and myocardial oxygen supply ($\dot{M}Do_2$). Threats to myocardial oxygen balance by either an increase in myocardial oxygen demands or a decrease in myocardial oxygen supply can result in myocardial ischemia and ventricular dysfunction.

tility, as well as those of myocardial oxygen supply ($M\dot{D}o_2$). In light of this, it is apparent that hemodynamic monitoring of the determinants of both myocardial oxygen supply and demand is vital to assessment and management of the postoperative cardiac patient.

A major objective after cardiac surgery is the restoration of hemodynamic and ventilatory independence from supportive assistance while ensuring adequate tissue perfusion and gas exchange. Thus maintenance and monitoring of both cardiovascular and pulmonary parameters are equally essential. Incorporation of data from clinical assessment as well as hemodynamic monitoring, pulmonary function, and clinical laboratory studies provides the most accurate management of the patient after cardiac surgery.

Many immediate outcomes or postoperative problems can be anticipated on the basis of the patient's preoperative status. A patient with a low cardiac index, elevated left-sided pressures, and/or an ejection fraction of less than 50% preoperatively will be more likely to have problems with left ventricular dysfunction following surgery. There should be few surprises in the postoperative period if the clinician knows the patient's preoperative cardiac status.

A patient with single vessel coronary artery disease and no previous infarction or episodes of cardiac failure will most likely experience no significant postoperative complications. However, the patient with multiple coronary artery lesions, previous infarction, and decreased ejection fraction will likely have slower recovery and will need pharmacologic support of cardiac output.

The patient with valvular heart disease and a hypertrophied ventricle, as might be seen with preoperative aortic stenosis, is prone to hyperdynamic states postoperatively in which the generation of excessive cardiac output and hypertension might be problematic. Such a state markedly increases the demand for oxygen. Inotropic support is certainly not indicated for the patient whose ventricle is hypertrophied and generating cardiac outputs over 8 L/min. Instead, afterload reduction is appropriate to decrease SVR and thereby reduce hypertension, left ventricular work requirements, and myocardial oxygen consumption. Care must be taken to monitor the *pulse pressure* of the patient who is receiving vasodilator therapy rather than relying entirely on the mean airway pressure (MAP). A blood pressure of 175/45 mm Hg produces a MAP of 88 mm Hg that at first glance seems acceptable. However, this represents a pulse pressure of 130 mm Hg and an increased work requirement to support the high systolic pressure. At the same time, diastolic perfusion pressure is quite low and may be inadequate for coronary perfusion to meet energy requirements of a hypertrophied ventricle. In contradistinction, a blood pressure of 135/68 mm Hg represents a pulse pressure of 67 mm Hg and an MAP of 90 mm Hg. Although the mean pressure is essentially the same as in the previous example, the systolic work requirement is appreciably lower, and diastolic perfusion pressure is enhanced. This manipulation of blood pressure can be achieved with appropriate use of vasodilator therapy and careful monitoring of arterial blood pressure.

Volume requirements for this patient must also be considered in light of the hypertrophic state. A hypertrophied ventricle is stiff and less compliant. Large, sudden increases in volume may cause marked elevation of pulmonary venous pressure that may result in pulmonary edema. In the noncompliant ventricle, small changes in left ventricular volume result in larger changes in LVEDP and LA or PAW pressure (see Fig. 5-5). These measured values may overestimate left ventricular diastolic volume in a patient with a hypertrophied ventricle. Protecting the left ventricle from excessive oxygen demands is the key feature in the postoperative care of the patient with pure ventricular hypertrophy.

Diseases of valvular insufficiency with chronic volume overload result in dilatation of the ventricular chamber. Although concomitant ventricular hypertrophy may also occur, the dilatation completely alters the hemodynamic profile. This patient is more prone to low cardiac output states and hypotension postoperatively. Even after surgical correction of the valve, the patient may require increased left ventricular volumes. Preload monitoring with LA, PAW, or PAed pressures is useful in this situation to assess volume requirements and responses in cardiac output and SVR. In contrast to the patient with hypertrophy, this patient will demonstrate smaller increases in LA and PAW pressures with larger increases in volume. These pressures may therefore underestimate left ventricular diastolic volume. The optimum filling pressure for this patient should be determined by monitoring LA or PAW pressure response to volume therapy and measuring cardiac output to determine which filling pressure range produces optimum cardiac output according to the ventricular function curve. Actual plotting of the individual patient's ventricular function curve is very helpful in assessing optimum preload levels.

In low cardiac output states, particular attention must be given to SVR. Since MAP is a function of both cardiac output and SVR, MAP alone may not reflect the adequacy of cardiac ouput. If cardiac output begins to fall, SVR will most likely increase to maintain blood pressure. Monitoring MAP alone may not illustrate early hemodynamic changes in the patient. The key features in the care of this patient will be to determine and maintain adequate filling pressure and to assess the need for pharmacologic support of cardiac output with positive inotropic and/or afterload-reduction therapy.

EFFECTS OF ANESTHESIA AND SURGERY

Proper interpretation of postoperative monitoring data also requires knowledge of the effects of cardiac surgery and anesthesia on the cardiovascular and pulmonary systems. Myocardial depression occurs during the intraoperative phase and may extend into the postoperative period. Although there are multiple causes of myocardial depression, periods of intra-operative myocardial ischemia are most common.

Induction of anesthesia can be a particularly vulnerable time for the patient with cardiac disease. The physiologic stress of intubation can potentially cause a rapid release of catecholamines with resultant hypertension and tachycardia. Such an episode might precipitate significant ischemia and even infarction in the patient with coronary artery disease. This alone is a major reason for maintaining patients on prescribed beta-blocking agents until the time of surgery. This same catecholamine response can result in serious falls in cardiac output in patients with minimal cardiac reserve. Another contributing factor in such a patient is relative hypovolemia caused by chronic diuretic therapy and fluid restriction preoperatively. Resulting hypotension can again produce serious myocardial ishcemia. The anesthesiologist will take care to ensure that patients are adequately hydrated and sedated before induction to avoid such complications.

The optimum time for placement of monitoring lines is before induction of anesthesia. If the high-risk patient can be identified, it is desirable to have baseline hemodynamic parameters available, so that problems can be detected early and treated before the development of significant hypotension or hypertension that might result in ischemia. Monitoring is initiated with the placement of ECG leads, CVP catheter, an arterial pressure catheter, and in some patients a PA catheter. In some instances, a direct LA pressure catheter may be inserted during surgery in lieu of the PA catheter. This catheter demands extreme care to prevent air or clot embolization in the arterial system. To avoid this potentially lethal complication, the LA catheter is always aspirated before it is flushed or connected to the infusion line. It should also be clearly marked so that it is never used for withdrawal of blood samples or administration of any fluid or medication. Insertion of a urinary catheter before surgery is desirable because it allows continuous intraoperative and postoperative monitoring of urinary output. This continuous monitoring permits indirect assessment of cardiac output and renal function and precludes bladder distention.

Many anesthetic agents result in cardiac depression; however, with appropriate selection of the type of anesthetic agent and method of administration, this effect can be minimized. One approach is to administer large IV doses of morphine sulfate and diazepam while the patient inhales nitrous oxide. This method minimizes cardiac depression but causes respiratory depression, which may last several hours postoperatively, necessitating support with a ventilator and careful monitoring of oxygenation.

Another major cause of myocardial depression is the myocardial ischemia that is produced by cross-clamping of the ascending aorta to allow valve replacement or other intracardiac repairs. Aortic cross-clamping excludes perfusion to the coronary arteries, resulting in myocardial ischemia and ventricular dysfunction. Some protection may be afforded by myocardial hypothermia, coronary perfusion, and cardioplegia, but this protection is not complete. When the aorta is not cross-clamped, long periods of induced ventricular fibrillation during surgery may result in subendocardial ischemia and ventricular dysfunction. In addition to depressing myocardial function and contractility, ischemia may aggravate or cause arrhythmias.

Whole-body hypothermia (30° to 32° C) is used during cardiopulmonary bypass to reduce body metabolism and oxygen demand. This reduction in temperature causes vasoconstriction and increased SVR, which may extend into the postoperative period. As rewarming occurs, vasoconstriction decreases and the vascular space increases, resulting in relative hypovolemia and hypotension. Since this hypotension is caused by hypovolemia, it can be recognized hemodynamically by a low CVP or PAW pressure and appropriately managed by blood or fluid replacement.

If cardiopulmonary bypass is prolonged, widespread systemic effects may occur. Microemboli, consisting of blood-cellular elements, fat aggregates, and protein breakdown products, may form in the pump and embolize to the lungs, heart, brain, and kidneys. Embolization and occlusion of the capillary beds of these or-

Sample postoperative ICU advance information sheet

Patient name _____

Age _____ Preoperative weight _____

Diagnosis _____

Other health problems _____

Surgical procedure _____

Operative problems _____

(Check or complete the following)

A. Respiratory (please notify Inhalation Therapy)
1. Ventilator requested? _____ Type? _____
   Anticipated tidal volume? _____ PEEP? _____ cm H_2O
2. T-piece system requested (no ventilator needed)? _____
3. Patient will be extubated? _____
4. Humidified mask oxygen? _____

B. Monitoring
1. Arterial catheter? _____ Location _____
2. CVP catheter? _____ Location _____
3. PA catheter? _____ Location _____
4. LA catheter? _____

C. Intravenous infusions presently in use
Dopamine _____ Epinephrine _____ Nitroglycerin _____
Dobutamine _____ Calcium chloride _____ Lidocaine _____
Isoproterenol _____ Nitroprusside _____
Others _____

D. Please prepare a fresh infusion of _____
_____ Standard _____ Double _____ Other

E. Special information
1. Left ventricular device in use
   _____ Intra-aortic balloon
   _____ Other
2. Request cardiac outputs early postoperatively _____
3. Miscellaneous _____
   _____

F. Laboratory studies drawn in OR and time drawn
Coagulation panel _____ Potassium _____
Hematocrit, platelets _____ Enzymes _____
Blood gases _____ Other _____

Estimated time of arrival in ICU _____ AM _____ PM

gans result in decreased perfusion, which may lead to focal necrosis. With modern cardiopulmonary bypass techniques and improved oxygenators and filters, however, this problem has been minimized. Prolonged cardiopulmonary bypass, with extended periods of low perfusion pressure, increases the risk of tissue ischemia and the incidence of coagulation abnormalities. Other sources of myocardial ischemia during surgery include inadequate analgesia causing catecholamine release, prolonged hypotension, prolonged hypertension, arrhythmias, and hypoxemia.

At the conclusion of cardiopulmonary bypass, two mediastinal tubes are inserted to prevent accumulation of blood and to monitor blood loss. One tube is positioned anterior to the heart in the midline, and another right-angle chest tube is positioned from the superior aspect of the diaphragm to the posterior pericardium. If the right pleural space were opened during the surgical procedure, a chest tube would also be inserted at this time.

The orotracheal or nasotracheal airway established for the anesthetic is left in place in practically all patients. This provides for assisted ventilation in the early postoperative period when respiratory depression from anesthesia may be present. A safer, smoother transition from anesthesia and surgery can be achieved when sedation can be maintained during the rewarming phase, a period of great potential hemodynamic instability.

TRANSFER TO INTENSIVE CARE UNIT

A critical period in the patient's postoperative course occurs during the transfer from the operating room to the intensive care unit. Serious arrhythmias, volume changes, and blood pressure changes can occur during this relatively short period of time. The goal is to optimize conditions for a smooth transition from the operating room to the intensive care unit. Staff in the intensive care unit should know what to expect and be prepared for the patient's arrival to minimize inefficiency that is inherent in confusion. One method of facilitating a smooth transfer is via communication with the operating room team. The box on p. 363 illustrates a written report format that can be sent by the anesthesiologist as the patient's chest is being closed. This is generally around 45 minutes to 1 hour before arrival. The report is brief but outlines the monitoring and pharmacologic support to be expected. Also included are approximate ventilator settings, so that time is not wasted preparing the ventilator for the patient after arrival in the ICU. Any problems that developed during surgery can also be outlined. This allows extra time to set up additional monitoring systems and to secure extra staff if necessary. A quick "on-the-way" call from the operating room staff just before the patient's departure also ensures optimum readiness to admit the patient to the intensive care unit.

When the patient is connected to the monitoring equipment in the intensive care unit, priorities should be established to minimize problems and confusion. One approach follows:

1. Connect the ECG monitoring leads for immediate monitoring of the heart rate and detection of arrhythmias or cardiac arrest. During this time, blood pressure may be monitored by an anaeroid manometer previously connected to the arterial pressure line (p. 172) or simply estimated by palpation of the femoral or brachial artery.

2. Connect the ventilator to the patient's airway. Adequate ventilation can be checked by watching the patient's chest move during respiration. Air movement into both lungs must be confirmed by auscultation of both the right and left sides of the chest. Since serious errors may occur when reliance is placed solely on spirometer tidal volume measurements, adequacy of venti-

lation is accurately determined by arterial oxygen saturation measurements. To avoid hypoxia, ventilation is initiated with 80% oxygen; the percentage of oxygen is then decreased as guided by Pao_2 determinations.

3. Connect the pulse oximeter sensor to the oximeter.

4. Connect venous and pulmonary artery pressure lines to their appropriate transducers, IV infusion systems, and oximeter, if appropriate. At this time, after noting mean arterial pressure, clarify volume and drug infusion rates as well as hemodynamic parameters desired by the physician. This is also a good time to quickly note the amount of drainage in the chest tube drainage system.

5. Connect the arterial pressure line to its appropriate transducer and IV infusion systems.

6. Milk or strip the chest tubes, record the amount of drainage, and connect them to the vacuum source if suction is to be applied.

7. Measure and empty urine drainage from the operating room and begin hourly urine output monitoring.

8. Insert a nasogastric tube to prevent abdominal distention from positive pressure ventilation.

9. Insert a rectal temperature probe.

10. Clarify expectations, potential problems, and unique features for the care of the patient with the attending physician.

11. Institute rewarming measures such as the use of warm blankets or blood warmers.

12. Once the patient is hemodynamically stable and ventilation is adequate, obtain a chest x-ray film with portable equipment. This film serves several purposes: it establishes a baseline from which to compare subsequent changes in mediastinal or cardiac size; it rules out pneumothorax; and it identifies the location of the endotracheal tube, nasogastric tube, and intracardiac monitoring catheters. It is particularly important to ensure that the endotracheal tube is positioned neither near the larynx nor in the right or left bronchus. The optimum location of the endotracheal tube tip is 1 to 2 cm above the carina. The examination also serves to monitor changes in pulmonary vascularity, which can reflect abnormalities in cardiac function and fluid balance. At this time, also obtain blood samples for arterial blood gases, serum potassium, hematocrit, and coagulation studies, if warranted.

13. Obtain a 12-lead ECG to serve as a baseline from which to interpret any changes.

EARLY POSTOPERATIVE MONITORING
Assessment of Cardiac Output

Since low cardiac output is the most common immediate postoperative problem, it is crucial to carefully assess and measure cardiac output. The thermodilution technique of cardiac output measurement is most commonly used in the critical care setting (see the discussion in Chapter 7). However, because of the severe hypothermia that is often present in the immediate postoperative phase, it may be necessary at times to use ice-temperature rather than room-temperature injectate to measure the cardiac output. A minimum of 12° difference between the injectate and the core temperature is necessary to reliably measure ensuing temperature differences.

If serial thermodilution cardiac outputs are not measured postoperatively, arterial pressure monitoring may be used as the hemodynamic parameter reflecting cardiac output. Systemic hypotension always suggests the possibility of a low cardiac output and inadequate tissue perfusion. Additional, less direct evaluation of tissue perfusion may be obtained by monitoring changes in the peripheral circulation. Peripheral perfusion can be assumed to be adequate if extremities are warm and have rapid capillary filling and full peripheral pulses (radial, dorsalis pedis, and posterior tibial). A urinary output greater than 40 ml/hr also usually indicates an adequate cardic output.

Although low cardiac output in the postoperative setting may be because of preoperative or perioperative factors, hypovolemia, decreased myocardial contractility, and cardiac tamponade are the three most likely causes of low cardiac output and hypotension postoperatively. However, assessment of intravascular volume and vascular resistance during rewarming is also crucial and plays a major role in providing early hemodynamic stabilization. Alterations in cardiac output postoperatively must be assessed and interpreted with regard to the determinants of cardiac output, namely preload, afterload, and contractility (see Table 14-1).

Preload, the ventricular filling volume (or pressure), is clinically measured by the RA, LA, or PAW pressures. Decreases in filling volume, or hypovolemia, in the postoperative setting may occur as a result of actual blood loss or as a result of fluid shifts from the vascular space to the interstitial spaces. The use of mannitol during cardiopulmonary bypass also increases diuresis after bypass, which can further reduce vascular volume. However, the most common cause of decreased filling, or hypovolemia, postoperatively relates to the increase in vascular space that occurs as the patient rewarms following induced hypothermia. As the peripheral vessels begin to dilate with temperature rise, the vascular space and thus the requirements for additional volume increases. This requirement should be anticipated and appropriate vasodilators and volume administered to establish adequate circulation volume before this occurrence.

Careful monitoring and maintenance of optimum ventricular filling pressures allow time to recognize and treat developing hypovolemia before the development of serious hypotension. For this reason, MAP should always be evaluated along with the CVP and heart rate response. It is initially possible for the MAP to remain relatively unchanged because of SVR changes in spite of decreases in intravascular volume. An increase in heart rate with a downward trend in CVP should alert the clinician to the possibility of developing hypovolemia, even though MAP has not dropped markedly. Right- and left-sided filling pressures that are both low (less than 8 and 12 mm Hg respectively) provide confirmation of hypovolemia. Changes in right-sided pressures appear later than left-sided changes because of the more compliant nature of the venous system.

Another less common cause of relative hypovolemia resulting from changes in the vascular space is an allergic reaction. An antigen-antibody response from drug or transfusion reactions can result in decreased SVR caused by histamine release. The resultant hypotension is caused by insufficient volume to fill the increased vascular space. The change in preload requirement will result in decreased CVP and LA or PAW pressures. Temporary support of blood pressure can be achieved with vasopressors until the causative factor is removed or treated and vascular volume has been restored.

The fluid replacement of choice varies from institution to institution. There is a trend in most centers to maintain patients in a state of normovolemic anemia. Minimal blood replacement decreases the risk of hepatitis transmission and conserves valuable blood products. Maintenance of the hemotocrit at 30% is acceptable for most patients. Transfusion of blood for hematocrits below this level is indicated. This, of course, would not apply to any patient who is seriously bleeding. Iron therapy can be initiated in the postoperative period to aid in the restoration of a normal hematocrit. For individuals with significant left ventricular dysfunction, a lower hematocrit may not be indicated. Lower oxygen-carrying capacity will necessitate an increase in heart rate or cardiac output to maintain adequate oxygen delivery to tissues. This extra demand might outweigh the benefits of normovolemic anemia. Care must also be taken to monitor such a patient for arrhythmias that could be hypoxic in origin. Volume replacement for the majority of patients will most likely be either crystalloid (normal saline), colloid (albumin), Hep-starch, or a combination of these.

Decreased afterload or resistance may occur postoperatively secondary to anaphylaxis (a reaction to blood, protamine, or drug allergy) or in the presence of sepsis.

Ventricular contractility, another determinant of cardiac output, is almost always depressed immediately after cardiac surgery as a result of the affects of anesthesia and hypothermia as well as ventricular ischemia. Calculation of the stroke work index of the left and right ventricles is used as a reflection of their contractile state (see Table 10-1).

Afterload, in the clinical setting, is reflected by the resistance to ventricular ejection (SVR for the left side, PVR for the right side) (see Table 10-1). Since afterload is inversely related to cardic output, it is an important hemodynamic parameter to monitor and effectively manipulate to improve flow. Increased afterload manifested by elevated SVR is commonly seen postoperatively as a result of hypothermia, increased circulating catecholamines, and surgical stimulation. High afterload may exist despite normal arterial blood pressures if cardiac output is reduced (Pressure = Flow × Resistance). Therefore, calculation of the SVR is clinically necessary to evaluate afterload of the left side of the heart.

Case 1

A 50-year-old man underwent an uncomplicated aortic valve replacement. On arrival in the ICU, he was still well sedated (not yet able to be aroused) and hypothermic. A pulmonary artery catheter inserted before induction remained in place. Initial vital signs demonstrated elevated MAP and SVR. Immediately after arrival, nitroprusside therapy was begun to control hypertension. Over the next 2 hours, right- and left-sided filling pressures gradually decreased as heart rate increased. Cardiac index also fell despite reductions in SVR. After 2 hours, the patient's temperature had risen to 36° C. Vasodilation had occurred from both rewarming and nitroprusside therapy, creating a state of relative hypovolemia. Hemodynamic stability was achieved in this patient with adequate fluid administration.

During hypothermia, SVR can be quite elevated, and this greatly increases the oxygen demand of the heart. This is a period in which patients are also prone to

Case 1

	Arrival	30 min	1 hr	90 min	2 hr	3 hr
HR (beats/min)	92	90	94	100	110	80
MAP (mm Hg)	110	100	90	85	70	85
PAW (mm Hg)	8	8	7	5	4	8
CVP (mm Hg)	10	10	10	8	7	10
CI (L/min/m^2)	3.4	—	3.2	—	2.8	4.0
SVR dynes/sec/cm^{-5}	2000	—	1600	—	1100	1100
Temperature (°C)	34	34	35	35	36	36
Rx	—	0.5 µg/kg/min nitroprusside	1 µg/kg/min nitroprusside	1.5µg/kg/min nitroprusside	1 µg/kg/min nitroprusside; volume therapy	1 µg/kg/min nitroprusside; 400 ml saline; 250 ml albumin

hypertension. Excessive pressure elevation places stress on new suture lines, increasing the risk of potential tears in the suture line with resultant hemorrhage. Vasodilators are used to treat hypertension by reducing vascular resistance and to enhance peripheral perfusion. When vasodilator therapy is begun, great care must be taken to watch for changes in preload requirements. The rewarming process will almost always require additional fluid administration.

If the right- and left-sided filling pressures rise after fluid replacement but hypotension and low cardic output persist, *myocardial failure* with decreased contractility must be considered. In this case positive inotropic agents may be required to improve cardiac output and blood pressure. Cases of severe myocardial depression may require a combination of positive inotropic agents and vasodilators to optimize cardiac output. In this instance it is essential to use serial cardiac output determinations with calculation of SVR to maintain the proper balance of inotropic agents and vasodilators for maximal cardiac output.

Case 2

A 47-year-old woman underwent uncomplicated mitral valve replacement for recurrent mitral stenosis. Following surgery, she remained in a state of low CO even with the administration of IV dopamine. Four hours postoperatively, the patient's cardiac index was 1.45 L/min/m^2 and the SVR was 2350 dynes/sec/cm^{-5}. The addition of IV nitroprusside with concomitant volume therapy resulted in a significant increase in cardiac index to 2.21 L/min/m^2 and a decrease in SVR to 1370 dynes/sec/cm^{-5} (Fig. 14-2).

Left ventricular failure is recognized by decreasing peripheral perfusion, which is usually seen in the form of decreased pulses, capillary refill, skin temperature, and urine output. Forward flow of blood is impaired by depressed contractility. As blood flow backs up in the pulmonary vasculature, rales will be evident when breath sounds are assessed. A rise in SVR is predictable as a result of an attempt to maintain blood pressure. The resulting increase in afterload further compromises

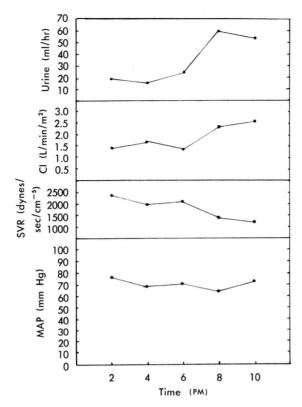

Fig. 14-2. Improvement in cardiac index associated with reduction of systemic vascular resistance in response to intravenous nitroprusside therapy. The slight decrease in mean arterial pressure suggests that the reduction of excessive systemic vascular resistance is responsible for the increase in cardiac index. *MAP,* Mean arterial pressure; *SVR,* systemic vascular resistance; *CI,* cardiac index.

cardiac performance. The left ventricle's inability to handle volume will also be reflected by an increase in left-sided filling pressures (mean LA or PAW pressures).

Ventricular contractility may also be excessive in the later postoperative period. This is more commonly seen in patients with preexisting ventricular hypertrophy (such as in AS, IHSS, or systemic hypertension) as well as in conjunction with positive inotropic agents. Increased contractility markedly increases myocardial oxygen consumption and causes systemic hypertension which endangers suture lines and grafts and can cause hemorrhage. Reductions in contractility, if necessary, can be achieved with the use of beta-blocking agents or calcium channel blockers possessing negative inotropic effects.

The persistence of inadequate cardiac output after correction of hypovolemia may also be caused by *cardiac tamponade.* This complication is also manifested by a markedly elevated venous pressure and low arterial pressure. The diastolic pressures of both the right and the left sides of the heart tend to equilibrate because of the constriction of the heart by the accumulation of blood in the pericardial space. There may also be a characteristic pattern to the RA or RV pressure (Chapter 5).

An excessive output of blood through the chest tubes (greater than 300 ml/hr) before the development of systemic hypotension may suggest impending cardiac tamponade. Although a paradoxical pulse (fall in systolic pressure over 10 mm Hg during inspiration) is usually present in cardiac tamponade, the use of a positive pressure ventilator obscures these signs. Their absence therefore does not rule out the complication of cardiac tamponade. Significant mediastinal widening, as determined by serial chest x-rays provides strong evidence that cardiac tamponade may be responsible for a low cardiac output. Surgical removal of the clotted blood is the definitive management of cardiac tamponade. However, fluid replacement to ensure adequate filling (despite already high filling pressures) and administration

Table 14-1. Evaluation of inadequate cardiac output

Findings	Causes	Correction
BP or MAP ↓ CVP and left-sided filling pressure ↓ Urine outut ↓ Peripheral circulation ↓	Hypovolemia	Expansion of volume
BP or MAP ↓ CVP and left-sided filling pressure ↓ Peripheral circulation adequate Urine output adequate	↓ Peripheral vascular resistance Allergic response	Expansion of volume Alpha-adrenergic drugs (for example, methoxamine)
BP or MAP ↓ CVP ↓ and left-sided filling pressure ↑ Peripheral circulation ↓ Urine output ↓	Left-sided heart failure LA thrombus Intraoperative myocardial infarction Valve malfunction	Inotropic agents; afterload reduction Surgical correction Inotropic agents: diuretics; afterload reduction Surgical correction
BP or MAP ↓ CVP ↑ and left-sided filling pressure ↓ Urine output ↓ Peripheral circulation ↓	Right-sided heart failure Pulmonary embolism Valve malfunction	Inotropic agents Heparin; vasopressors; possibly surgery Surgical correction
BP or MAP ↓ CVP and left-sided filling pressure ↑ Urine output ↓ Peripheral circulation ↓	Cardiac failure Cardiac tamponade	Inotropic agents: diuretics Surgical correction
Arrhythmias	Hypoxemia Hypokalemia Hypocalcemia Drug-induced Surgical trauma Other (idiopathic)	Maintenance of adequate Pao_2 Potassium replacement Calcium replacement Withholding of further medication Additional measures (pharmacologic treatment, electroversion)

of inotropic agents to optimize cardiac contractility are important adjuncts in preparing the patient for reoperation.

Case 3

A 60-year-old woman underwent distal right coronary endarterectomy with saphenous vein bypass grafts from the aorta to the distal right, left anterior descending, and circumflex coronary arteries because of preinfarction angina resulting from coronary artery disease. Postoperatively, hypotension slowly developed and persisted even though the filling pressures (CVP and PAW) increased to 15 mm Hg after blood replacement (Fig. 14-3). Her extremities remained cool. Comparison of the chest x-ray film taken immediately postoperatively (Fig. 14-4, *A*) with that taken 5 hours postoperatively (Fig. 14-4, *B*) revealed marked

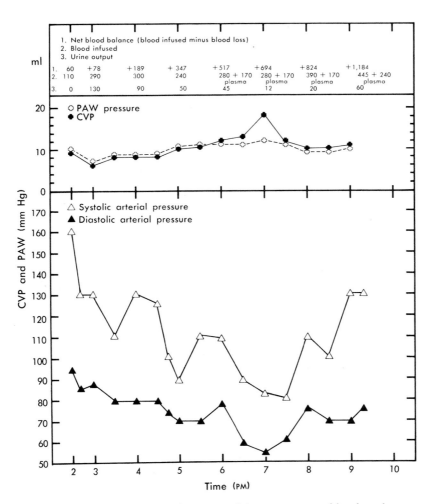

Fig. 14-3. Changes in vital signs with time and in response to blood replacement and dopamine. Although the CVP and the PAW pressure rise during fluid replacement, the arterial pressure falls until the blood balance is significantly increased and dopamine is added. At the time of the patient's return to surgery, the blood replacement is 1184 ml more than the measured loss, and the patient is given an additional 750 ml of plasma. The fluid replacement, along with the dopamine, results in an arterial pressure of 130/70 mm Hg.

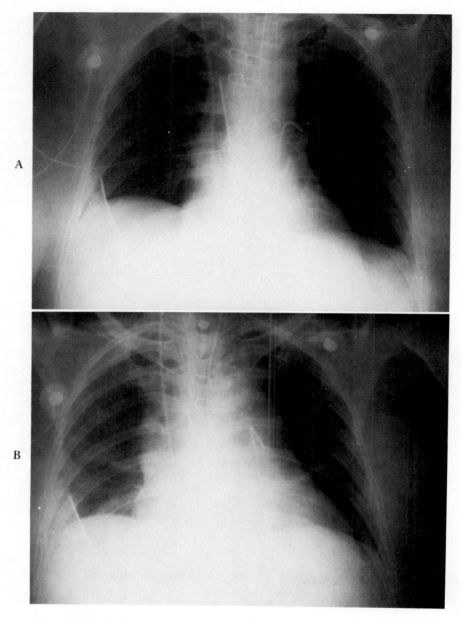

Fig. 14-4. A, Chest roentgenogram taken immediately after the patient's arrival in the intensive care unit. The mediastinum is not widened, and there is no apparent fluid collection in the pleural spaces. The chest tubes in the right pleural space and in the mediastinal space are apparent. Swan-Ganz catheter is visualized in the left pulmonary artery. A nasogastric tube is present in the esophagus and stomach. **B,** Chest roentgenogram taken 4½ hours later. There is considerable mediastinal widening, consistent with cardiac tamponade.

mediastinal widening. Cardiac tamponade was suspected, and reoperation was immediately performed. At surgery blood clots surrounding the heart were removed, and bleeding was controlled. Following this surgery, arterial pressure and tissue perfusion returned to normal without the use of vasopressors.

Abnormal heart rates and rhythms may also cause decreases in cardiac output (CO = HR × SV). Very slow heart rates, which can be seen postoperatively as a result of excessive hypothermia, can reduce cardiac output despite relatively normal stroke volumes. Augmentation of the heart rate via the implanted atrial or ventricular pacing wires, or by pharmacologic means may be necessary to augment cardiac output. Tachycardias are frequently seen postoperatively in the presence of hypovolemia. Excessive heart rates (>120 bpm) may reduce cardiac output and coronary filling time as well as increase myocardial oxygen consumption. If the heart rate remains rapid after adequate volume restoration, pharmacologic intervention with calcium channel blockers or beta-blockers may be necessary to reduce the rate and improve the oxygen supply and demand balance.

The immediate detection and accurate diagnosis of *arrhythmias* is important because of the potentially adverse effect of arrhythmias on cardiac output caused by impaired diastolic filling time. Ventricular extrasystoles may indicate myocardial irritability and the increased probability of more serious arrhythmias to follow. Hypoxemia, hypokalemia, and cardiovascular drugs are frequent causes of arrhythmias in the postoperative patient. These contributory causes should be carefully looked for and treated when arrhythmias are present. In the absence of specific etiologic factors, antiarrhythmic treatment, cardioversion, or both are used.

Other causes of low cardiac output postoperatively include inadequate prosthetic valvular function or residual RV or LV outflow obstruction. Abnormal valve sounds during auscultation of the heart may indicate prosthetic valvular malfunction, but right- or left-sided heart catheterization with angiography must be performed to confirm the diagnosis. LA thrombus formation is a rare and extremely serious complication, causing low cardiac output. It is most often seen after mitral valve replacement in association with atrial fibrillation. Unrecognized coronary artery disease or intraoperative myocardial infarction may also cause low cardiac output and hypotension. Serial monitoring of cardiac enzymes and ECGs assist in the diagnosis.

CARDIOVASCULAR EFFECTS ASSOCIATED WITH RESPIRATION

Since tissue perfusion and gas exchange are essential for cellular metabolism, monitoring pulmonary function and oxygenation is an essential adjunct to monitoring the cardiovascular system. For example, inadequate ventilation will result in carbon dioxide retention and hypoxemia. If this inadequate ventilation persists, respiratory and metabolic acidosis in conjunction with hypoxemia will depress cardiac function. This negative inotropic effect is aggravated by a depressed response to inotropic agents because of acidosis and hypoxia, and the result is progressive cardiac failure.

Continuous measurement of mixed venous oxygen saturation (Svo_2) is very helpful in assessing the adequacy of cardiac output and oxygen delivery to the tissues (see the discussion in Chapter 8). Declines in Svo_2 to 60% or less indicate a decrease in oxygen supply or an increase in oxygen demand and frequently precede any other hemodynamic change. Assessment of the components of oxygen delivery (cardiac output, hemoglobin, and arterial oxygen saturation) should be made whenever the Svo_2 falls 5% to 10%. Svo_2 has been shown to be a sensitive indicator of overall or global tissue oxygenation.

After cardiac surgery the primary concerns regarding respiration are the work of breathing, gas exchange, and maintenance of acid-base balance. A normal, resting individual requires 2% to 4% of the basal energy for cardiorespiratory function, whereas this requirement markedly increases postoperatively. Several factors responsible for the increased work of ventilation postoperatively are the following:

1. A decrease in chest wall compliance resulting from thoracotomy and pain-induced muscle spasm.
2. A decrease in lung compliance resulting from a reduction in pulmonary surfactants (Left-sided heart failure of any cause results in pulmonary venous congestion, further reducing lung compliance. Chronic preoperative pulmonary edema will also render the lungs less compliant in the postoperative period.)
3. Increased production and retention of airway secretions resulting in elevated airway resistance
4. Postoperative shivering causing decreased chest wall compliance

To decrease the work of breathing, all postoperative patients receive mechanical ventilatory assistance. Experience has shown that this practice also reduces the incidence of arrhythmias and cardiac arrest. Assisted ventilation via an endotracheal tube is used for 48 to 72 hours after surgery. Low-pressure, high-volume cuffs on contemporary endotracheal tubes allow maintenance of intubation for periods of up to 1 week without damaging effects to the trachea.

Ventilatory assistance via a closed airway requires careful control and monitoring of ventilation and oxygenation, including respiratory rate (with or without triggering by the patient), tidal volume, and percentage of inspired oxygen. Minute-to-minute adequacy of ventilation is estimated by observing the degree of excursion of the patient's chest wall during ventilation. Auscultation of the lungs for bilateral inspiratory sounds affords additional evidence of ventilation adequacy. Spirometer measurement alone should not be relied on for ventilation adequacy. Apnea alarms and equipment to continuously monitor end-tidal carbon dioxide and flow rates can provide for further respiratory function monitoring in the critically ill patient.

During ventilator assistance, continuous monitoring of arterial oxygen saturation (Sao_2) is used to determine the adequacy of ventilation (Table 14-2). Adjustments in ventilatory management are frequently necessary to maintain arterial oxygen saturations at 95% or more. Frequent blood gas analyses are also necessary to assess CO_2 production and pH.

Ideally, the minute volume of ventilation is adjusted by varying the respiratory rate, tidal volume, and dead space to obtain a $Paco_2$ of 40 mm Hg. In practice, maintaining the $Paco_2$ at exactly 40 mm Hg requires inordinate time and attention. Therefore, it is easier to slightly hyperventilate the patient to maintain a $PaCO_2$ in the 30 to 40 mm Hg range. This slight respiratory alkalosis has minimal impact on the cardiovascular system.

Table 14-2. Evaluation of arterial blood gases

Findings	Cause	Correction	
		On ventilator	Extubated
Pa_{CO_2} ↑ Sa_{O_2} or Pa_{O_2} ↓ or NL* pH ↓ or NL	Inadequate ventilation Rewarming with shivering ↑ Secretions	↑ Tidal volume ↑ Respiratory rate ↓ Dead space Aspiration of secretions	↓ Sedation Respirator Coughing, deep breathing Nasotracheal suctioning
	Pneumothorax Bronchospasm Respirator malfunction	Chest tube Bronchodilator Correction of respirator	Chest tube Bronchodilator
Sa_{O_2} or Pa_{O_2} ↓ Pa_{CO_2} ↓ or NL pH NL	Pulmonary AV shunting Pulmonary edema	↑ Fi_{O_2} Inotropic agents PEEP Diuretics Correction of underlying cause	↑ Fi_{O_2} via mask or cannulas Inotropic agents, diuretics Possibly ventilator with PEEP Correction of underlying cause
	Cardiac failure Atelectasis	See Table 14-1 Pulmonary physiotherapy Bronchoscopy, if severe and intractable	See Table 14-1 Coughing, deep breathing Physiotherapy Possibly bronchoscopy
Sa_{O_2} or Pa_{O_2} ↑ or NL Pa_{CO_2} ↓ pH ↑ or NL	Pain, anxiety causing hyperventilation Metabolic alkalosis	Decrease in minute volume Addition of dead space Replacement of electrolytes, fluid	Sedation Replacement of electrolytes, fluids

*NL: Normal; PEEP: positive end-expiratory pressure.

Oxygen administration is determined by Sa_{O_2} and Pa_{O_2} assessment. In general, the inspired oxygen (Fi_{O_2}) is increased to whatever level necessary to maintain an Sa_{O_2} above 95% and a Pa_{O_2} in the normal range of 90 to 100 mm Hg. An Fi_{O_2} greater than 60% for more than 3 to 4 hours has been associated with oxygen toxicity; however, since the harmful effect of hypoxemia may surpass the potential of adverse effects from oxygen toxicity, the Fi_{O_2} is increased to whatever level necessary to maintain a Pa_{O_2} above 50 mm Hg. A higher Pa_{O_2} may be required if there is anemia, increased tissue demand caused by fever, or a low cardiac output. Repeated assessment of pH from arterial blood gas analyses is essential for complete cardiorespiratory monitoring.

The rewarming phase is a crucial time, requiring close monitoring of the postoperative patient. During hypothermia, carbon dioxide production and oxygen use are decreased. As the patient begins to warm, metabolism increases. As a result, carbon dioxide production and oxygen use increase. Therefore it is prudent to maintain slight respiratory alkalosis with a Pa_{O_2} over 100 mm Hg during rewarming. A Pa_{CO_2} of 40 mm Hg and a Pa_{O_2} of 80 mm Hg will rapidly result in respiratory acidosis with hypoxemia as the patient's temperature elevates from 34° C to 37° C. Anticipation of this process when blood gas results are assessed will prevent serious acid-base imbalance and hypoxemia. Control of any shivering during this time is also important since shivering further increases carbon dioxide production and oxygen use because of the intense metabolic activity. In addition, shivering impairs mechanical ventilation, further complicating the situation.

POSTOPERATIVE MONITORING AFTER 24 TO 48 HOURS

In the majority of patients, vital signs stabilize within the first 24 to 48 hours after surgery. Drainage from the chest tube stops, and blood replacement is no longer necessary. Ventilatory support usually is not required, and removal of the endotracheal airway is well tolerated. Oxygen can be delivered by mask or nasal cannula, if required. At this point, arterial, PA, and/or LA pressure lines are removed. Usually, a CVP line is left in place for up to 48 hours postoperatively to permit blood sampling and drug administration. ECG monitoring is continued for the duration of the period in the intensive care unit, usually for 48 to 72 hours, or longer if arrhythmias have been present.

Tables 14-3 and 14-4 present some guidelines regarding this type and frequency of monitoring of the postoperative patient.

As the patient's condition stabilizes and improves, monitoring consists of less frequent recording of temperature, respiratory rate, pulse, and blood pressure by cuff measurement. Daily measurement of intake and output and patient's weight is continued. Assessment of circulatory adequacy, including vital signs, observation, and examination, is performed as deemed necessary by the patient's condition and the amount of pharmacologic support. Routine laboratory tests consist of CBC, se-

Table 14-3. Monitoring guidelines for the postoperative patient

Monitored parameters	Postoperative period (hr)			
	1 to 24	24 to 72 (with pharmacologic support)	24 to 72 (without pharmacologic support)	72 to 120
NONINVASIVE				
ECG	Continuous	Continuous	Continuous	Daily and prn
Cuff blood pressure	—	q 1 to 2h	q 2 to 4h	q 4h
Respiratory rate	q 15 to 20 min	q 1 to 2h	q 2 to 4h	q 4h
Temperature	q 15 to 20 min	q 1 to 2h	q 4h	q 4h
Peripheral circulation	q 15 to 20 min	q 1 to 2h	q 2 to 4h	q 4h
Intake and output	q 1h	q 1 to 2h	q 8h	q 8h
Chest x-ray	Immediately and prn	Daily and prn	Daily and prn	Daily and prn
INVASIVE				
CVP	q 15 to 20 min	q 1 to 2h	q 2 to 4h	prn
Arterial pressure	q 15 to 20 min	q 1 to 2h	q 2 to 4h	prn
LA pressure	q 15 to 20 min	q 1 to 2h	q 2 to 4h	prn
Chest tube drainage	q 15 to 20 min	prn	prn	prn

Table 14-4. Laboratory analysis guidelines for the postoperative patient

Laboratory analysis	Postoperative period (hr)		
	1 to 24	24 to 72	72 to 120
Arterial blood gas	Immediately and q 4h	prn	prn
Chemistry panel	q 8h	Daily and prn	Daily and prn
Hematocrit	Immediately and q 4h	Daily	Daily
Potassium	Immediately and q 4h	Daily and prn	Daily and prn

rum electrolytes, arterial blood gas analyses, BUN, creatinine, ECG, and chest x-rays. In most cases daily determinations suffice, but more frequent assessments are made when indicated. During this later postoperative period, the more important monitoring goals include detection of hypotension, respiratory distress, and arrhythmias. Even more important is the capability to immediately detect and respond to unexpected cardiac arrest.

MONITORING FOR OTHER POSTOPERATIVE COMPLICATIONS

Some of the more common postoperative problems have already been discussed. Others occur frequently enough to be looked for in each patient's postoperative course.

Hemorrhage

Excessive bleeding after cardiac surgery necessitating reoperation occurs in approximately 1% to 5% of patients. Thus the CVP or PA pressure, as well as the arterial pressure, should be closely monitored. External blood loss is monitored every 15 minutes by measuring chest tube drainage. Clotting of the chest tube may occur, so that measured blood loss may be less than the actual loss. For this reason assessment of the blood loss must be correlated with the arterial pressure, ventricular filling pressures, and chest x-rays. The definition of excessive blood loss is somewhat arbitrary. An accepted figure for total average blood loss is 400 ml/m^2 BSA. General guidelines for reoperation for hemorrhage are bleeding in excess of 300 to 400 ml/hr for the first 2 hours, 250 ml/hr from 3 to 6 hours, and over 200 ml/hr for the next 4 hours. Excessive bleeding may also be related to a coagulopathy and should be confirmed by clotting studies.

Embolization

Systemic arterial emboli during or after cardiac surgery are infrequent but may occur any time. The most usual source is from a thrombus on prosthetic cardiac valves. Other sources are from a clot on suture lines on the left side of the heart, LA thrombi, calcium from the aortic or mitral valve, or thrombus from a left ventricular aneurysm. A rare cause is tumor embolization occurring at the time of surgery for removal of an LA myxoma or other left-sided cardiac tumor. To detect embolization, the most important systems to monitor are the central nervous system (mental status), kidneys (renal function), mesenteric arteries (acute abdominal pain), and peripheral arteries (loss of distal pulse). Central nervous system effects are extremely diverse, ranging from slight changes in cerebration to coma or hemi-paralysis. Pulmonary embolization may cause respiratory distress. An abnormally low Pao_2 is the most reliable bedside parameter for diagnosing the problem. Pulmonary embolization can be suspected by an increase in PA pressure with a normal PAW or LA pressure and confirmed by a lung scan and angiography. If the embolus is large, a fall in cardiac output and hypotension may occur.

Renal Failure

Postoperative renal failure is associated most commonly with long periods of cardiopulmonary bypass with low flow rates or prolonged low cardiac output after surgery. Current trends toward more liberal fluid administration in the postoperative period have decreased the incidence of postoperative renal failure. Maintenance of adequate intravascular volume and cardiac output are paramount in the prevention of renal failure. Renal failure must be recognized as early as possible to prevent fluid and electrolyte overload. Inadequate renal function will be evident by a decrease in urine sodium and decreased creatinine clearance. A patient at risk or who appears to be developing acute renal failure will benefit from early assessment of these studies. Creatinine clearance will decrease long before marked elevations in serum creatinine occur, thus providing an early, more specific indicator of renal function. Monitoring hourly urine output in conjunction with frequent serial potassium and BUN or creatinine determinations will provide other valuable information regarding renal function.

Central Nervous System Complications

Postoperative complications involving the central nervous system are frequent and require diligent monitoring of the patient's motor or sensory abilities and mental status. Diffuse cerebral dysfunction most frequently occurs in the older patient after a period of hypotension, either intraoperatively or postoperatively. Air or particulate material embolization may also cause these changes. More focal central nervous system abnormalities usually result from emboli or from hypotension in association with occlusive disease of the carotid, vertebral, or intracranial arteries.

Postoperative delirium or psychosis is another central nerous system complication. Its exact cause remains undetermined, but diffuse microembolization of the intracranial arteries during cardiopulmonary bypass may be a factor. Other possibilities include deprivation of sleep and sense of time during intensive postoperative care. The diagnosis is established by recognition of the inability to concentrate, hallucinations, and paranoid or delusional psychotic behavior. To a great degree it can be prevented by affording adequate opportunities for the patient to sleep, allowing the patient access to both a clock and calendar, and assisting in orienting the patient to time. Most patients are aware of their hallucinations, which is a source of tremendous anxiety to them. These patients require a significant amount of reassurance that they are not "losing their minds" and that the hallucinations will pass. It might also be helpful to discuss the effects that narcotics might have in contributing to their condition. This will help reinforce the fact that the situation is only temporary. If psychotic behavior does occur, it almost always disappears before or shortly after discharge from the hospital.

Cardiac Arrest

One of the most important goals of monitoring after cardiac surgery is the immediate detection of cardiac arrest. Only by immediate detection and resuscitation can the patient's life be spared and the central nervous system's function be optimally preserved. The primary mode of detection of cardiac arrest is continuous ECG monitoring and arterial pressure monitoring. Caution must be used in placing total reliance on electronic monitoring for detection, since dislodgment of the ECG leads may result in an oscilloscopic pattern closely resembling asystole or ventricular fibrillation. Before resuscitation (and especially before defibrillation) is begun, absence of effective cardiac activity should be confirmed by palpation of the brachial or femoral arteries. Palpation of the carotid arteries may interfere with cerebral circulation or stimulate the carotid sinus nerves and should be avoided. Without continuous electronic monitoring, cardiac arrest is recognized by a sudden loss of consciousness and loss of brachial and femoral artery pulses. Even though cardiac activity may be present or detected by observation of the chest wall or stethoscopic examination of the heart, resuscitation measures should be instituted if the brachial and femoral pulses are absent or inadequate.

REFERENCES

Bodai BI, and Holcroft JW: Use of the pulmonary arterial catheter in the critically ill patient, Heart Lung 11:406-416, 1982.

Connors JP, and Avioli LV: An update on cardiac surgery, Heart Lung 10:323-328, 1981.

Cosgrove A et al: Blood conservation in cardiac surgery, Cardiovasc Clin 12:165, 1981.

Fernando H et al: Late cardiac tamponade following open heart surgery: detection by echocardiography, Ann Thorac Surg 24:174-177, 1977.

Futral J: Postoperative management and complications of coronary artery surgery, Heart Lung 3:477-486, 1977.

Harken D: Postoperative care following heart-valve surgery, Heart Lung 3:839, 1974.

McCauley KM, Brest AN, and McGoon DC: McGoon's cardiac surgery: an interprofessional approach to patient care, Philadelphia, 1985, FA Davis Co.

Norback CR, and Tinker JH: Hypothermia after cardiopulmonary bypass in man, Anesthesiology 53:277-280, 1980.

Palmer PN: Advanced hemodynamic assessment, Dimens Crit Care Nurs 1:139-144, 1982.

Ream AK, and Fogdall RP: Acute cardiovascular management, Philadelphia, 1982, JB Lippincott Co.

Reddy PS: Hemodynamics of cardiac tamponade in man. In Reddy PS, Leon DF, and Shaver JA, (editors): Pericardial disease, New York, 1982, Raven Press.

Seifert PC: Protection of the myocardium during cardiac surgery, Heart Lung 12:135-142, 1983.

Sladen RN: Management of the adult cardiac patient in the intensive care unit. In Ream AK and Fogdall RP: Acute cardiovascular management: anesthesia and intensive care, Philadelphia, 1982, JB Lippincott Co.

Thurer RL, and Hauer JM: Autotransfusion and blood conservation, Curr Probl Surg 19:97-156, 1982.

Viljoen JF: Anesthesia and monitoring techniques for open heart surgery in the adult, Surg Clin North Am 55:1217-1228, 1975.

Weeks KR et al: Bedside hemodynamic monitoring: its value in the diagnosis of tamponade complicating cardiac surgery, J Thorac Cardiovasc Surg 68:847-856, 1974.

Wilson RS, Sullivan SF, Malm JR, and Bowman FO, Jr: The oxygen cost of breathing following anesthesia and cardiac surgery, Anesthesiology 39:387-393, 1973.

Woods SL (editor): Cardiovascular critical care nursing, New York, 1983, Churchill Livingstone.

Young LC: Coronary artery surgery: commonplace yet complicated, Crit Care Nurse 1:15-24, 1981.

Chapter 15

Hemodynamic Monitoring During Critical Care Transport

JANET LASSEN MOHS AND ALVIN HACKEL

The concept of transporting critically ill patients is not new. As early as 1834 an elementary form of ambulance was used in sections of England, and in 1870 French citizens and wounded soldiers were evacuated in Paris by hot air balloon. Concurrently, the physiologic effects of high altitude were being investigated and the birth of aviation medicine occurred. Since that time, technologic advances in neonatal, pediatric, and adult critical care have necessitated the development of critical care transport programs. Through the efforts of both military and civilian health care personnel, it is now possible to transport critically ill patients over long distances while providing a high level of intensive care.

The goal of critical care transport is to provide a high level of care similar to that in the ICU during interfacility transfer. This service is a crucial link in optimum patient care as regionalized medical programs, such as trauma and perinatal care, become more widespread.

Medical transport programs throughout the world vary greatly. Many programs are hospital based, whereas others are operated by privately owned companies. Team selection differs, but most programs use some combination of physicians, nurses, respiratory therapists, and paramedics. The mode of transportation may be ground ambulance, helicopter, fixed-wing aircraft, or a combination. Services are usually initiated by a physician-to-physician referral, but some programs merely require a telephone call from a family member. In spite of these differences in program organization, the principles governing patient care remain unchanged.

The principles of critical care transport are based on the characteristics of and interaction between three entities within the transport environment (Fig. 15-1). The people in the environment, including team members, patients, and vehicle operators, are dependent on both the equipment and transport vehicle for optimum patient outcome. Conversely, the vehicle and equipment are only as efficient as the people operating them. The physical laws that exist in the aeromedical transport

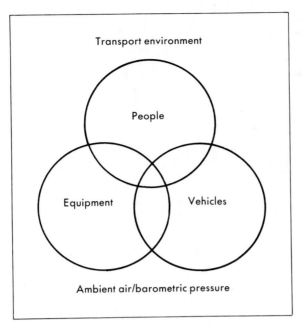

Fig. 15-1. Transport environment.

environment influence all of the entities within that environment. Dalton's law describes the characteristics of ambient air at altitude, and Boyle's law states the effects of barometric pressure on volume. Maximal integration and understanding of these factors in the transport environment optimize the efficiency, safety, and quality of patient care.

TYPES OF PATIENTS TRANSPORTED

The appropriateness of a patient for critical care transport is not determined solely by diagnosis but is assessed on an individual basis. A retrospective study of transported critically ill adults by our program revealed diagnoses including cardiovascular disease (arrhythmias, myocardial infarction, congestive heart failure, aneurysm), respiratory disease (pneumonia, adult respiratory distress syndrome, respiratory insufficiency, pulmonary embolism), renal disease, neurologic disease, trauma, and all types of shock. Therefore the deciding factor is not the patient's diagnosis but rather the patient's current hemodynamic stability and anticipated stability during transport.

TRANSPORT ENVIRONMENT
Aviation Physiology

To appreciate the effects of the transport environment on both the patient and the team, the physiologic effects of altitude must be understood. Two physical laws govern these phenomenons. The first law, Boyle's law, states that the volume of a dry gas is inversely proportional to its pressure when the temperature remains constant. In other words, as altitude increases and barometric pressure decreases, the volume of a gas will expand. The effect of increasing altitude on volume of gas follows*:

Altitude (ft)	Expansion factor
Sea level	0
5000	1.2
10,000	1.5
18,000	2

This law has significance when a gas is totally or partially trapped. As the gas begins to expand because of decreasing ambient pressure, the trapped pressure rises, causing tension on the structure's walls. Structures with flexible walls will expand proportionately. The trapped increased pressure will attempt to equalize to the lower ambient pressure by seeking the area of least resistance, such as a small opening or weakness in the structure's wall. This pressure difference has significant clinical implications in transport.

Dysbarisms, or pressure-induced changes in the body, result from an increase or decrease in ambient barometric pressure. Body structures that contain partially or completely trapped gas, that is, the lungs, gastrointestinal tract, middle ear, and sinuses, are at risk for compromise. At a cabin altitude of 8000 feet, a 30% gas expansion occurs. A small undetected pneumothorax at sea level can result in respiratory distress at altitude. The expansion of trapped gas in the gastrointestinal tract may result in abdominal distention, causing respiratory embarrassment, stress on suture lines, and pain. Aerotitis media results from the effects of the pressure differences on the middle ear. During ascent, air in the middle ear expands; the pressure is vented through the eustachian tube into the throat. During descent, however, the air in the middle ear contracts. If air cannot reenter via the eustachian tube, pain and trauma to the middle ear result. Similarly, barosinusitis results from the inability of the sinuses to adjust to ambient pressure differences and can cause severe discomfort if pressures are not equalized.

The second gas law affecting the patient at altitude is Dalton's law. This law states that the partial pressure of a gas in a gas mixture is the pressure that this gas would exert if it occupied the total volume of the mixture in the absence of other components. In other words, a gas contributes its share of the total pressure of a mixture in proportion to its percentage of the mixture. Thus oxygen always contributes 21% of the partial pressure in atmospheric air. However, when the total pressure of the mixture changes, as with altitude, so will the partial pressure of a gas. For example, the percent of oxygen in air is 21%, and sea level barometric pressure is 760 mm Hg; therefore 760 mm Hg $\times$ 0.21 = 160 mm Hg, which is the partial pressure of oxygen (Po_2) at sea level. At an altitude of 8000 feet, the barometric pressure decreases to 565 mm Hg. However, the proportion of oxygen in the air remains constant, and therefore 565 mm Hg $\times$ 0.21 = 119 mm Hg. The Po_2 is now reduced to 119 mm Hg at 8000 (Fig. 15-2).

---

*From Ferrara A, and Harin A: Emergency transfer of the high-risk neonate, St Louis, 1980, The CV Mosby Co.

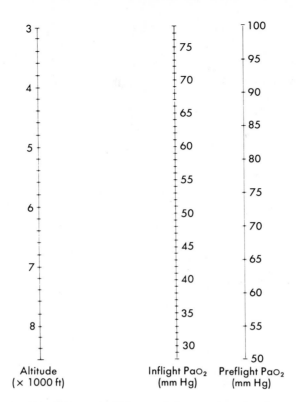

Fig. 15-2. Nomogram for predicting in-flight arterial oxygen tension from cabin altitude and preflight arterial oxygen tension. (From Henry JN, Krenis LJ, and Cutting RT: Hypoxemia during aeromedical evacuation, Surg Gynecol Obstet 136:49-53, 1973. By permission of Surgery, Gynecology & Obstetrics.)

The concern in the aeromedical transport of patients is the availability of oxygen at the alveolar level. As normal respiration occurs, not every molecule of air entering the respiratory tract has contact with alveoli and participates in gas exchange. Of each 500 cc of air inhaled, approximately 150 cc remains behind in the anatomic dead space. This phenomenon reduces the Po_2 at the alveolar level to approximately 100 mm Hg. The pressure difference between the alveolar Po_2 (PAo_2) and the arterial Po_2 (Pao_2) in the pulmonary capillary determines the oxygen diffusion rate across the blood-gas barrier. As the PAo_2 decreases as a result of reduced barometric pressure, the alveolar-arterial gradient decreases and less oxygen is diffused, resulting in a lowered Pao_2. For example, in a normal person at an altitude of 8000 feet, the barometric pressure at 565 mm Hg, and the Po_2 at 119 mm Hg, the PAo_2 is reduced to 65 mm Hg and the Pao_2 to 56 mm Hg with an oxygen saturation of 89%. In a person with any type of respiratory embarrassment, the Pao_2 would be further reduced. To avoid or minimize these problems in aeromedical transports, two prophylactic measures are practiced. First, supplemental oxygen is given at a percentage necessary to maintain an acceptable Pao_2 (Fig. 15-3). Second, the air carrier cabin is pressurized to near sea level when possible.

Because of the changes in ambient oxygen and barometric pressure in aeromed-

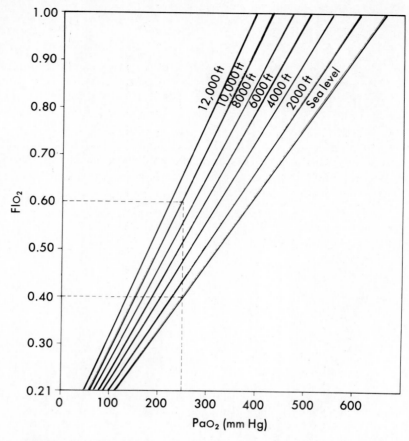

Fig. 15-3. Relationship between FIo_2, pressure altitude, and Pao_2. This graph shows that if an FIo_2 of 0.4 is required to maintain a Pao_2 of 250 mm Hg at sea level, then an FIo_2 of 0.6 will be required at an altitude of 9000 ft to maintain the same Pao_2. (From Ferrara A, and Harin A: Emergency transfer of the high-risk neonate, St Louis, 1980, The CV Mosby Co.)

ical transport, certain clinical conditions deserve careful consideration. One set of conditions includes those in which even mild hypoxia is detrimental, such as severe anemia, severe cardiac disease, respiratory disease, or glaucoma. A second set of conditions includes those in which a volume of gas is trapped within a body cavity, such as pneumothorax, penetrating eye injury, bowel obstruction, recent bowel surgery, or air within the central nervous system. Although these conditions do not absolutely contraindicate transport, they deserve special attention.

Transport Environment: Different from ICU

Within the transport environment, a level of care similar to that of the ICU is performed safely and efficiently; however, the transport environment has certain characteristics that are different from the usual intensive care setting. These characteristics must be initially recognized, thoroughly understood, and incorporated into the plan of care.

Gravitational forces and turbulence

When an aircraft changes speed (as in landing and taking off) or turns, the body experiences a force of gravity as measured by the g-force. A *g* is defined as a unit of force exerted on a body at rest that is equal to the force exerted by gravity; it is experienced when there is a change in velocity, that is, rate and direction. Turbulence is experienced when there are rapid changes in wind speed and direction, either horizontally or vertically. Both of these factors have implications for patient care and team comfort, with safety being a top priority. People or equipment that are not secured quickly become projectiles when an increased g-force or turbulence is encountered. For this reason, all passengers are always secured to their seat or stretcher, and all equipment is secured or stored in accordance with Federal Aviation Administration (FAA) regulations.

A speculative effect of the g-force is a transient blood-fluid redistribution. For instance, during aircraft takeoff, the acceleration force would be from the front to back of the plane. If the patient were lying supine, with the head to the aft of the cabin, a transient increase in venous return could occur from redistribution of blood from the legs. This phenomenon would be desirable in a patient with shock but contraindicated in a person with congestive heart failure, increased intracranial pressure, or an eye injury. During landing, the effects would be the reverse: the deceleration force would be from back to front. Although the practical application of this phenomenon has not been investigated, it bears consideration in aeromedical transport.

Turbulence is probably most annoying for the transport team. Not only does patient care become more difficult, but the symptoms of motion sickness may also become manifest. Motion sickness, caused from vestibular stimulation, often results when the horizon becomes unstable or when a person sits facing backwards or sideways. Symptoms include headache, nausea, vomiting, diaphoresis, and pallor. The steps that can be taken to minimize symptoms include (1) restriction of head movement, (2) visual fixation on a stationary object, (3) loosening of restrictive clothing, (4) good ventilation, and (5) medication. However, the best treatment is prevention.

Vibration

Mechanical vibration is experienced to varying degrees in both ground and air ambulances. Vibration levels in ground ambulances have been measured in the low-frequency range from 3 to 18 Hz, which exceeds tolerance limits for adults, especially for long transports. The biologic effects of mechanical vibration have been investigated primarily in military personnel. Such effects as changes in arterial blood pressure, altered respiratory function, and decreases in body temperature with changes in peripheral nerve conduction time have been documented. Probably more applicable to the transport team are the symptoms of headache, motion sickness, and general fatigue. Vibration can also cause monitor artifacts, making ECG and hemodynamic interpretation difficult.

Noise

The effects of noise in ICUs have been well documented. However, the noise in the transport environment has a different impact. The decibel level in ICUs has been recorded between 60 and 70 dB, whereas the decibel level in an aircraft is between 85 and 110 dB. High decibel noise over a span of time can create such symptoms as general physical discomfort, headache, and fatigue. In time, without proper protection, a small but detectable hearing loss can occur. Fatigue is often not noticed during the time of transport but is experienced once the noise stops. The FAA recommends wearing snug ear plugs whenever flying.

The high noise level also affects patient care. As the noise level increases, conversation becomes difficult and communication is impeded. Monitor beepers and alarms are of little value, since they are too soft to hear. In addition, blood pressure, breath sounds, and heart sounds cannot be auscultated, since the transmission from a stethoscope is inadequate. Alternative methods of assessment include visual inspection, monitors with digital displays, and invasive monitoring when necessary.

Limited space and decreased lighting

The interior of air and ground ambulances are configured in many different ways, but they all have one characteristic in common—limited space. A common configuration is that of having the stretcher on one side of the vehicle, a bench large enough for three people opposite it, and a single seat at the head of the patient. There is very little space between the bench and the stretcher, so it is not possible to move around the patient. In addition, there is no room to stand up. Patient care must be delivered sitting at the patient's side with supplies within an arm's reach.

Most transport vehicles have limited lighting sources. Indirect lighting is sometimes available along the sides of the vehicle and through the window as sunlight. Most vehicles have spot lighting that is more intense but limited in area. At night the problem increases, since sunlight is not available. Patient assessment becomes more difficult as visual acuity decreases. It is advisable to bring a portable, light-weight, external light source such as a flashlight to aid in visualization.

Limited electrical power and oxygen supply

When planning the care of a patient during transport, it must be remembered that the inexhaustible power sources in the hospital are indeed exhaustible resources during transport.

Some type of electrical power is a necessity for most types of monitoring equipment. When transferring patients from hospital to vehicle or from vehicle to vehicle, it is imperative to have a continuous source of power. There are two common methods by which to meet these challenges. With the first, the transport vehicle is equipped with some type of rechargeable battery system. Currently, most monitors have gel cell or Nicad batteries with a life of 2 to 3 hours. This situation allows for continuous monitoring during entrance to or exit from the transport vehicle or during any time when electrical power is not possible. The second method is the use of an inverter system installed in the transport vehicle. The inverter converts electrical power from the vehicle's power source to power that is usable by the transport equipment. A common inverter provides 110 V of AC power at 60 Hz.

Most patients who are transported require some type of oxygen therapy, whether by mask, ventilator, or AMBU bag. Since the patient is moved from place to place, a portable oxygen source is imperative. A standard E cylinder with regulator and flow meter is small, easy to move, and adequate in volume. Equally as efficient is the Linde Walker liquid oxygen system, which is lightweight and holds approximately 1000 L of oxygen. Frequently, a larger, nonportable oxygen system, such as an H or M tank, can be permanently installed in the transport vehicle. This option is highly desirable for long transports or when high gas consumption is anticipated.

To ensure that an adequate amount of oxygen is taken on transport, it is essential to calculate the amount of oxygen to be used before departure. The equation for calculating the amount of time a cylinder will last is

$$\text{Duration (min)} = \frac{\text{Gauge pressure (psi)} \times \text{Gauge factor}}{\text{Liter flow}}$$

The gauge pressure, indicated in pounds per square inch (psi) on the gauge dial, represents the pressure of the compressed gas in the cylinder. As the volume of gas in the cylinder decreases, so does the pressure. It is also known that, for every liter loss in cylinder volume, there is a proportional drop in gauge pressure. In others words, the ratio between the volume in the cylinder and the gauge pressure reading remains constant. This number is known as the gauge factor. The liter flow is defined as the rate in liters per minute that oxygen is leaving the cylinder. Therefore the number of minutes that oxygen will flow until the tank is empty is equal to the gauge pressure multiplied by the gauge factor divided by the liter flow per minute. Standard tank sizes with corresponding gauge factors follow:

Common tank sizes	Gauge factors
E	0.28
G	2.41
M	1.57
H & K	3.14

EXAMPLE: If an E cylinder has a gauge pressure reading of 1800 psi and a 6 L/min liter flow is needed, the cylinder would last 84 minutes.

$$\frac{\text{Gauge pressure (psi)} \times \text{Gauge factor}}{\text{Liter flow}} = \text{Duration}$$

$$\frac{1800 \text{ psi} \times 0.28}{6 \text{ L/min}} = 84 \text{ min}$$

When calculating the amount of oxygen to be taken on a transport vehicle, it is important to remember five variables: (1) the patient may be more critical than reported and hence require more oxygen; (2) the patient will require more oxygen at altitude than on the ground; (3) the patient's condition may deteriorate during transport and require more oxyen; (4) there may be unexpected travel delays necessitating a longer use of oxygen; and (5) equipment may fail, causing an unnecessary loss of gas. To avoid the potential problems associated with these variables, it is advisable to carry twice the amount of oxygen anticipated. In all cases a self-inflating AMBU bag should be carried in the event of a total oxygen supply depletion.

TECHNIQUES IN MONITORING
Effects of Altitude on Equipment

The physical laws present in the transport environment not only affect the patient and the team but also are a consideration with equipment. Boyle's law is of the most concern. Briefly restated, as altitude increases and barometric pressure decreases, the volume of a gas will expand. This law has a direct impact on any equipment with trapped air space, including Foley catheter balloons, endotracheal tube cuffs, air splints, PA catheter balloons, IV bottles, and pneumatic trousers.

Intravenous solutions in plastic bags rather than glass bottles are suggested for use on transport for several reasons. First, the flow rate with glass bottles alters considerably because of the pressure changes during aircraft ascent or descent. Second, glass bottles break easily during turbulence or movement. Finally, glass bottles are difficult to pack and require more space in supply boxes. The use of plastic IV bags alleviates these problems.

Special precautions are also necessary for other equipment with air-filled spaces. Pneumatic trousers, air splints, and Foley catheter balloons must be deflated on reaching altitude and inflated on landing. Circulation should be carefully assessed throughout the transport.

Endotracheal tube cuffs pose a special problem. Since cuff expansion at altitude can cause tracheal mucosal damage, a slight cuff deflation is necessary on ascent. However, during descent, an endotracheal tube leak may result, which is inaudible because of the loud background noise. Endotracheal tubes with high–residual volume cuffs and those with foam cuffs overcome these concerns.

PA catheter balloons require the injection of approximately 1 to 1.5 cc of air for placement in the wedge position. If the balloon is inflated during ascent to 10,000 feet, this amount of air will expand 1.5 times, or from 1.5 to 2.25 cc, possibly causing balloon rupture and PA damage or rupture. Therefore it is important that the balloon of the catheter be completely deflated and the pulmonary artery waveform be continuously monitored during ascent.

Criteria for Choosing Types of Equipment

The criteria against which transport equipment is evaluated are somewhat different from those used in the ICU. Transport equipment must be capable of functioning in the rugged and unpredictable environment in which it is used. All transport equipment must be able to withstand severe mechanical, thermal, and electrical stresses, constant vibration, and changes in barometic pressure.

Four general guidelines can be used when evaluating equipment for critical care transport. The first guideline is that the equipment must be portable, since it is both moved from vehicle to vehicle and carried alongside the patient. A dependable battery is crucial for continuous, uninterrupted monitoring when AC power is unavailable or impractical. Similar to the first guideline, the second criterion maintains that the equipment be of a reasonable size and weight. Ease of movement remains important and allowance for the limited space within the transport vehicle is also considered. The third guideline provides that transport equipment have full intensive care monitoring capability. To provide continuous critical care services between institutions, intensive care standards must be maintained. Provision should be made for direct arterial pressure, PA pressure, and intracranial pressure monitoring and for cardiac output measurement and multiple drug infusions. Finally, transport equipment must be reliable and durable. Optimum care and safety of the patient depends on equipment that functions during all the events encountered during transport. Additionally, equipment must be durable enough to withstand the knocks and jolts that are inevitable on even the most routine transport. Proper equipment is vital to the effective transport of any patient; team members must have confidence in its reliability, a thorough knowledge of its operation, and an understanding of its limitations.

Equipment Options
Cardiac monitor

As alluded to earlier, the cardiac monitor used during transport must provide the level of hemodynamic monitoring necessitated by the patient's medical condition. To monitor arterial, PA, and venous pressures, a two-channel monitor with ECG should be used, complete with strip recorder and paper calibration capabilities. The oscilloscope and digital numbers must be easily read and impervious to vibration and movement that can cause annoying artifacts. Calibration and zeroing of the channels must be uncomplicated and quick. Finally, the battery must be reliable, have at least 2 hours of power, and require a minimal amount of recharging time once depleted.

Defibrillator

Congruent with critical care standards, electrical countershock should be available for all transported patients. In addition, a defibrillator with an oscilloscope can be used in place of the cardiac monitor when pressure monitoring is not necessary, thus decreasing the amount of equipment that is taken. The defibrillator should be simple to operate, require a minimal number of steps to energize the paddles, and have a strip recorder to document ECG tracings. The batteries must be easily interchangeable, easily stored, and of sufficient capacity to deliver 20 to 30 countershocks at maximal joules if necessary.

Perhaps no other physiologic system is affected by the transport environment as acutely as the respiratory system. Recent technologic advances in pulse oximetry have made it possible to monitor respiratory stability through continuous monitoring of arterial oxygen saturation. The pulse oximeter is now a mandatory addition to any transport team's equipment. It must be lightweight, require a reasonable amount of battery power, and be minimally affected by vibration and movement. Both adult and pediatric sensors should be available. (See Chapter 8 for a further discussion of pulse oximetry.) The monitor can be conveniently positioned, either permanently or temporarily, on top of the cardiac monitor for accessibility.

Pneumatic suit

A pneumatic suit, also known as a MAST (military anti-shock trousers) suit, is an airfilled trouser used for attaining and maintaining hemodynamic stability in states of shock when other methods are not available and for short periods of time (less than 6 hours).

Physiology. As the pressure from the inflated compartments of the pneumatic suit is exerted on the legs and abdomen of the patient, approximately 750 to 1000 ml of blood from the peripheral circulation is diverted to the vital organs. This results in an increase in venous return, an increase in aortic and carotid flow and pressure, and an increase in vital tissue perfusion. Cardiac output remains unchanged, however, as increased stroke volume is accompanied by decreased heart rate. The suit also decreases bleeding through internal pressure and external tamponade. Internal pressure is achieved as the external compression of the suit on the lower body is transmitted to the internal vasculature, causing an increase in intraperitoneal pressure, a decrease in the radius of the arteries, and a rise in MAP. External tamponade is a reflection of the direct pressure of the suit over the tissues, thereby decreasing direct bleeding. Fracture immobilization is a secondary benefit of the use of the pneumatic suit.

Indications. The pneumatic suit should be included on any transport in which (1) hypovolemic shock or hemorrhage is suspected or anticipated, (2) neurogenic shock is a possibility, or (3) multiple fractures of the lower body exist. These indications would include patients with a diagnosis of multiple tauma, suspected intra-abdominal bleeding, or possible dissecting abdominal aneurysm. It is wise to anticipate hemorrhage or shock by bringing extra crystalloid or colloid fluid for stabilization at the referring hospital or during transport, but as an additional option it is prudent to apply the suit but not inflate it unless needed on the trip back. The indications and contraindications for the use of the pneumatic suit follow:

Indications	Contraindications
Hypovolemic shock	Cardiogenic shock
Neurogenic shock	Congestive heart failure
Lower extremity or pelvic fracture	Pulmonary edema
Internal or external hemorrhage of abdomen or lower extremities	Tension pneumothorax

Procedure

ASSESSMENT

1. General
   a. Past medical history
   b. Present medical history
   c. General systems review with special attention to possible bleeding sites or sites of further injury
2. Respiratory
   a. Breath sounds
   b. Symmetry of chest movement
   c. Rate and quality of respiration
3. Neurologic
   a. Level of consciousness
   b. Movement and sensation of all four extremities
4. Cardiovascular
   a. Vital signs

    b. Quality of arterial pulses (carotid, brachial, radial, femoral, popliteal, dorsalis pedis)

    c. Skin temperature and color

INFLATION (FIG. 15-4)

1. Unfold the suit completely and lay it flat on the stretcher.
2. Position the patient supine on the opened suit. Palpate the lowest rib and position the upper border of the suit just below that point.
3. Fasten both trouser legs around the patient's legs by securing the Velcro straps. Repeat the procedure for the abdominal section (contraindicated in cases of pregnancy, diaphragmatic hernia, or evisceration).
4. Attach the foot pump to inflation deflation-valves (stopcocks) and open them (stopcock handles are parallel to the tubing).
5. Inflate the leg compartments by closing the stopcocks (stopcock handles are perpendicular to the tubing) to the abdominal compartment.
6. Depress the foot pump until the suit compartmental pressure reaches 20 to 30 mm Hg. Check the patient's vital signs.

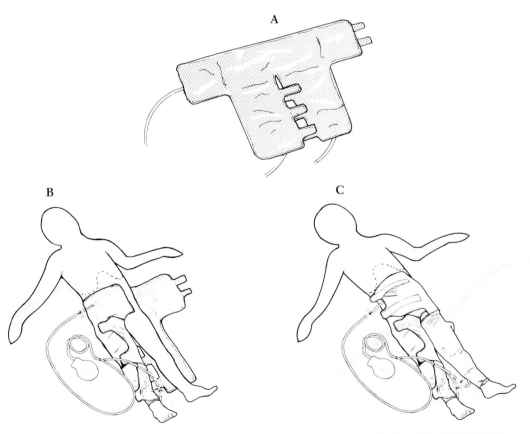

Fig. 15-4. Application of pneumatic suit. **A,** Lay the pneumatic suit flat on the stretcher. **B,** Position the patient on the suit and wrap the suit around the patient's legs and abdomen by securing the Velcro straps. **C,** After checking baseline vital signs and attaching the foot pump, inflate the suit to the appropriate pressure.

7. Continue to inflate the legs until one of the following occurs (NOTE: The suit inflation pressure should not exceed 100 mm Hg.):
   a. An acceptable blood pressure is reached.
   b. Leg sections indent with firm pressure.
   c. Pop-off valve releases.
   d. Velcro straps slip.
8. Close the stopcocks to the leg compartments.
9. If an acceptable blood pressure has not been reached by inflating the leg sections, inflate the abdominal compartment by using the procedure described in steps 6 to 8.
10. Make sure all stopcocks are closed and disconnect the foot pump. Keep it readily available, since inflation is sometimes necessary.
11. Begin therapy for shock and/or bleeding.
12. Monitor vital signs every 5 minutes.

DEFLATION. It is absolutely imperative that deflation be done by persons familiar with the use of the pneumatic suit.

1. Check the patient's cardiovascular status (heart rate, blood pressure, respirations). Check the blood pressure frequently throughout the procedure.
2. Ensure that at least two large-gauge IV lines are in place and that adequate volumes of fluid or blood are available in case rapid infusion is needed.
3. Make sure all the stopcocks are in the closed position and access tubing is removed. This is necessary for air to escape.
4. Deflate the abdominal compartment first. Turn the stopcock slightly to remove air intermittently. Blood pressure should decrease no more than 5 mm Hg. Check vital signs. Watch for both an increase in heart rate and a decrease in blood pressure.
5. Hold suit pressure stable for about 10 minutes as long as vital signs remain stable. Give volume as needed. When blood pressure remains stable, replacement is probably adequate. If deflation is not possible despite volume replacement, further definitive treatment should be considered.
6. Continue deflating the abdominal compartment in this manner, carefully watching the vital signs.
7. Deflate the legs using the same procedure.
8. Leave the suit in place for at least an hour to ensure stability before removal.

Cardiac output computer

At times a patient will have a PA catheter in place or the patient's medical condition will warrant the insertion of one before transport. As efforts toward medical stability are made, the information supplied by cardiac output data may prove invaluable. Therefore there are three reasons a cardiac output computer is indicated for transport. First, a small referral hospital may not have the capability for inserting and using PA catheters and therefore would not own a cardiac output computer. In this situation it would be essential to bring all supplies that might be needed to insert a PA catheter. Second, a cardiac output computer might not be readily available. For instance, perhaps the number of patients requiring this type of monitoring is very small, so two hospitals have co-ownership of one computer.

When the transport team wants to do cardiac output measurements, the computer might be at the other hospital. Finally, it may happen that the referral hospital's catheter and the team's computer are not compatible. In this case a new catheter would be inserted.

The technique involved in measuring cardiac output by the thermodilution method has been described in Chapter 7. The technique used during transport is similar to that used in ICUs. Special attention is needed to avoid making measurement during turbulence or extreme vibration.

Drugs and supplies

Medications and supplies must be complete enough to provide for every situation encountered during transport yet be light enough to be easily carried. In addition, they must be packaged in an organized fashion. Many companies manufacture supply boxes that are both versatile and durable. Unlike in the ICU, supplies during transport are completely expendable, so every effort is made to conserve.

Monitoring Equipment Setup

IV lines

The critically ill patient who is transported often has a number of intravenous lines into which drugs or fluids must flow accurately. Even with "keep-open" lines, constant infusion must be maintained to ensure accuracy. When the patient is moved from place to place or when the IV fluid must be hung a short distance above the patient, as in an aircraft or ambulance, constant and accurate infusion is difficult with standard methods. The following methods prevent this problem.

Method I: use of pressure bag

INDICATIONS
1. "Keep-open" lines
2. Lines through which rapid amounts of fluid can be given

SUPPLIES
1. Pressure bag
2. IV bag of fluid
3. IV tubing with minidripper or macrodipper
4. Luer-Lok extension tube
5. Dial-A-Flow (optional)

PROCEDURE
1. Connect IV fluid with tubing and extension tube. Flush system. Fill drip chamber approximately one-third full.
2. Connect IV to patient and ensure patency of IV. Regulate rate.
3. Put pressure bag over IV bag and pump up until it is snug around bag. It does not have to be tight, since it is overcoming venous pressure. Regulate the rate by adjusting the IV roller clamp or by adding a Dial-A-Flow distal to the extension tube.

The IV bag can now be placed anywhere close to the patient, including on the stretcher, as long as the drip chamber is half full and remains in a dependent position.

Method II: use of an infusion pump

INDICATIONS
1. When accurate or limited infusion is indicated
2. Drug infusions

SUPPLIES
1. IV bag
2. IV tubing with minidripper or macrodipper with or without volutrol
3. Stopcocks as needed for entry ports
4. Luer-Lok extension tubing
5. Holter pump

PROCEDURE
1. Assemble IV system in the following order: IV bag, IV tubing, Holter pump tubing, stopcock, extension tubing.
2. Flush system and connect to IV catheter. Ensure IV patency.
3. Place the Holter pump tubing in the Holter pump by first engaging the small, white rectangular fittings in the slots in the pump chamber block near the inflow and outflow arrows. Stretch the tubing around the rotor assembly. Check to make sure the direction of flow is *from* the IV bag *to* the patient.
4. Completely open the IV roller clamp and turn the Holter pump on.
5. Regulate the infusion rate by turning the rate selection dial. Once the rate is attained, lock the rate selection dial.

The IV bag can now be placed anywhere around the patient as long as the drip chamber remains half full and is in a dependent position. (NOTE: Watch the IV site carefully. The Holter pump will continue to infuse even if an IV infiltration occurs. The Holter pump is only one type of infusion pump. A thorough investigation of all available infusion pumps should be made before selection.

Method III: use of an auto syringe

INDICATIONS
1. When accurate or limited infusion is indicated
2. Drug infusions

SUPPLIES
1. IV bag
2. Penthothal pin
3. Multiple 35 ml or 60 ml syringes
4. Luer-Lok extension tubing

PROCEDURE
1. Prepare proper IV solution
2. Insert Penthothal pin into IV bag
3. Withdraw necessary amount of fluid into syringe and attach to Luer-Lok extension tubing.
4. Purge the extension tubing of air and insert into auto syringe, following manufacturers' guidelines.
5. Connect extension tubing to IV catheter and set infusion pump at desired rate.

Secure the infusion pump close to the patient. Keep IV bag and additional syringes in an accessible location for necessary refills.

Arterial catheter

Arterial pressure monitoring during transport is similar to that in the ICU. The catheter must be well secured to avoid accidental dislodging during frequent movement or turbulence. The infusion system can be varied, although is similar to the setup described in Chapter 6. The infusion must be continuous or intermittently flushed to ensure catheter patency. Continuous infusion must use either a pressure bag or Holter infusion pump. If intermittent manual flushing is done, the infusion pump and tubing are deleted and a syringe is attached to the distal stopcock. The syringe is manually filled from the IV bag and the catheter flushed with 1 to 2 ml of fluid as necessry to maintain patency.

In either method the transducer reference port must be kept at RA level for accurate measurement. Taping the transducer reference port to the patient's side is one method of securing it. The Holter pump is most often used in pediatric patients, whose infusion rates must be minimal and accurate. Fig. 15-5 demonstrates the setup for arterial pressure monitoring with a Holter pump.

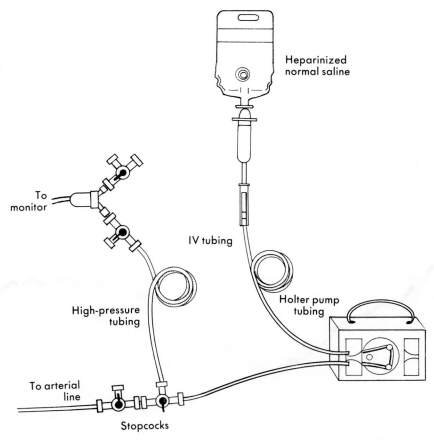

Fig. 15-5. Arterial monitoring with Holter pump infusion system. This system can be used for venous infusions by deleting the transducer, high-pressure tubings, and one stopcock and attaching an extension tube distal to the remaining stopcock.

PA pressure, arterial pressure, and CVP monitoring

Comprehensive monitoring during transport frequently requires the use of a PA catheter and an arterial catheter. The methods, techniques, and problems associated with using these catheters have been thoroughly discussed elsewhere in this book; these facts certainly apply during transport. The main difference in transport, however, is the system setup. Multiple pressure monitoring systems must be kept simple because of decreased space and increased movement of the patient. Therefore, when monitoring CVP, PA pressure, and MAP, the manifold system provides both simplicity and accessibility to the pressure parameters needed for optimum care.

Supplies
1. 250 ml IV bag of heparinized normal saline (1 unit heparin per milliliter of fluid)
2. Nonvented IV tubing
3. Three 4-foot high-pressure tubings
4. Two disposable transducer domes
5. Five Luer-Lok stopcocks
6. Manifold
7. 10 ml syringe for flush

Equipment setup
1. Insert the nonvented IV tubing in the IV bag and connect to manifold stopcock 3 (Fig. 15-6).
2. Attach transducer domes to each end of the manifold. Attach stopcock to the free port of the dome (for venting to atmospheric air when calibrating).
3. Connect a 4-foot high-pressure tubing to manifold stopcocks 1, 2, and 5.
4. Attach a stopcock on the free (proximal) end of each tubing.
5. Place a 10 ml syringe in manifold stopcock 4.
6. Open the roller clamp on the IV bag and flush the entire manifold system through the transducer domes (making sure they are free from air bubbles) and the pressure tubings. Close all stopcocks when the system is flushed.
7. Place several drops of sterile IV fluid on the head of the transducers, attach the transducers to transducer domes, and zero and calibrate the monitor according to specifications.
8. Connect the PA, CVP, and arterial catheters to stopcocks on the pressure tubing, opening the stopcocks after they are secure.

Procedure for monitoring
1. Secure the manifold near the patient's RA level but keep it accessible.
2. Keep catheters patent by manually flushing every 10 to 15 minutes. Open manifold stopcocks 3 and 4 to one another and aspirate 10 ml of flush from IV bag into syringe. Close manifold stopcock 3. Manually flush appropriate line(s) with small amount of fluid.
3. Arterial pressure may be monitored continuously by closing manifold stopcock 5 to the syringe, thereby opening it to the arterial line and transducer.
4. PA pressure may be monitored by closing manifold stopcock 1 to stopcock 2, thereby opening it to the PA lumen of the catheter and the transducer.
5. Monitoring CVP is accomplished by closing manifold stopcock 1 to the PA

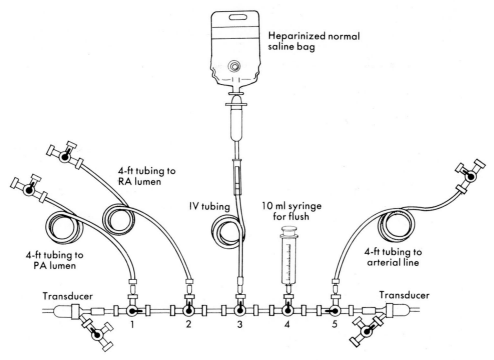

Heparinized normal saline bag

4-ft tubing to RA lumen

IV tubing

10 ml syringe for flush

4-ft tubing to PA lumen

4-ft tubing to arterial line

Transducer

Transducer

1   2   3   4   5

Fig. 15-6. Setup for monitoring arterial, PA, and RA pressures using manifold system. System is manually flushed by aspirating normal saline from the IV bag into the 10 ml syringe in stopcock 4 and injecting it into the appropriate catheter. Arterial pressure can be continuously monitored by turning stopcock 5 off to stopcock 4 and open to the transducer. The PA and RA pressures cannot be monitored simultaneously. In this illustration, stopcock 2 is turned off to the RA lumen. Stopcock 1 is turned off to stopcock 2 and open to the transducer for continuous monitoring of the PA pressure.

catheter and closing manifold stopcock 2 to manifold stopcock 3, which opens the system to the CVP line and the transducer.

6. The PA pressure and CVP cannot be monitored simultaneously. On some monitors the channels must be adjusted for waveform and digital number viewing when changing from one pressure reading to another.

Patient Care

Preparation for transport begins at the time of the referral of the patient. The first issue to be resolved is whether or not the patient should be transported. The answer is obtained after a direct consultation between the referring and receiving physicians and the physician responsible for the patient during the transport. The variables involved include the following: (1) the severity and acuteness of the patient's illness, (2) whether or not the patient can be stabilized before transport, (3) the modes of transport and the types of transport carriers avaliable, (4) the anticipated interhospital transport time, and (5) the capability of the available transport team. Present-day hospital-based transport programs have the capability of transporting any patient who can be stabilized before transfer. The physiologic factors relating to air and surface transport discussed earlier in this chapter need to be considered as well. Vibration and noise increase fatigue and contribute to all types of shock, particularly hypovolemic shock. Changes in barometric pressure increase the severity of cardiac and pulmonary insufficiency. Nevertheless transport programs do exist that regularly transport patients over interhospital distances of more than 1000 miles. The effects of transport on the patient can be compensated, provided the transport program personnel are aware of their existence and manage them properly.

The patient should be under the care of the transport team during the entire transport process. Transfer of patient care responsibilities under other circumstances, for example, at an airport after deplaning, is strongly discouraged.

Providing intensive care in a moving environment is the major challenge facing the transport team. The basic philosophy is simple. The transport team brings the therapeutic modalities of the critical care unit to the patient's bedside in the referring community hospital. The care established is continued during transport. The team spends as much time as is needed in the community hospital to prepare the patient for transport. Except in the most unusual circumstances, the patient can be stabilized with the initial major therapy provided in that hospital. Usually, dramatic therapy does not have to be initiated during the transport. Patients suffering from cardiogenic shock and/or severe and unstable respiratory insufficiency will not tolerate movement well. If the major therapy cannot be done in the community hospital, it should not be attempted during transit unless it is absolutely essential to do so.

Patient stabilization before transport includes the following: (1) the treatment of shock with the administration of blood and other replacement parenteral solutions and the use of cardioactive agents; (2) the treatment of respiratory insufficiency with the initiation of endotracheal intubation and assisted ventilation; and (3) the insertion of indwelling arterial, venous, and PA catheters.

Serious consideration should be given to inserting an endotracheal tube before transport in patients who (1) are in borderline respiratory insufficiency requiring oxygen by mask or prongs or (2) have a compromised cardiac output resulting from increased work of respiration. With the endotracheal tube in place, assisted ventilation can be controlled more easily. Insertion of an endotracheal tube in a moving environment with limited working space is fraught with problems. Clinical judgment will have to be exercised in those conditions in which intubation may create iatrogenic problems. Two examples are croup and asthma. In both cases, medical management at the referring hospital may improve the clinical condition of the patient enough to preclude the need for intubation. If there is a borderline situation, however, in which the patient will need intubation if the clinical condition worsens, intubation should be performed.

The multifactor respiratory influences of oxygenation, ventilation, and the work of breathing on the cardiovascular and neurologic systems mandate that patients requiring assisted ventilation be carefully assessed before transport. Because the transport team frequently has to change the ventilator settings during their initial management of the patient in the referring hospital, patients with severe respiratory insufficiency, central nervous system disease, or an unstable cardiovascular system may require further stabilization measures before transport. The team should be prepared for this situation and not leave the referring hospital in haste;

spending a minimum of 1 hour preparing the patient for transport can be expected.

The same considerations taken into account for an endotracheal tube also apply to the insertion of central venous and arterial lines. These lines should be inserted before leaving the referring hospital whenever there is anticipated need. Dependable and secure means of providing intravenous fluids and monitoring the cardiovascular system are essential during transport; patient risk increases considerably in the absence of these means. It is essential that flow through these lines must be free enough to withstand the frequent changes in gravity that occur in the transport environment as a result of movement of the patient in and out of ambulance carriers and through hospitals. A continuous infusion system ensures the patency of the lines. In addition, all lines must be securely taped at the insertion site and at the connection points to prevent dislodgment or disconnection. These lines experience a greater amount of tension than most. Accurate labeling of IV bags and IV tubing close to the patient decreases confusion in limited space.

Critically ill patients are prone to be unstable almost by definition. It is therefore essential that they be observed closely for signs of clinical change (specifically deterioration) from the moment the actual transport begins to the time the patient's care is transferred to another team within a hospital facility. The clinical changes of particular concern relate to the cardiovascular and pulmonary systems.

Patients in shock can become hypotensive when moved. Cardiac arrest is not uncommon under such circumstances if the shock state has not been carefully evaluated and pretreated before movement. Continuous monitoring of the ECG and direct arterial pressure is essential in such patients. Measurement of the CVP and/or PA pressures is also important.

Respiratory insufficiency can easily be accentuated during transport by (1) inadvertent changes in assisted ventilation, (2) changes in the ambient oxygen concentration that are not compensated for, (3) catastrophic changes such as endobronchial intubation or pneumothorax, or (4) gravitational factors and factors associated with surface and airplane movement. Patients with respiratory insufficiency are prone to changes in their clinical state even if transport is not underway because of the dynamic state of their pathophysiologic condition.

Patient assessment in the transport environment, although somewhat different than in the ICU, is not impossible. A thorough baseline clinical assessment and reliable monitoring techniques are essential. Monitors with digital displays and portable supplemental light sources help to overcome the problem of decreased lighting. Although a high noise level precludes the use of auscultation, meaningful data can be obtained by palpation and visualization. For example, since breath sounds cannot be heard, increased respiratory effort is assessed by visualizing the respiratory muscles and feeling chest expansion. Recognizing the limitations of the environment and planning for them decrease many potential problems.

Placement of the patient, the transport team, and the equipment in the transport vehicle must allow for the appropriate care of the patient. It is useless to take a full complement of team members if they all cannot participate in patient care during transport. Potential nursing and medical problems must be anticipated before loading the vehicle. This assessment will dictate where specific people and equipment will be placed. A patient with recurrent ventricular tachycardia would certainly have a defibrillator and antiarrhythmic drugs located close by. The team member most proficient at airway management would sit at the head of a patient with respiratory insufficiency. Oxygen, suction, and ventilatory support would be located nearby. Basically, the patient's needs should dictate the environmental requirements rather than vice versa.

In essence, critically ill patients must be treated with utmost care during transport. The pathophysiology of their clinical condition and the impact of transport on their disease state(s) must be understood. By precise preparation in the referring hospital and careful monitoring and attention to patient care during transport, the necessary quality of patient care can be delivered.

REFERENCES

Alfaro R: Pneumatic anti-shock trousers: when and how to use them, Dimens Crit Care Nurs 1:9, 1982.

Armstrong HG: Principles and practices of aviation medicine, Baltimore, 1979, Williams & Wilkins.

Barger J: Strategic aeromedical evacuation: the inaugural flight, Aviat Space Environ Med 57:613-616, 1986.

Bureau of Medicine and Surgery: United States naval flight surgeon's manual, ed 2, Washington, DC, 1978, US Government Printing Office.

Clark JG et al: Initial cardiovascular response to low-frequency whole body vibration in humans and animals, Aerosp Med 38:464-467, 1967.

Dhenin G: Aviation medicine: health and clinical aspects, London, 1978, Tri-Med, Ltd.

Dhenin G: Aviation medicine: physiology and human factors, London, 1978, Tri-Med, Ltd.

Egan DF: Fundamentals of respiratory therapy, ed 3, St Louis, 1977, The CV Mosby Co.

Ehrenwerth J, Sorbo S, and Hackel A: Transport of critically ill adults, Crit Care Med 14:543-547, 1986.

Ernsting J: Prevention of hypoxia: acceptable compromises, Aviat Space Environ Med 49:495-502, 1978.

Floyd WN, Brodersen AB, and Goodno JG: Effect of whole body vibration on peripheral nerve conduction time in the rhesus monkey, Aerosp Med 44:281-285, 1973.

Hackel A (editor): Critical care transport, International Anesthes Clinics 25(2), 1987.

Hansen PJ: Air transport of the man who needs everything, Aviat Space Environ Med 51:725-728, 1980.

Hart HW: The conveyance of patients to and from the hospital, 1720-1850, Med History 22:397-407, 1978.

Henry JN, Krenis LJ, and Cutting RT: Hypoxemia during aeromedical evacuation, Surg Gynecol Obstet 136:49-53, 1973.

Hoffman JR: External counterpressure and the MAST suit: current and future roles, Ann Emerg Med 9:419-421, 1980.

Icenogle TB, Smith RG, Nelson R, and Davis B: Long distance transport of cardiac patients in extremis: the mobile intensive care (MOBI) concept, Aviat Space Environ Med 59:571-574, 1988.

Johnson A: Treatise on aeromedical evacuation, I. Administration and some medical considerations, Aviat Space Environ Med 48:546-549, 1977.

Johnson A: Treatise on aeromedical evacuation, II. Some surgical considerations, Aviat Space Environ Med 48:550-554, 1977.

McNeil EL: Airborne care of the ill and injured, New York, 1983, Springer-Verlag New York, Inc.

McSwain N: Pneumatic trousers and the management of shock, J Trauma 17:719-724, 1977.

Noise, hearing damage, and fatigue in general aviation pilots, AC No. 91-35, Washington, DC, 1972, Department of Transportation, Federal Aviation Administration.

Oxer HF: Carriage by air of the seriously ill, Med J Aust 64:537-540, 1977.

Parsons CJ, and Bobechko WP: Aeromedical transport: its hidden problems, Can Med Assoc J 126:237-243, 1982.

Poulton RJ, and Kisicki P: Physiologic monitoring during civilian air medical transport, Aviat Space Environ Med 58:367-369, 1987.

Shenai JP, Johnson GE, and Varney RV: Mechanical vibration in neonatal transport, Pediatrics 68:55-57, 1981.

Shenai JP: Sound levels for neonates in transit, J Pediatrics 90:811-812, 1977.

Spearman C, and Sheldon R: Egan's fundamentals of respiratory therapy, ed 4, St Louis, 1977, The CV Mosby Co.

Stoner DL, and Cooke JP: Intratracheal cuffs and aeromedical evacuation, Anesthesiology 41:302-306, 1974.

United States Naval Flight Surgeon's Manual, ed 2, The Bureau of Medicine and Surgery, 1978.

West JB: Respiratory physiology: the essentials, ed 2, Baltimore, 1979, Williams & Wilkins.

Appendix A

Abbreviations

Ao	Aorta
Ao dp/dt	Rate of aortic pressure rise (mm Hg/sec)
AV	Atrioventricular
BA	Brachial artery
CI	Cardiac index
CO	Cardiac output
CVP	Central venous pressure
FA	Femoral artery
FO	Foramen ovale
IVC	Inferior vena cava
LA	Left atrium
LLSB	Lower left sternal border
LV	Left ventricle
LV dp/dt	Rate of left ventricular pressure rise (mm Hg/sec)
LVEDP	Left ventricular end-diastolic pressure
MI	Myocardial infarction or mitral insufficiency
$M\dot{V}o_2$	Myocardial oxygen consumption
PA	Pulmonary artery
PAW	Pulmonary artery wedge
PDA	Patent ductus arteriosus
PMI	Point of maximal impulse (of left ventricle on precordium)
PVR	Pulmonary vascular resistance
RA	Right atrium
RV	Right ventricle
SEP	Systolic ejection period (sec/min)
SET	Systolic ejection time (sec/beat)
SV	Stroke volume
SVC	Superior vena cava
SVR	Systemic vascular resistance

Standard abbreviations in pulmonary medicine

Cao_2	Oxygen content in arterial blood
Cvo_2	Oxygen content in venous blood
$CvSo_2$	Oxygen saturation in central venous blood
Fio_2	Fractional concentration of oxygen in inspired gas
$Paco_2$	Partial pressure of carbon dioxide in arterial blood
Pao_2	Partial pressure of oxygen in arterial blood
PAo_2	Partial pressure of oxygen in alveolus
Sao_2	Oxygen saturation of hemoglobin in arterial blood
Svo_2	Oxygen saturation of hemoglobin in venous blood
$TcPao_2$	Transcutaneous partial pressure of oxygen in arterial blood
$\dot{V}o_2$*	Oxygen consumption per minute

*Dot indicates per unit of time.

Appendix B

Normal Resting Values

Site	Pressure range	Oxygen saturation
Superior vena cava (*a*/*v*/m)*	<8/<8/2 to 6	60 to 75%
Right atrium (*a*/*v*/m)	<8/<8/2 to 6	60 to 75%
Right ventricle (sys/dias/end-dias)	15 to 30/0 to 5/2 to 6	60 to 75%
Pulmonary artery (sys/dias/m)	15 to 30/10 to 15/10 to 20	60 to 75%
Pulmonary artery wedge (*a*/*v*/m)	<12 to 15/<12 to 15/4 to 12	99%
Left atrium (*a*/*v*/m)	<12 to 15/<12 to 15/4 to 12	95 to 99%
Left ventricle (sys/dias/end-dias)	100 to 140/0 to 5/5 to 12	95 to 99%
Aorta (sys/dias/m)	100 to 140/60 to 80/70 to 100	95 to 99%

Measurement	Units	Range
Cardiac output	L/min	4 to 8
Cardiac index	L/min/m^2	2.5 to 4
Stroke volume	ml/beat	60 to 130
Stroke index	ml/beat/m^2	35 to 70
Oxygen consumption	ml/min	200 to 300
	ml/min/m^2	125
Arteriovenous oxygen difference	vol %	3 to 5.5
Pa$_{O_2}$	mm Hg	95 to 100
Pv$_{O_2}$	mm Hg	40
Pa$_{CO_2}$	mm Hg	38 to 42
Plasma HCO$_3$	mEq/L	23 to 25
pH	—	7.38 to 7.42
Pulmonary vascular resistance	units	<2
Systemic vascular resistance	units	15 to 20
	dynes/sec/cm^{-5}	900 to 1400
Ca$_{O_2}$	vol%	18 to 20
Cv$_{O_2}$	vol%	14 to 16
Ejection fraction	%	58 to 75
Sa$_{O_2}$	%	95 to 100
Sv$_{O_2}$	%	60 to 75

*a, a wave; v, v wave; m, mean pressure; sys, systolic; dias, diastolic; end-dias, end-diastolic.

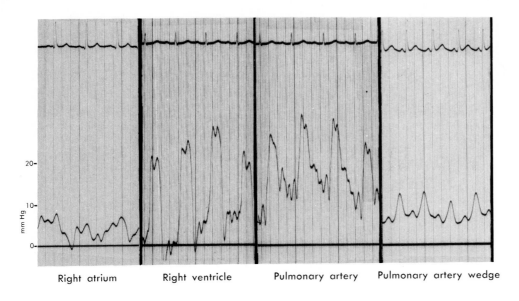

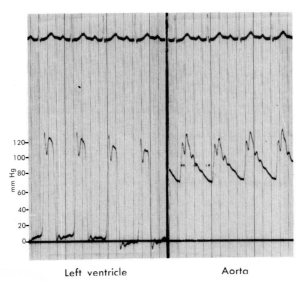

Fig. B-1. Normal hemodynamic pressure tracings of a person at rest.

Appendix C

Dubois Body Surface Charts

Body Surface of Adults

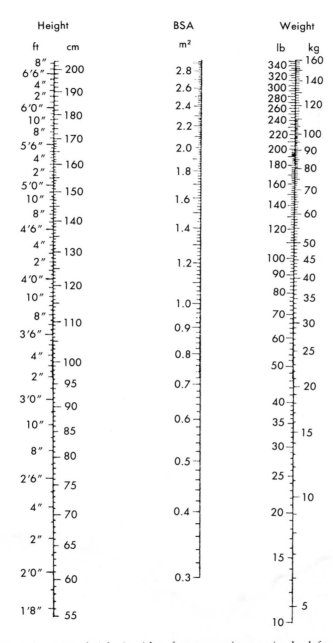

Fig. C-1. Find the patient's height in either feet or centimeters in the left column and the patient's weight in pounds or kilograms in the right column. Connect these two points with a ruler. The BSA is indicated at the point where the ruler crosses the middle column. (From DuBois EF: Basal metabolism in health and disease, ed 3, Philadelphia, 1936, Lea & Febiger.)

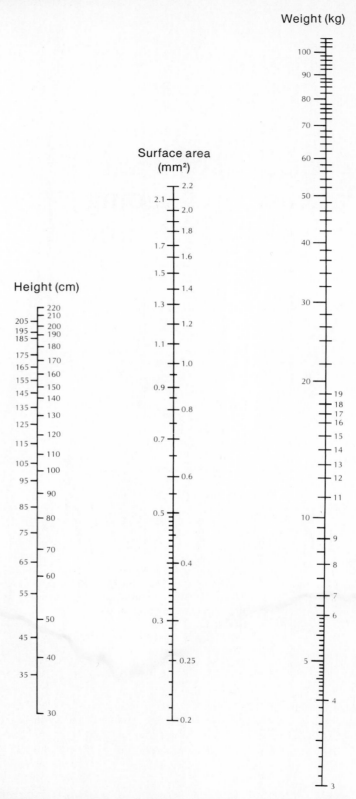

Fig. C-2. Nomogram to determine body surface area. Redrawn from Cole, CH, editor: The Harriet Lane handbook, Chicago, 1984, Year Book Medical Publishers, Inc. Based on data from Gelian, EA, and George, SL: Estimation of human body surface area from height and weight, Cancer Chemother Rep 54:225, 1970.

Appendix D

Nursing Diagnoses and Patient Care Plans for Patients Undergoing Hemodynamic Monitoring

1. Decreased cardiac output

GOALS	NURSING INTERVENTION(S)	RATIONALE
Patient will demonstrate optimal hemodynamic function by: CI 2.5 - 4 L/min/M^2 PAEDP/PAWm or LAm 15-20 mm Hg RAm 4-8 mm Hg MAP 70-80 mm Hg HR 50-100 bpm without ectopy SVR < 1400 dynes/sec/cm^{-5} PVR < 250 dynes/sec/cm^{-5} Normal arterial blood gases Normal hemoglobin level Urinary output ≥ 40 ml/hr Svo$_2$ 60%-77% Oxygen delivery to tissues of ≥ 900 ml/min	Monitor preload (RA and PAEDP, PAW or LAm) and administer appropriate medications and fluids as ordered. Measure CO and CI and calculate SVR and/or PVR. Administer appropriate medications as ordered. Plot ventricular function curves. Calculate LVSWI and/or RVSWI. Administer appropriate medications as ordered. Monitor ECG for rate, rhythm, and ectopy, and determine patient's hemodynamic response to changes in rate or rhythm. Treat according to protocol. Implement emergency measures as necessary. Physically assess patient (vital signs, heart and lung sounds, skin color and temperature, fluid balance, mentation, and jugular vein distention) and report any significant changes. Measure arterial blood gases and hemoglobin levels and report significant changes. Administer appropriate RX as ordered. Measure hourly urine output and report if < 30 ml/hr	Optimize preload to ↑ systolic ejection according to Starling's Law. High LVSWI or RVSWI → ↑ heart work and O$_2$ need (MVo$_2$). Very fast heart rates may ↓ SV by ↓ing LV filling. Very slow heart rates (< 50) may produce inadequate CO (CO = HR × SV). Arrhythmias reduce CO. Baseline heart and lung sounds necessary to determine onset of new sounds associated with cardiac pathology; ↓ mentation or ↑ restlessness may be early indication of ↓ CO Optimize O$_2$ delivery by maintaining CO, Sao$_2$ and Hgb. at normal levels. To determine renal perfusion and function and prevent dysfunction resulting from ischemia.

1. Decreased cardiac output

GOALS	NURSING INTERVENTION(S)	RATIONALE
	Measure Svo_2 and report reductions of 10% for 2-3 min or if < 60%.	Decrease in Svo_2 indicates inadequate tissue perfusion. Svo_2 < 60% associated with poor prognosis
	Reduce patient's activity and stress	Reduced activity and stress will decrease O_2 demands

2. Altered peripheral tissue perfusion related to: compromised circulation associated with invasive monitoring

Patient will demonstrate: optimal skin integrity normal skin color and temperature equal arterial pulses in all extremities	Assess catheter insertion site daily; cleanse site, apply iodophor ointment and new sterile dressing	Inflammation at catheter insertion site associated with infection and/or thrombophlebitis.
	Assess skin color, temperature and sensitivity in area around catheter insertion site. Report any significant changes.	Alteration in tissue perfusion may result in ↑ in skin temperature below catheter site. An ↑ in skin temperature with pain or tenderness is associated with thrombosis or thrombophlebitis.
	Palpate and compare pulses in each extremity. Report any changes.	A ↓ or loss in arterial pulsations distal to catheter insertion site is associated with arterial insufficiency 2° thrombus formation.
	Assess catheterized extremity for evidence of edema by measuring like extremities at the same anatomic location.	Edema is characteristic manifestation when tissue perfusion is a result of venous interference.

3. Potential for infection: related to invasive monitoring

Patient will be free of infection as demonstrated by: normal temperature normal WBC negative cultures of blood or catheter tip	Check patient's temperature every 4 hr and as needed, and report any significant changes.	Increase in patient's temperature associated with infectious process.
	Change catheter and catheter site every 4 days.	Risk of infection increases with duration of catheter placement > 5 days.
	Change IV fluid, tubing, stopcocks and disposable transducer every 48-72 hr.	Static fluid potential source for bacterial growth.
	Inspect and cleanse catheter insertion site every day and apply iodophor ointment and clean sterile dressing.	Skin and old blood are potential sources for infection. Iodophor ointment reduces bacterial growth.
	Do not use IV solution containing glucose.	Glucose solutions promote growth of bacteria.
	Place sterile dead-ender caps on all stopcocks.	Open stopcock port allows bacteria to enter.
	Use aseptic technique when withdrawing from, or flushing the catheter.	Prevent contamination of open system.
	If reusable transducers used, sterilize transducer before patient use.	Minute flaws in disposable transducer domes allow contact between infusing fluid and transducer contaminating IV fluid.

GOALS	NURSING INTERVENTION(S)	RATIONALE
	Carefully remove all traces of blood from stopcock ports after obtaining blood sample from catheter.	Old blood promotes growth of bacteria.
	Use sterile plastic catheter sleeve over PA catheter.	Maintain external portion of catheter sterile to permit catheter advancement, if necessary.

4. Potential for injury related to: A) Hemorrhage
   B) Thromboemboli
   C) Venous air embolism
   D) Pulmonary infarction or hemorrhage
   E) Cardiac arrhythmias or conduction disturbances

A) Patient will remain without hemorrhage	Keep all catheter connecting sites visible and observe frequently for possible hemorrhage.	Major blood loss can occur without notice from stopcocks or loose connections that are hidden beneath dressings or bed linens.
	Tighten all catheter connecting sites and stopcocks every 4 hr and as needed.	Plastic connections become loose over time and leakage can occur.
	Restrain patient, if necessary.	A restless or confused patient may pull catheter out, or connecting tubing apart.
	After removal of arterial catheter, apply firm pressure to insertion site for 10 min before checking and applying pressure dressing.	Allow clot to form at insertion site to seal vessel opening.
	Discontinue systemic heparinization several hr before catheter or sheath removal.	
B) Patient will remain without thrombus as evidenced by: patent catheter unimpeded infusion or flush undamped waveform	Use heparinized IV solution with continuous flush device to continuously infuse all catheter ports and sideport of sheath, if used.	Continous forward flow and use of heparin is associated with ↓ thrombus formation at catheter tip or around catheter in sheath.
	Always aspirate and discard before gently flushing any catheter. If unable to aspirate, do not flush catheter. Periodically aspirate and manually flush catheter or activate flush device (every 4-6 hr).	Remove any fibrin or clot from within or at tip of catheter to prevent injection of clot material. Forward movement of heparinized fluid prevents clot formation.
	Do not fast flush arterial catheter longer than 2 seconds; manually flush arterial catheter by gently tapping plunger of flush syringe with no more than 2-4 ml fluid.	Vigorous flushing of arterial catheter with large amounts of fluid can result in cerebral embolization.
	Maintain 300 mm Hg pressure on IV cuff.	300 mm Hg ± required to maintain forward flow of heparinized solution via flush device.
	Remove all traces of blood from catheter, tubing, and stopcocks after withdrawing blood; flush completely.	Residual blood in catheter, tubing, or stopcock can form small clots which can occlude catheter or be injected into patient.

	GOALS	NURSING INTERVENTION(S)	RATIONALE
C)	Patient will remain without venous air embolism	Tighten all catheter connecting sites and stopcocks every 4 hr and as needed; check frequently.	Plastic connections become loose over time permitting intake of air into system.
		Place dead-ender caps on all stop cock ports.	Open or vented ports permit intake of air.
		Keep all connections or possible openings into vascular system below level of heart.	Air intake more likely to occur through loose connection or open port when patient is in an upright position and takes a deep breath.
		Remove all air from IV solution bag.	Air in bag and solution enters tubing and catheter.
		Have patient hum or suspend respirations when vascular system is open and near or above heart level.	Air intake through open port occurs during inspiration.
		After removal of venous catheter which was in place for a long period of time, apply Vaseline and occlusive dressing to insertion site.	Air intake can occur through the open tract formed by long-dwelling catheter, especially in thin person with little subcutaneous tissue.
D)	Patient will be free of pulmonary infarction or hemorrhage as evidence by: normal respirations no hemoptysis normal ABG's	Continously monitor PA waveform at distal tip of PA catheter.	Forward migration of catheter into a wedged position will be evidenced by PAW waveform.
		Inflate balloon to wedge catheter briefly (< 20 sec).	Minimize cessation in blood flow to reduce risk of pulmonary ischemia or infarction.
		Leave balloon of PA catheter deflated with stopcock open and syringe removed.	Open stopcock with syringe off permits passive deflation should any air remain in balloon.
		Monitor PAedp instead of PAW (if close relationship).	Reduce risks caused by inflation of balloon and cessation of blood flow in branch of PA.
		Check location of catheter tip after insertion and as needed via PA chest film.	Catheter tip migrates forward along with blood flow into a wedge position (particularly during first 24 hr).
		Continuously observe waveform during *slow* balloon inflation; stop inflation at first appearance of PAW waveform. Do not inflate 7 F catheter with more than 1.5 cc air.	Overinflation of balloon can cause rupture of vessel.
		Do not inflate balloon with air if resistance is met.	Catheter may be in a small branch of the PA and already mechanically wedged, or ballon may already be inflated.
E)	Patient will remain free of life-threatening arrhythmias or conduction disturbances	Continuously monitor waveform from distal port of catheter.	Appearance of RV waveform indicates catheter tip has fallen into RV and could cause ventricular arrhythmias.
		Monitor daily chest film.	Check for coiling of catheter in RV or RA which could cause arrhythmias.

GOALS	NURSING INTERVENTION(S)	RATIONALE
	If RV waveform appears, quickly inflate balloon of catheter.	Catheter tip in RV can produce ventricular arrhythmias; with balloon inflation, catheter should float to PA.
	To remove catheter, deflate balloon actively and completely with syringe and quickly remove catheter.	Rapid removal of catheter with fully deflated balloon should result in few, if any, arrhythmias.
	Follow emergency protocols for occurrence of life-threatening arrhythmias.	

5. Anxiety related to: fear of technologic equipment and procedures associated with hemodynamic monitoring

Patient will: verbalize feelings demonstrate a relaxed manner verbalize familiarity with hemodynamic monitoring procedures and equipment	Intitiate interventions to reduce anxiety	Readiness to learn facilitates meaningful learning and retention of knowledge
	Assess ability and readiness to learn the following, when appropriate: reasons for hemodynamic monitoring function and purpose of hemodynamic monitoring equipment explanation of procedures related to hemodynamic monitoring	Knowing rationale and purpose of hemodynamic monitoring reduces anxiety
	Instruct patient in relaxation techniques	Use of energy release techniques helps reduce anxiety.
	Listen attentively, encourage verbalization, and provide a caring touch	Reassurance to patient that he or she is not alone.

6. Sleep Pattern Disturbance: related to invasive monitoring procedures

Patient will have undisturbed sleep	Do not awaken or reposition patient to obtain hemodynamic parameters.	Hemodynamic measurements may be obtained with patient in supine, R or L lateral positions, or 45° semi-fowler's position as long as air-reference stopcock is adjusted to mid-RA level and transudcer is re-zeroed.
	Instruct in relaxation techniques.	Energy release techniques help relax patient and aid in sleep.
	Provide quiet, dimly lit environment.	Quiet, dark environment more conducive to sleep.

Glossary

afterload Tension developed by the ventricle during systole. The arterial systolic pressure best reflects this parameter.

autoregulation Local control of blood flow by the blood vessels not mediated by neural activity.

Bowditch's law An increase in heart rate resulting in an increase in the contractile tension developed.

cardiac reserve Ability of the cardiac muscle to increase its cardiac output under stress (normally 300% to 400% over resting values).

carotid body (chemoreceptor) Cells adjacent to the carotid sinus that regulate respiration by responding to changes in P_{O_2}, P_{CO_2}, and pH.

carotid sinus (baroreceptors) Pressure or stretch receptors at the carotid bifurcation that maintain blood pressure via reflex mechanisms.

central venous pressure Pressure in the superior vena cava.

central venous return Venous blood flowing into the right atrium.

chronotropic Relating to the heart rate.

contractility Force of contraction when preload and afterload are held constant.

counterpulsation Action of circulatory assist pumping device synchronized counter to the normal action of the heart.

damping Diminished amplitude of vibrations of pressure waves.

diastolic augmentation Increase in arterial diastolic pressure produced by counterpulsation of a circulatory assist device. This increase results in increased retrograde blood flow into the aortic root and coronary arteries.

diastolic filling pressure Pressure in the ventricle during diastole.

dp/dt Rate of pressure rise per unit of time. Another index of contractility but difficult to measure at the bedside.

ejection fraction (EF) Proportion of blood ejected from the ventricle per beat compared with end-diastolic volume.

Frank-Starling law The response to an increase in ventricular volume is an increase in myocardial fiber length, resulting in an increase in tension developed. This increase in tension results in an increase in the contractile force of the next beat and an increased stroke volume.

inotropic Relating to the force of a muscle contraction.

Kussmaul's sign Paradoxical rise in venous pressure and neck vein distention during inspiration seen in constrictive diseases.

La Place relation Tension of a wall of a sphere directly related to the pressure inside the cavity and to its radius; the tension is inversely related to the wall thickness.

mean pressure Time-averaged pressure, sometimes indicated by a dash over the value.

oxygen consumption Amount of oxygen in milliliters per minute used by the body to maintain aerobic metabolism.

preload Initial stretch of the myocardial fiber at end-diastole. The ventricular end-diastolic pressure and volume reflect this parameter.

pulmonary vascular resistance (PVR) Resistance to forward blood flow through the lungs.

pulsus alternans Alternating strong and weak pulses caused by alterations in stroke volume.

pulsus bisferiens Double peaked pulse associated with hypertrophic cardiomyopathy or aortic regurgitation.

pulsus paradoxus Decrease of more than 10 mm Hg in systolic blood pressure during normal inspiration.

pulsus parvus Small pulse associated with low pulse pressure.

stroke volume Amount of blood ejected by the ventricle per heartbeat.

systemic vascular resistance (SVR) Resistance to arterial blood flow.

systolic ejection period Time spent in systole per minute.

transducer Device that converts one type of energy into another.

Index

ALSO AVAILABLE!

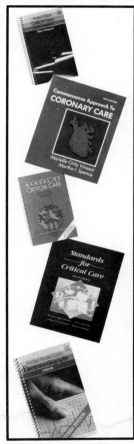

POCKET GUIDE TO CRITICAL CARE ASSESSMENT
by Laura A. Talbot, R.M., C., M.S.; Mary Meyers Marquardt, R.N., B.S.N., CCRN.
POCKET GUIDE TO CRITICAL CARE ASSESSMENT is the only reference on the market to focus on assessment of critically ill patients. This portable, practical assessment tool is designed for quick access to pertinent information at the bedside. Organized by body systems and using an outline format, this guide presents detailed information on critical care assessment covering history taking, the physical examination, and diagnostic studies.
■ Presents complete and detailed assessment guidelines related to specific diagnostic procedures and disease entities to enhance nursing care of the critically ill patient.
■ Includes special considerations for the older adult
■ Provides information on bedside monitoring, including quick-reference tables on respirator setting, blood gas determination, ECG interpretation, assessing patient monitoring systems, and diagnostic studies.

COMMONSENSE APPROACH TO CORONARY CARE, 5th Edition
by Marielle Ortiz Vinsant, R.N., M.S.; Martha Inglis Spence, R.N., M.N., CCRN.
COMMONSENSE APPROACH TO CORONARY CARE, 5th Edition is useful whether you are a beginning or advanced student, or practitioner. This popular text incorporates the latest information on quality care for patients with coronary artery disease or related problems, and encourages you to think through clinical problems rather than memorize solutions.
■ Includes coverage of: arrhythmia and 12-lead ECG assessment, fluid and electrolyte balance, blood gases, hemodynamics, diagnostic studies, drug therapy, and pacemakers.
■ NEW! Chapter on the patient without coronary artery disease in the coronary care unit that covers: Torsades de pointes, Wolff-Parkinson-White Syndrome, cardiomyopathies, mitral prolapse, and malignant arrhythmias unrelated to CAD.
■ Includes the newest antiarrhythmic agents: Tonocard, Mextil, Enkaid, Tambocor, Cardarone; beta blocking agents: Breviblock, Normodyne/Trandate, IV Lopressor; inotropic agent: Incor; and thrombolytic agent: Activase.

MANUAL OF CRITICAL CARE: Applying Nursing Diagnoses to Adult Critical Illness
by Pamela L. Swearingen, R.N.; Marilyn Sawyer Somers, R.N., M.A., CCRN; Kenneth Miller, R.N., Ph.D., CCRN.
MANUAL OF CRITICAL CARE: Applying Nursing Diagnosis to Adult Critical Illness is a unique care planning guide that applies nursing diagnoses to specific critical care disorders. The authors, all clinical experts, give the latest hands-on tips, facts, and findings for critical care nurses and students.
■ Applies NANDA-approved nursing diagnoses to more than 70 specific critical care dysfunctions.
■ Includes for each dysfunction: pathophysiology, assessment, diagnostic tests/medical management, nursing diagnoses, desired outcomes, nursing interventions, rehabilitation, and patient-family teaching.
■ Organizes dysfunctions by body systems, and stresses nursing responsibilities.

STANDARDS FOR CRITICAL CARE, 3rd Edition
by Brenda Crispell Johanson, R.N., M.A., Ed.M., CCRN; Sara Jeanne Wells, B.S.N., M.N.; Denis Hoffmeister, R.N., M.A., C.N.R.N.; Consuelo Urtula Dungca, R.N., M.A., Ed.M.
STANDARDS FOR CRITICAL CARE, 3rd Edition is perfect for establishing or reinforcing critical care standards in the clinical setting. This exciting new edition takes a problem-oriented approach to a wide range of conditions, integrates nursing diagnosis terminology, states care goals specifically, and expands introductions wherever appropriate.
■ Provides in each standard: an introduction (pathophysiology as well as diagnostic and therapeutic modalities), assessment parameters, goals of care, and a chart of nursing activities (nursing diagnoses/patient problems, expected outcomes, and nursing interventions).
■ Includes new standards for: cardiac transplantation, ultrafiltration, autotransfusion, multilumen catheters, enteral feeding, chest trauma, abdominal trauma, spinal cord trauma, and intracranial pressure monitoring.
■ Follows a consistent format to deliver essential information as efficiently as possible.

UNDERSTANDING ELECTROCARDIOGRAPHY: Arrhythmias and the 12-Lead ECG, 5th Edition
by Mary Boudreau Conover, R.N., B.S.
UNDERSTANDING ELECTROCARDIOGRAPHY: Arrhythmias and the 12-Lead ECG, 5th Edition completely surveys the heart, heart electrophysiology, arrhythmia genesis, types and classifications of arrhythmias, interpreting ECG tracings, electrical safety, pacemakers, and arrhythmic drugs. Mary Conover shares state-of-the-art information and current, well-referenced guidelines for using the ECG as a superior diagnostic tool.
The new edition includes:
■ new ECG criteria for the differential diagnoses of broad and narrow QRS tachycardia to help readers distinguish aberrancy from ectopy and identify patients with symptomati movement tachycardia;
■ all forms (overt, concealed, or nonevident) of Wolff-Parkinson-White syndrome so that examiners can recognize this syndrome's life-threatening, yet treatable, arrhythmias;
■ a simplified approach to locating myocardial infarction;
■ discussion of coronary circulation and AV nodal reentry with concise, clinically useful illustrations.